Women's Health Research

A Medical and Policy Primer

Women's Health Research

A Medical and Policy Primer

Society for the Advancement of Women's Health Research

Florence P. Haseltine, Ph.D., M.D., Editor
Beverly Greenberg Jacobson, Executive Editor

Lynne Beauregard
Elizabeth Fee, Ph.D.
Marya Grambs, M.S.
Janet B. Henrich, M.D.
Beverly Greenberg Jacobson
Tracy L. Johnson, M.A.
Ruth B. Merkatz, Ph.D., R.N., F.A.A.N.
Sharon Monsky, M.B.A.
Lesley Primmer, M.A.
Ruth Anne Queenan, M.D.
Estelle Ramey, Ph.D.
Esta Soler
Elyse I. Summers, J.D.
Donna L. Vogel, M.D., Ph.D.
Nancy Fugate Woods, Ph.D., R.N.

Washington, DC
London, England

Note: This book is an educational resource and does not provide medical advice. Therefore, with regard to medical advice, it is recommended that readers follow the advice of a physician who is directly involved in their care or the care of a member of their family.

Books published by the American Psychiatric Press, Inc., represent the views and opinions of the individual authors and do not necessarily represent the policies and opinions of the Press or the American Psychiatric Association.

Copyright © 1997 Society for the Advancement of Women's Health Research
ALL RIGHTS RESERVED
Manufactured in the United States of America on acid-free paper
First Edition   00   99   98   97   4   3   2   1

American Psychiatric Press, Inc.
1400 K Street, N.W., Washington, DC   20005

Library of Congress Cataloging-in-Publication Data
Women's health research : a medical and policy primer / Society for
   the Advancement of Women's Health Research ; Lynne Beauregard . . .
   [et al.]. — 1st ed.
       p.   cm.
   Includes bibliographical references and index.
   ISBN 0-88048-791-7
   1. Women—Health and hygiene—Research.   2. Women—Health
and hygiene—Research—Government policy—United States.
   I. Beauregard, Lynne.   II. Society for the Advancement of Women's
Health Research.
       [DNLM: 1. Women's Health—United States.   2. Research—
United States.   3. Health Policy—United States.   WA 309 W8743 1997]
RA564.85.W686   1997
616'.0082—dc20
DNLM/DLC
for Library of Congress   96-43828
                                                                          CIP

British Library Cataloguing in Publication Data
A CIP record is available from the British Library.

Contents

Part 1
Introduction and History

Part 2
What We Know

Contributors

Lynne Beauregard
Director, Health Programs and Publications
Alliance for Aging Research
Washington, DC

Elizabeth Fee, Ph.D.
Chief, History of Medicine Division
National Library of Medicine
National Institutes of Health
Bethesda, MD

Marya Grambs, M.S.
Senior Program Director
Family Violence Prevention Fund
San Francisco, CA

Florence P. Haseltine, Ph.D., M.D.
Co-founder and President, Board of Directors
Society for the Advancement of Women's Health Research
Washington, DC

Janet B. Henrich, M.D.
Associate Professor of Medicine
and Obstetrics and Gynecology
Director, Women's Health Program
Yale University School of Medicine
New Haven, CT

Beverly Greenberg Jacobson
Free-lance writer and editor
Co-author of The Healing Diet *(Macmillan, 1995)*
and The Woman's Guide to Good Health
(Consumer Reports Books, 1991)
Shelburne, VT

Tracy L. Johnson, M.A.
Doctoral Candidate
Johns Hopkins University
School of Hygiene and Public Health
Evergreen, CO

Ruth B. Merkatz, Ph.D., R.N., F.A.A.N.
Senior Advisor to the Commissioner
Food and Drug Administration
Associate Professor
Albert Einstein College of Medicine
Rye, NY

Sharon Monsky, M.B.A.
Chairman, Board of Directors
Scleroderma Research Foundation
Santa Barbara, CA

Lesley Primmer, M.A.
President and Founder, Women's Policy, Inc.
Former Executive Director, Congressional Caucus
for Women's Issues
Washington, DC

Ruth Anne Queenan, M.D.
Fellow
Department of Obstetrics and Gynecology
Northwestern University School of Medicine
Chicago, IL

Estelle Ramey, Ph.D.
Professor Emeritus, Physiology and Biophysics
Georgetown University School of Medicine
Bethesda, MD

Esta Soler
Executive Director
Family Violence Prevention Fund
San Francisco, CA

Elyse I. Summers, J.D.
Special Assistant to the Director
Office of Women's Health
U.S. Food and Drug Administration
Rockville, MD

Donna L. Vogel, M.D., Ph.D.
Medical Officer
Reproductive Sciences Branch
Center for Population Research
National Institute of Child and Human Development
National Institutes of Health
Rockville, MD

Nancy Fugate Woods, Ph.D., R.N.
Director, Center for Women's Health Research
School of Nursing
University of Washington
Seattle, WA

Foreword

Florence P. Haseltine, Ph.D., M.D.
President, Society for the Advancement of
Women's Health Research

One of the most interesting aspects of women's health research has been the way it has evolved from a rather narrow definition into a new and much broader paradigm. In the past, research on women's health focused primarily on the reproductive system. If women's health grabbed the headlines, the topics that caught the attention of the public and the research community were prenatal care, fertility, "The Pill" and other contraceptives, breast cancer, premenstrual syndrome, and the politics of abortion. Scientists and physicians who wanted to study other women's health conditions were handicapped by the belief that women's menstrual cycles were difficult to deal with and understand. This argument went unchallenged for decades, long after feminists and scientists realized that most women live a third of their lives after menopause, a time when hormonal changes cease to be an issue but when chronic medical illness becomes an increasingly dominant factor in women's lives.

Despite the centrality of reproduction to women's health, the politicalization of reproductive concerns made inadequate funding for gynecological and obstetrical research inevitable. Thus, the shift from reproductive health to more general health issues was a direct result of the deficiencies in gynecological research. Part of this history is personal; as director of the Center for Population Research at the National Institutes of Health (NIH), I was the only gynecologist in a senior management position and one of only a handful of permanent staff members.

Therefore, when projects were being designed that needed the scientific and medical input of gynecologists, there simply were not enough of us to lobby our point of view effectively. This was the situation we had to correct—if our profession was to improve the care we gave women. But NIH had been experiencing a belt-tightening, and it was impossible for me to create change within the system.

In fact, the 1980s and early 1990s altered NIH dramatically—as Congress started to manage the Institutes and special interest groups exerted their considerable influence. For example, the acquired immunodeficiency syndrome (AIDS) lobby—through its political and media activism—affected the amount of time and money devoted to this disease in a major way. Following the AIDS lobby example and that of other groups, such as breast cancer activists, I began to work with women who knew how to affect legislation. We found there was a pressing need for a much broader framework, one that went beyond the lack of gynecological research at NIH. We decided to expand into menopause. The joke at the time was that I had a hot flash and declared it a national emergency. That was the personal part—but the real pragmatic issue was that we needed to find a way to separate research on women's health from reproductive health issues because abortion was a problem that always came up whenever women's health concerns were raised. Because pregnancy is rarely a problem for women older than 50, abortion becomes irrelevant. In fact, so does a woman's sexuality. By a strange kind of logic, if a woman cannot get pregnant, questions surrounding sexual activity, promiscuous behavior, and their impact in destroying families are no longer part of society's concern. In effect, the politically powerful groups that worry about sexual control of teenagers and young women have basically neutered menopausal women; therefore, older women now have different rights than they had when they were younger. Menopause turned out to be a safe issue.

As our own discussions continued, we realized that there were a large number of female policy makers, with an incredible fund of knowledge, who were all worried about menopause. This knowledge helped to launch our attempt to make menopause the next focus of an expanded research agenda. It was a matter of luck and timing that the idea caught on, but its importance cannot be overstated. This was the first time that a women's health issue was separated from reproductive functioning.

There has always been a vital tie between a woman's freedom over her sexual rights and her ability to control whether and when she will become pregnant. That is why it was so crucial to sever the link between women's sexual functioning and the new and important women's health research issues that were trying to emerge. Once that was accomplished it became much more difficult to try and reconnect the two.

We also were helped by demographics. The fact that a large portion of the female population in the United States, thanks to the baby-boom generation, will shortly be peri- and then postmenopausal gave older women additional clout. But we still had a major problem: how to make a specific scientific area of research, such as women's health, exciting to the media, the general public, politicians, and, of course, scientists. We took a page from the book created by AIDS activists and studied how they had made AIDS a national issue and how that had led to huge amounts of money going into AIDS research and therapy. The first thing we understood was that AIDS is a disease involving graphic visual imagery, which our memories can reproduce with great accuracy and detail—namely, the picture of many young people dying early and agonizing deaths. Second, because AIDS is a disease that develops slowly, most of those who are infected live a relatively long time and thus can become spokespersons for their disease. The result has been that, over a 10- to 15-year period, these activists have captured and held national attention.

The same approach worked for breast cancer, which has become the focus of a tremendous amount of recent attention from the media, the public, Congress, and now, investigators. It is hard for politicians to stare down a woman who has lost one or both breasts to cancer and is determined that her daughters and granddaughters will have better options. The vocal and determined breast cancer lobby, by impressing legislators with the urgent need for research, not only got Congress to increase the National Cancer Institute's (NCI) breast cancer research funds by about 300%, but also, using fiduciary imagination, to add money to the defense department's budget to start a research effort there. The fact that the U.S. Army received more than 2,000 applications for funding shows how this imaginative thinking allowed scientists to expand their research efforts into breast cancer. Similarly, when NIH put out a contract to study postmenopausal therapies in the large multicentered study called the Women's Health Initiative, hundreds of applications arrived. Both of these developments demonstrate two important trends—that there is a wellspring of ideas and talent that can be devoted to women's health if the opportunity and funding exist and that the medical profession is now ready to accept that it is worth studying diseases important to women, an immensely exciting development given the neglect of women's health issues in the past.

Americans believe that research is fundamental to changing how we care for people. Therefore, the public and Congress are influenced by research needs that are clearly defined and explained by authorities they respect. But there are limits to how much money can be poured into any investigative area—both by budgetary constraints and by public awareness. For example, for a new or newly realized public health threat, the amount of money allocated can rise exponentially at first, but when the total amount approximates $1 billion, as has happened with cancer and AIDS research, the nation realizes a saturation point has been reached and additional funding efforts will not be successful. In current phraseology, the topic has hit the budget makers' "radar screen" and therefore becomes more vulnerable to challenges. Moreover, as the evolution of a new topic develops, the research into that topic starts to overlap traditional investigational areas.

In the first two chapters of this book, we define women's health research and explain how the movement developed. Women's health research issues, and actions to find answers raised by those issues, have grown and expanded dramatically since 1990. For example, when the Government Accounting Office (GAO) tried to determine if NIH was implementing its own 1986 policy to include women in clinical trials, it discovered that NIH had no uniform definition of what constituted research on women's health and, indeed, had a hard time identifying research that was related to this issue. Therefore, we needed individuals who could explain what women's health research is. Over time, two clear ideas have emerged. The first idea is the concept of diseases found only in women. The second idea concerns diseases that present differently in women than in men; that is, conditions with a higher prevalence in women or that develop disparate symptoms. We have expanded these concepts in detail in Chapters 5, 6, and 7. Each of these definitions has provided investigators with valuable insights that helped them understand how the research support system works and how to use that understanding to get funding for their research.

Clarifying everything that constitutes women's health research is, of course, an evolving challenge. For example, early in our efforts, difference itself was a defining factor. If an investigator identified a hormone receptor that acted differently in the female system than in the male system, that was considered research on women. But today we are more sophisticated and mature; we want to study the *process* by which that hormone acts differently. It has been exciting to see how creative scientists have gone from thinking that the complications introduced by gender differences, such as menstrual cycling, were what made research on women so much harder, to the realization that the effects of menstrual cycling on various conditions represent the real and important reason for studying a disease in the first place. Obviously, we need to know how the menstrual cycle affects the disease process itself as well as how it affects the drugs and other therapies used to treat the disease. Thinking this way has expanded the range of topics we can cover.

Let us consider some of the consequences of how we define women's health research. First, let us look at diseases that affect women only. These conditions stem from a woman's ability to have children. Illnesses that influence childbearing involve functions of the brain, the reproductive tract, and, of course, the breast. But there is the secondary influence of reproduction on other physiological systems, which this primary definition automatically covers, opening possibilities for ever-expanding patterns of investigation. Other areas that now look like bona fide women's health research issues include lifestyle factors. The factors range from occupational exposure to toxins to the environmental hazards that society faces. Some cancer activists, for example, believe that environmental degradation is a major cause of the current breast cancer epidemic (see Chapter 8). This kind of thinking means that behavioral research that can answer questions of how best to change negative lifestyles should be added to the future agenda of women's health research.

Lung cancer is a disease that illustrates graphically some of the difficulties involved in lifestyle changes. Lung cancer kills more women than breast cancer, yet there is no dramatic public outcry. Why? Is it because women are locked into and made mute by the disabilities lung cancer imposes on them, or is it because the women's magazines publish smoking ads, as some consumer groups argue? Is it because women with lung cancer are older and the disease is rapidly fatal? Or is it because lung cancer is now seen as a preventable disease, and, even though we did not know the connection five decades ago when women started smoking in earnest, there is a blame-the-victim component? We have all seen that, for a condition to develop an effective political lobby, the people who have it must become articulate, and they must live long enough to make their case. With lung cancer, for which there is rarely a cure, prevention is our major tool, particularly because studies have shown it is much harder for women to stop smoking than it is for men. But preventive research is behavioral research, and funding for this type of inquiry is not easy to obtain.

We have seen how women's health research has grown from its early emphasis on reproduction to a much more sophisticated arena. Now we are looking at a wide variety of women's health issues—everything from the effects of the menstrual cycle on diseases and their treatments, to illness and health in older women, to environmental causes of disease, to behavioral research. The next great area of expansion will be in research on gender differences. I have more to say about this in the conclusion.

Acknowledgments

This is my favorite part of writing or editing a book. All the footnotes have been checked, the typos have been corrected, the book is at the final stages, and the person in charge of getting everything neatly wrapped up is after me to write the acknowledgments. Of course, the acknowledgments must be written last because until the book is almost ready to be printed, it is hard to know which people along the way have helped.

My acknowledgments are not limited to this book but also include the birth of the Society for the Advancement of Women's Health Research and its critical role in encouraging the changes we are witnessing today. *Women's Health Research: A Medical and Policy Primer* was conceived almost 6 years ago in Washington, DC, and well before the past three national elections and several major changes in the political landscape. The exact date when I said, "We need a book to serve as both a survey of the field and a history of the movement," is hidden in memory and, unfortunately, not recorded in writing. Many of the people who were first involved with the undertaking have gone on to other projects, and many may not remember their original involvement. If I do not mention their contributions, I apologize.

Some time in 1990 or 1991, I asked a friend, Mrs. William McCormick Blair, Jr. (Deeda), to help identify sources of support for a fledgling organization, the Society for the Advancement of Women's Health Research, that was dedicated to improving women's health through research. She had been advising me on the effort since 1988 and had offered her recognizable name and gracious introductions to many of her hundreds of friends and acquaintances.

One of those letters of introduction was to Dr. Robert Gussin, corporate vice president, science and technology, Johnson & Johnson. He listened to my ideas at a lunch to which he brought his wife, Patricia Stewart, vice president, research and development, worldwide consumer pharmaceuticals, Johnson & Johnson. We had lunch at the Cosmos Club, a scholarly refuge in Washington, DC, that had only recently begun to admit women. Dr. Gussin left the lunch saying that he was interested in the society's mission but that he would feel most comfortable supporting a specific project, perhaps a book. (More than 5 years later, I was honored to attend a dinner at which Dr. Gussin received the 1996 Presidential Medal for Science and Technology on behalf of Johnson & Johnson and was most pleased to be able to tell him about the progress of his idea.)

Within a year of my meeting Dr. Gussin, the book was outlined with the help of Joanne Howes and Pat Morgan. Pat, one of those wonderful behind-the-scenes people who gets things done, was in charge of the book publishing section of the American Association for the Advancement of Science (AAAS).

I then asked Dr. Gussin whether he thought the outlined book would be an appropriate project for funding by Johnson & Johnson. He said yes, and we were on our way. Johnson & Johnson was enormously helpful, especially the support of two people, Dr. Do Won Hahn and Ruth Edelson. It is with great pleasure that I acknowledge the support of the Johnson & Johnson Corporate Contributions Committee. This book literally would not have been possible without Johnson & Johnson.

I had worked with a skilled medical writer and editor, Beverly Greenberg Jacobson, on another book. Her professionalism is most remarkable, and she was engaged to edit the entire volume and make the language flow.

Unfortunately, our publisher, the AAAS, closed its book division before we were ready to print. Dr. Carol Nadelson, president and chief executive officer of American Psychiatric Press, Inc. (APPI), a division of the American Psychiatric Association, agreed to publish *Women's Health Research*. We owe Dr. Nadelson and everyone at APPI a special debt of gratitude for the acceptance of our work and their diligent efforts at shepherding us through their editorial process.

Those events added to the time we (I should say Bev Jacobson) spent writing and rewriting the book to keep it updated.

In the meantime, the Society for the Advancement of Women's Health Research was acting behind the scenes to foment the women's health revolution. Many of the original and early board members of the society were instrumental in this effort. They are mentioned here because their names may not appear elsewhere in the book. They are Joanne Howes, Marie Bass, Dr. Mary Lake Polan, Dr. Susan Blumenthal, Chris DeVries, Nancy Vreeland, Irene Pollen, Gerald Peal, Lynne Cutler, and especially Phyllis Greenberger, the society's current executive director, who has taken us through the most amazing times. Some of these people have risen to prominent positions in the women's health community. Others are engaged in the less visible yet equally important work of educating the public, the medical community, and the government on women's health.

In addition, I want to thank Lesley Primmer, who was director of the Congressional Caucus on Women's Issues and is now the president of Women's Policy, Inc. Also deserving of special mention is a former employee of the caucus, Cynthia de la Fuentes. In the spring of 1989, Cynthia listened to concerns that no clinical center for women currently existed at the National Institutes of Health (NIH). She asked several leaders of the society how much it would cost to create a center for women's health that had an obstetrical and gynecological service. Dr. Mary Lake Polan, then an associate professor of obstetrics and gynecology at Yale University, put together the answer over a weekend and faxed the response to Cynthia. That original budget was guided by the Office for HIV/AIDS Research to include building a new outpatient and inpatient facility and to develop an extramural section. When we later heard that in negotiations with NIH the main point of the discussion was whether the entity should be called an office or a center, I knew we had achieved our goal. Unfortunately, the budget was meager; we never did get a full-fledged intramural component, and a separate women's center has not been included in the plans for the new NIH clinical center.

Another major contributor to the society's success was a board member, Lisa Burns, who did a phenomenal job of organizing the initial work with the press. She ensured that they were present at the June 18, 1990, congressional hearing on what is now known as "the GAO Report" and formally as *National Institutes of Health: Problems in Implementing Policy on Women in Study Populations.* The press was at the hearing and armed with the material they needed to tell the story because of the efforts of the society and Lisa Burns.

On a personal note, because several members of the society's first board were government employees and our livelihood was directly related to that employment, we needed help to ensure that we obeyed the laws. Being a government bureaucrat challenged us all. Help was forthcoming from many sources, but the perspective on public service came chiefly from the advice of Drs. Duane Alexander and Mary Clutter. Many government employees gave me advice, usually involving clever stratagems on how to both obey the law and be an advocate. I am sure they definitely would not like to see their names and their role acknowledged in print.

Other board members and consultants to the society, not employed by the government, worked with the staff of the Congressional Caucus on Women's Issues (CCWI) to identify areas that needed to be addressed and to craft the requisite legislative language. These board members and consultants worked in cooperation with the CCWI to address many details of the future Office for Research on Women's Health at NIH and the language requiring the inclusion of women and minorities in clinical studies.

Three unique men particularly helped me make this book possible. They are William T. Golden, a man to whom many in the science world owe the realization of their dreams; the late William McCartney-Cooper, who while being treated for AIDS and working hard on behalf of research in AIDS gave the society $25,000; and Dr. Warren Pearse, who is well-known to most obstetrician/gynecologists. If you are not an obstetrician/gynecologist, you should know that he is an angel to women and their health. He had faith in the goals of the society and gave us the first check to open our bank account for the society.

Special thanks go to the present members of the society's board of directors: Claudia Baquet, M.D., M.P.H.; Enriqueta (Queta) Bond, Ph.D.; Kathy Bryant, J.D.; Lisa Burns; Maria Bustillo, M.D.; James H. Cavanaugh, Ph.D.; Colleen Conway-Welch, Ph.D., R.N.; Rosemary Berkel Crisp, R.N.; John Fletcher, Ph.D.; Freda Lewis-Hall, M.D.; Irma Mebane-Sims, Ph.D.; Gloria E. Sarto, M.D., Ph.D.; Susan K. Sudman, M.S.; Anne Colston Wentz, M.D.; and Nancy Fugate Woods, Ph.D., R.N.

Finally, I must acknowledge society staff members Anita Bollt, Beverly Reece, and Lynne Beauregard, who played significant roles in moving and completing this project.

Florence P. Haseltine, Ph.D., M.D.

Part 1

Introduction and History

1

Women's Health Research: An Introduction

Tracy L. Johnson, M.A.
Elizabeth Fee, Ph.D.

W omen have been excluded from health research for decades. Although the National Institutes of Health
(NIH) attempted to remedy this situation in 1986 with
a policy statement encouraging the inclusion of women in clinical research trials, a study by the General Accounting Office (GAO) in 1990
found that "little progress" had been made.[1] In fact, GAO was unable to
establish with any certainty just how much of the total NIH budget had
been spent on women because of decentralized and nonautomated
recordkeeping methods. Because NIH is the largest source of public funds
for health research, with a budget of 10 billion tax dollars in 1993,[2] the
failure to include women in research studies discriminates against women
in general and female taxpayers in particular.

This chapter is reprinted with permission from Women in Clinical Studies, Volume 2,
Workshop and Commissioned Papers. Copyright 1994 by the National Academy of
Sciences. Courtesy of the National Academy Press, Washington, DC.
Note: The authors acknowledge the contribution of Susan Blumenthal, M.D., M.P.A.,
to this chapter as a source of information and perspective. All comments and conclu-
sions, however, are solely those of the authors.

Although the omission of women from medical research has been documented across the board, several of the best known examples deal with cardiovascular research. The Harvard Physicians Health Study, for example, looked at the relationship between moderate aspirin use and heart disease. Its sample population included 22,071 men and no women. The study found that taking an aspirin every other day may reduce the risk of heart disease in men. It is not known conclusively if these results apply to women.[3]

The Multiple Risk Factor Intervention Trials (MR. FIT) was another major research initiative on heart disease that excluded women. This national study of 15,000 men examined how cholesterol levels, blood pressure, and smoking affect the development of heart disease.[4] The cardiovascular benefit of lowered cholesterol levels through a low-fat diet was first demonstrated in MR. FIT, but only for men, not for women.

Omitting women from the Physicians Health Study, MR. FIT, and other research on cardiovascular disease is particularly unfortunate in view of the associated mortality rates in women. Heart disease kills more women than any other condition—approximately 500,000 of them annually.[5] Another 88,220 women die from strokes annually.[6] Hypertension, a major risk factor for cardiovascular disease, is more common among African American women than among white men and women. Nevertheless, diagnostic tools, nutritional guidelines, and antihypertensive agents used to treat this condition have been developed based predominantly on studies of white male populations (Blumenthal SJ, Johnson TL: *Women's Health Research: A Historical Perspective.* Unpublished manuscript, Washington, DC, 1993).

Defenders of NIH's record on women's health point to the Nurses' Health Study, which followed more than 87,000 registered nurses for 6 years, as evidence that women's concerns have not been ignored. The study reported in 1991 that women taking between one and six aspirin weekly experienced a 25% reduction in the risk of a heart attack (myocardial infarction) compared with those who took no aspirin.[7] However, unlike the Physicians Health Study, the Nurses' Health Study was an observational investigation, not a more costly, randomized clinical trial. A "randomized clinical trial" means that participants are assigned to either a treatment or "control" (comparison) group by a computer or another "random" method. Those in the treatment group receive the medication being studied while those in the control group take a placebo, a pill that looks like the medication but has no medicinal effect. Most clinical trials involve "blinding." When the participants do not know whether they receive medication or placebo, it is called a single-blind study. In a double-blind study, neither the person giving the medicine nor the participant knows who is receiving treatment and who is in the control group. The purpose of random assignment and blinding is to eliminate conscious or unconscious bias among researchers and participants. Randomization also helps to ensure that the only difference between the two groups is the one under study, in this case aspirin.[8]

In contrast, an observational study does not assign but rather observes two existing groups with different behaviors or "exposures" (aspirin takers versus non–aspirin takers) and notes any difference in observed symptoms or rates of disease. Observational studies are considered less rigorous than, and a precursor to, clinical trials because they lack randomization. Nurses who take aspirin regularly, for example, may be more health conscious generally—they may eat better or exercise more—than those who do not. Hence, their lower observed rates of heart disease may have more to do with these health behaviors than aspirin intake. Moreover, observational studies often rely on the unreliable method of self-reporting for dose measurements and determination of possible "confounding" variables— in this case, hypertension, elevated cholesterol, and obesity. According to the Nurses' Health Study investigators, the study's findings are promising but insufficient proof that low-dose aspirin protects women from heart attack. They conclude that a randomized trial is warranted.[9]

Public outrage after the GAO revelations of women's exclusion from NIH-funded research helped to win funding for a follow-up to the Nurses' Health Study. A randomized trial on the effect of aspirin use in women was approved in July 1991, funded by the National Heart, Lung and Blood Institute (NHLBI), a division of NIH. This research, to be conducted by the same team that did the Physicians Health Study, will follow 41,600 nurses older than 50 for 5 years.[10] This episode provided an early lesson for women's health advocates within the research community: public pressure can reorient funding priorities. The necessity of grassroots organizing and support to expedite a women's health research agenda is a theme explored throughout this book.

In addition to cardiovascular studies, women have been omitted from studies on aging. The National Institute on Aging's (NIA) Baltimore Longitudinal Study of Aging began in 1958, but women were not added to the study sample for 20 years. The 1984 report based on this research, "Normal Human Aging," is often considered definitive, even though it contains virtually no data on women.[11] This oversight is particularly significant when one considers that women represented 59% of those older than 65 and 72% of those age 85 and older in 1995.[12]

Women also have been excluded from research financed by private sources. Although pharmaceutical companies conduct most of their own drug research—at a cost of $10.9 billion in 1992[13]—the U.S. Food and Drug Administration (FDA) must approve new medicines before they can be marketed. Until recently, FDA guidelines governing clinical trials of new drugs required the exclusion of women capable of becoming pregnant from the early stages of most pharmaceutical research.

This policy had the unintended effect of excluding women from both the early and late stages of drug testing. For 60% of the new drugs that secured FDA approval between 1988 and 1991, the proportion of women in test populations was less than the proportion of women who had the disease being studied. A GAO survey found female representation to be particularly poor in cardiovascular drug trials, even though pharmaceutical companies acknowledge this is an area in which gender differences in drug response have been observed.[14] As a result of recent congressional and public scrutiny, FDA revised its "guideline" in July 1993, encouraging but not requiring drug companies to include appropriate numbers of women in their studies and to report to the agency significant gender differences in drug response. However, unlike a "regulation," a guideline does not carry the force of law.[15] (For a more detailed discussion of FDA and NIH regulatory history, see Chapters 2 and 12.)

What Is Women's Health Research?

Historically, clinicians, public health professionals, and researchers defined "women's health" narrowly as reproductive health. Even today, many associate women's health with the disciplines that focus on reproductive issues, such as maternal and child health, or on reproductive systems, such as obstetrics and gynecology. Indeed, applying the results of research done on predominantly male populations to women is consistent with the view of women's bodies as being essentially male, with the exception of their reproductive capacity. Increasingly, however, basic and social scientists, clinicians, and women themselves are questioning this tacit assumption of equity. Like pediatrics and gerontology before it, women's health may be emerging as a separate, specialized field within medicine.

This new discipline embraces an expanded definition of women's health and women's health research, one which incorporates cellular, systemic, individual, and societal perspectives. Each of these perspectives provides only a piece of the women's health puzzle; together they demonstrate a complete picture of women's health. Basic science focuses on fundamental biological questions, such as how cells in the human body function, both biochemically and physiologically. Clinical research aims to understand entire organ systems—cardiovascular, respiratory, circulatory, reproductive, and so forth—and their relationship to individual health. Social science, behavioral medicine, and public health look at health behaviors, social interactions, cultural factors, and environmental influences and study their impact on individuals and society.

Thus we need a women's health model that integrates basic and social sciences and describes the health of women across the life span—from birth, through childhood, adolescence, adulthood, maturity, and old age. Interdisciplinary research that facilitates this needed integration is only now emerging.

Although biological, clinical, and social science perspectives clearly overlap, disciplinary boundaries and academic hierarchies have prevented communication. Indeed, integration and collaboration represent a radical departure from the traditional medical model, which has considered the individual apart from society, the body apart from the mind, and body parts—organ systems and cells—apart from the whole. It is clear that we need interdisciplinary studies to provide information about the way physiological, individual, and cultural factors interact and influence each other. There are many questions to be answered, such as the extent to which cellular differences in men and women influence the health of individuals and their behavior across the life span. Do social forces—poverty, sexism, and racism—and life experiences—happiness, exercise, and optimism—affect men's and women's health, and, if so, how? How do women differ from one another, and what are the societal consequences of diversity at the cellular level, in the various organ systems, and of the total organism? These are issues that cannot be explored without an integrated understanding of women's health.

Why Is Research on Women's Health Needed?

Women's longevity may have led to the perception among the research community that women's health needs were less pressing than those of men. After all, the so-called weaker sex outlives the stronger by an average of 7 years. As this book shows, although women live longer than men, they do not live better.

A variety of studies have documented that older women experience more chronic illnesses, such as arthritis, osteoporosis, and incontinence, and higher rates of poverty and disability than men of similar ages.[16] Because men die earlier and choose younger partners, more older women than older men are widowed and living alone. Women also are more likely to care for a disabled spouse at home than are men. These factors contribute to the fact that three times as many women as men live in nursing homes.[17] Some experts estimate that 50% of all admissions to nursing homes are as a result of incontinence, a statistic that automatically makes this condition a women's health issue.[18] Research on the prevention of and effective treatments for incontinence might allow many women to live independently and reduce the cost of long-term care.

Whereas women's health includes all conditions and diseases that influence their health status, research needs have been concentrated in three main areas. The first is the traditional focus of obstetrics and gynecology on the conditions—menstruation, pregnancy, menopause—and the diseases—vaginal, cervical, ovarian, and breast cancer—that only affect women. The second includes health issues also experienced by men but that are much more prevalent in women—osteoporosis, depression, and autoimmune diseases. The third includes those illnesses that are expressed differently in men and women—heart disease, substance abuse, acquired immunodeficiency syndrome (AIDS), and violence.

The Breast Cancer Experience

Breast cancer is a good example of a women's disease that used to receive inadequate research attention. The American Cancer Society projected that the disease would kill 44,300 women in 1996. The incidence of this disease has risen dramatically in the past 30 years across all subgroups. In 1950 the lifetime risk was 1 woman in 20; according to the American Cancer Society, it is now 1 in 8. But computing lifetime risk assumes that all women have an equal chance of getting breast cancer and that all women will live to be 110. More realistically, breast cancer risk for the average 40-year-old woman is 1 in 1,000 annually (0.1%), and for the average 50-year-old woman, the figure doubles to 0.2%.[19] The annual bill in medical costs and lost productivity is $6 billion.[20]

Breast cancer death rates are higher among African American women than among white women, possibly because of their lower rates of early diagnosis. Easier and earlier access to medical care for minority women might help reduce this imbalance.

We need breast cancer research to identify risk factors and causes. For example, we do not understand the independent roles and interplay of genetics, oral contraceptives, hormone replacement therapy, diet, and environmental toxins in promoting breast cancer. Indeed, the known risk factors account for a relatively small proportion of breast cancer cases. We also need better methods of prevention and early detection, and we must discover and remove the barriers to regular screening (mammography and breast self-examination) among different groups of women. Finally, despite some diagnostic and treatment improvements, such as the stereotactic needle breast biopsy that is rapidly replacing surgical biopsy and the less disfiguring lumpectomy currently favored over mastectomy, the basic medical treatment options of removing cancerous cells with surgery or killing them with radiation and chemotherapy have not changed in decades. There is a compelling need for more effective and earlier diagnostic methods and much less disfiguring treatments.[21]

The Unknowns of Women's Biology

Major gaps exist in our understanding of women's biology, largely because male physiology has been the norm and women's hormonal cycles have been defined as abnormal, especially when they do not result in pregnancy. Few studies have traced the typical hormonal life cycle in women from menstruation through pregnancy to menopause. We have little idea about what is normal in menopause and therefore not the faintest notion of what is abnormal.

Without a clear understanding of what is normal, it is difficult to identify, much less explain, abnormalities. This lack of a "baseline" has clouded our understanding of premenstrual syndrome, pregnancy-induced hypertension, and menopausal symptoms such as hot flashes, night sweats, and vaginal thinning and dryness.[22]

Osteoporosis—weakening of the bones—affects large numbers of older women in the United States. Up to 50% of women older than 45 and 90% of women older than 75 have the disease. Thin, small-boned women of European or Asian descent are at especially high risk. This crippling condition causes more than 1.3 million fractures of the hip, wrist, and vertebrae and 50,000 deaths annually. Osteoporosis adds between $7 and $10 billion to the nation's annual medical bill.[23]

Research has demonstrated that osteoporosis is not solely the result of the inevitable effects of aging, but rather may be preventable. For example, medical anthropologist Yewoubdar Beyene points out that osteoporosis does not appear to be a problem among postmenopausal women in the rural Greek and Mayan communities she studied, possibly because of factors other than estrogen loss, such as adequate calcium in their diets, a great deal of physical activity, and the fact that these women accept menopause as a normal part of the life cycle and, particularly among Mayan older women, a welcome event that ends their continual pregnancies.[24] Several Western studies have demonstrated that estrogen replacement therapy slows bone loss in older women. However, we need to learn more about estrogen's role in calcium absorption, bone growth, and remodeling. Does a high-calcium diet during childhood, adolescence, and young adulthood increase bone density and lessen the risk of osteoporosis later in life? One study suggests that a high-calcium diet does lessen the risk of osteoporosis later in life (see

Chapter 6). Although moderate exercise, especially "weight-bearing exercise"—walking, running, weight training—early in life appears to build denser bones, other studies indicate that excessive exercise and certain common eating disorders are risk factors. What, then, is the optimal dietary and exercise regimen to reduce the risk of this condition? Why do African American women escape this disorder? We do not know because no research has been done in this area. Effective prevention strategies must await a better understanding of the risk factors for this disease.[25]

Osteoporosis is just one of many diseases that affect women disproportionately. Twice as many women as men have affective disorders, and nearly four times more women than men older than 65 experience depression. More women have Alzheimer's disease. Autoimmune thyroid diseases have a 15:1 ratio of women to men. Systemic lupus erythematosus (SLE) affects nine times as many women as men. Women experience systemic sclerosis four times as often as men and rheumatoid arthritis three times more frequently. Both diabetes mellitus and multiple sclerosis occur more often in women than men.[26] Violence against women has reached epidemic proportions in the United States; every 15 seconds, an American woman is beaten in her home.[27]

For certain conditions and diseases, there may not be a statistical difference in the number of women and men affected, or more men than women may have the disease. Nevertheless, these conditions should be viewed from the perspective of women's health because there may be gender differences in risk factors, symptoms, and treatments. Cardiovascular disease, for example, has been seen as a male disease because it kills more men than women. This view has led to the use of all-male populations to study heart disease. But cardiovascular disease is also the number one killer of women. After age 65, one woman in three has a clinically recognized form of cardiovascular disease. Nearly 90,000 (88,220) women die of stroke annually.[28] Studies have documented that women with heart disease are older, are diagnosed later, have more complicating conditions, and may be treated less "aggressively" than men[29] (see Chapter 7). Whereas 31% of men who have heart attacks die within a year, the figure for women is 50%.[30] Women's health advocates have questioned whether the perception of heart disease as a male disorder has led physicians to discount symptoms in women.

We need research on heart disease in women to clarify the protective role of natural and synthetic estrogen. Studies on the use of birth control pills and hormone replacement therapy are needed to explain the positive and negative effects of these agents and to explore the interactions of these hormones with antihypertensive drugs and other commonly prescribed medications. As with breast cancer and osteoporosis, we need to understand relative risk factors for women, including diet, lack of exercise, obesity, hypertension, smoking, poverty, isolation, battering, and occupational and environmental stress.

The Toll of Sexually Transmitted Diseases

Sexually transmitted diseases (STDs) represent another health concern in which gender differences are apparent. Women's and men's distinctive physiology, for example, yields variations in disease symptoms and effects. In addition, sexuality is perhaps the area most laden with cultural and gender stereotypes, giving rise to significant gender differences in behavior and risk factors. Yet we lack research that explores adolescent and adult attitudes about sexuality and sexual behaviors, information that is critically important if we are to address issues such as teenage pregnancy, STDs, sexual violence, and AIDS.

Six million American women, half of them in their teens, contract STDs annually.[31] This adds $5 billion to the nation's medical costs every year (interview, August 20, 1992, with P. Hitchcock, section head, STDs, National Institute of Allergy and Infectious Diseases). As a result, involuntary infertility and ectopic pregnancies have quadrupled. Another 15 to 20 million women are chronically infected with either genital herpes or human papillomavirus (HPV) infections. Two and one-half million women get chlamydial genital infections, and 1 million women are treated for pelvic inflammatory disease (PID) every year. Women are the fastest growing population with AIDS.[32] Although both sexes contract AIDS from intravenous (IV) drug abuse, the most likely infection route for women is heterosexual contact.[33] Women are more than twice as likely as men to become infected with the AIDS virus during heterosexual sex, according to an Italian epidemiological study reported in 1994.[34]

Summary

In short, research on women's health is necessary to improve women's health status, reduce disease, improve life expectancy, and enhance the quality of women's lives. Additional benefits may include decreased health costs through prevention and data from women's health research that benefit men. For example, the luteinizing hormone–releasing factor (LRF) analogues now used to treat prostate cancer were first identified in infertility research on women.[35]

Why Are Women Excluded From Medical Research?

One reason that women have been omitted from the study of many human diseases is that women's health has historically meant reproductive health. Although it is clear that the early women's movement initially stressed reproductive rights because women had to gain control over their bodies to attain equality of access to education and employment, it is somewhat ironic that this primary focus on reproductive rights strengthened the central role of reproductive health.[36] Thus early women's health research fell under the rubric of maternal health.[37] Arguably even maternal health is a misnomer when so many of the studies assessed fetal, infant, and child outcomes and neglected maternal results. For example, when diet and weight gain during pregnancy were studied, the gauge was what was good for the infant, not the mother. It is telling that, until women's health concerns were centralized through the NIH Office for Research on Women's Health in 1990, they were handled by the National Institute of Child Health and Human Development (NICHD), which failed even to mention mothers or women.

Reproductive health is, of course, a central issue, but it is not the only one. Linking the health research needs of women and children inevitably equates the value of women with bearing and caring for children. In fact, women must be appreciated on a much broader scale. Although maternal and child health concerns often overlap, particularly during pregnancy, women's health advocates question linking the two across the board, particularly when that linkage implies a tacit ranking of child concerns above maternal needs.

Clearly the research community has not kept pace with social, legal, and demographic changes that recognize many important roles for women apart from mothering. In just the past two decades, society has witnessed a remarkable shift in middle-class norms. A majority of women now work outside the home. Many of the legal barriers to women's employment—several of which rested on paternalistic assumptions about maternal and child health—have been challenged successfully. Pregnant women now work almost until delivery; businesses grant unpaid maternal and paternal leave for a new baby, a seriously ill child, or an ailing grandparent; shared jobs and flextime have helped women remain employed when their children are young; and many enlightened corporations have provided quality child care centers at work as a way of attracting and retaining employees.

Pro-choice activism at the grassroots level and access to legal and safe abortion have posed a strong challenge to the Freudian assumption that "anatomy is destiny." Moreover, a woman's longer life span, close to 80 years for a girl born today, means that the childbearing function takes up an increasingly smaller portion of her life. Many women work for a decade before they have children and live 30 to 40 years after their child-rearing duties have lessened or ceased.

A second reason for the exclusion of women has been researchers' desire for homogeneous study populations, with individuals in a study as similar to one another as possible. Women's cyclical hormonal changes were thought to confound research results.[38] Including women in research studies seemed to mean controlling for variables caused by hormonal fluctuations, such as the monthly rise and fall of estrogen and progestin. Test drugs might respond to these rising and falling levels in unpredictable ways. Yet the potential for gender differences is precisely why research on women is so desperately needed. Ironically, these same researchers—who excluded women to obtain uncomplicated study designs—have nonetheless applied information from their research on men to women, arguing that gender differences are uncommon and generally inconsequential.

In fact, women's and men's bodies differ in potentially significant ways (see Chapter 3). Such differences support the argument for the inclusion of women in clinical trials of human diseases, not their exclusion. The same cognitive leap that leads researchers to follow laboratory results with animal research, and to move from animal studies to human research, suggests that risk reduction strategies, diagnostic techniques, and treatments drawn from research on men should be tested before they are uniformly applied to women.[39]

Another argument, especially in this era of health care cost-consciousness, is that studies become more expensive when researchers must test gender-specific hypotheses or complete subgroup analysis by gender.[40] How convincing this argument is depends on which costs are considered. Certainly, it is true that an individual research project with an all-male study sample will be less expensive than a larger study that adds women. However, costs are associated with excluding women. For example, the Physicians Health Study on aspirin use and cardiovascular disease is now being duplicated using female nurses. Surely it would have been cheaper to include both genders initially. In addition, women experience more adverse drug reactions than do men, arguably because they have been excluded from drug testing. Adding these costs to the calculus may create a more positive cost-benefit ratio for including women in research.

Moreover, because women—who constitute 52% of the population—also are taxpayers, they ought to have an equal voice in the allocation of federally funded research dollars. Increasingly, women have found this voice and have questioned the practice of systematically ignoring their gender in human research studies to cut costs. It is interesting to speculate on the reaction of men if we suddenly decided that, with money in short supply, we would only do research on women's health needs.

Ways to minimize the cost of larger sample sizes do exist. Although the NIH Revitalization Act of 1993 mandates the inclusion of women in NIH-funded clinical trials, this does not automatically mean enormous study populations; instead it requires analysis by gender (which requires sample sizes of "statistical significance") only when the existence of gender differences is unknown.[41] If scientific evidence predicts no gender differences, women and men can be assumed to be homogeneous with respect to gender. In this instance, population samples will not need to be increased.

A recent Institute of Medicine report recommends developing guidelines for determining which research should address gender-related issues. Development of such guidelines will require a careful examination of existing scientific evidence with respect to gender differences—epidemiological evidence; data from basic studies; evidence from clinical studies, including drug trials; and postmarketing drug surveillance data. For example, a drug that is metabolized along pathways influenced by sex steroid hormones would clearly need gender analysis.[42] Undoubtedly, we will require more research to establish less obvious connections. Significant gender differences in efficacy observed during a measles vaccination project in Haiti, for example, have yet to be explained.[43]

Yet another reason for the lack of focus on women's research concerns has been scientists' belief that it is harder and more costly to recruit women because they often need help with child care and transportation.[44] This opinion is at odds with the observation that women have more annual contacts with health professionals than do men. Studies on patient "compliance" have indicated that women are more likely than men to follow clinical advice. Women who work at home may have more flexibility than their male counterparts, which may reduce the costs of clinical research. Perhaps women's particular needs when they are participants in research are merely different from those of men, not necessarily more "expensive."[45] Accommodation of women's child care and transportation requirements may pay off in terms of better protocol compliance.

Still another argument for excluding women from research studies has been the fear of harming pregnant women and their fetuses. This is a real public health concern, which became expensive when several drug companies were sued for fetal harm. It led researchers and policy makers to adopt protectionist policies that excluded not only pregnant women but also all fertile women. Restrictions on women's participation in research smacks of circular reasoning because the serious congenital malformations witnessed in diethylstilbestrol-[46] and thalidomide[47]-exposed children occurred as a result of maternal use of products *that had been inadequately tested in women.*

Protectionist policies tacitly assume that women are not willing or able to control their fertility. They also ignore the fact that many women—celibate, homosexual, and sterile women, for example—are unlikely to become pregnant and might be suitable study participants. Fetal harm represents a legitimate concern, but the virtual ban on re-search participation for all women of childbearing age is an excessive response. (For further discussion of protectionist policies, see Chapter 2.)

Finally, women's health has been neglected because of a pervasive if unconscious sense in the male-dominated research community that women's health issues were of secondary importance, especially in the case of health issues that had already been studied in men.[48] Scientists are often reluctant to repeat a successful study with a different demographic group—women instead of men, for example—because such studies may fail to meet the criteria of "original research" necessary for funding and subse-quent publication, particularly if the study should find no significant dif-ferences. Moreover, researchers strive to "break new ground." This "publish or perish" imperative has led many to avoid "repeat" studies, another subtle reason for the dearth of information about women. In fact, the interdisciplinary *Journal of Women's Health* was created in part to provide an academic venue for researchers with an interest in women's health and has already served as a repository for previously neglected "repeat" studies.[49] It is perhaps significant that the *Journal* was founded by women—two female researchers in the women's health field and one female publisher. Many have observed that the concern about androcentric bias in research emerged only as women began to occupy the more senior levels of scientific institutions and Congress.

Women and AIDS: A Case Study

The AIDS crisis represents a classic example of research priorities set according to the male model. Until recently, a review of the medical literature revealed a striking dearth of articles addressing the issue of AIDS in women.

The reasons for women's invisibility are complex and historical. AIDS was originally understood as a disease affecting homosexual men. Language and metaphors in the professional literature and the popular press reinforced this perception. For example, before the acronym AIDS was coined in 1982, the disease was known as GRID: Gay-Related Im-munodeficiency. Even when other modes of transmission were recognized, AIDS—like heart disease—maintained its reputation as a "male" disease. Until recently, the official Centers for Disease Control and Prevention (CDC) definitions of AIDS and AIDS-related complex (ARC) did not include gynecological symptoms.[50] As a result, clinical and social services, educational programs, and research targeted predominantly male populations.[51]

Globally, the World Health Organization (WHO) estimates of the number of women infected with the human immunodeficiency virus (HIV) in 1994 jumped to between 7 and 8 million from 3 million in 1990 (phone interview by B. Jacobson with Dr. Paloma Cuchi, Regional Advisor for Self Information Systems and Special Projects, World Health Organization AIDS Program, July 16, 1996). Young women of childbearing age represent the demographic group in which the incidence of AIDS is growing most rapidly. In certain (especially, sub-Saharan) African countries, seropositive rates among pregnant women range from 5% to nearly 30%. In those areas, women represent more than half the known cases of HIV infection.[52]

In the United States, AIDS is the fourth leading cause of death for women between ages 25 and 44 and *the primary cause of death* for women in this age group in 15 major United States cities.[53] Women with few financial resources, minority women, and sex workers are disproportionately represented in these statistics. AIDS has displaced injury as the leading cause of death for young women aged 25 to 29 in New York City.[54]

Institutional forces constitute an important explanation for women's invisibility in AIDS research priorities. Research agendas tend to reflect the health needs and priorities of policy makers. As noted, AIDS has taken the heaviest toll among women of color (Africans, African Americans, Latinas), sex workers, intravenous drug users (IDUs), and their sexual partners. Thus, much of the existing AIDS research on women tends to examine these "high-risk" categories of women. However, the definition of and focus on "risk groups" has a stigmatizing effect.[55] Women with AIDS, for instance, are viewed as transmitters of the disease to men and especially to children. Interventions targeting women—such as condom distribution to prostitutes—often aim to "protect" others from infection, yet women's personal needs for medical attention and social services often go unmet.[56]

Although a number of complex social and economic factors account for the uneven distribution of AIDS cases, the research community has demonstrated a long-standing lack of interest in pursuing nonbiological components of disease. AIDS affects the kind of women with whom many policy makers do not identify—sex workers, drug users, the companions of male drug users, and members of minority groups. Women and AIDS became a concern only when the disease threatened to "escape" from the ranks of the socially devalued and economically disenfranchised into the "general population."

In particular, NIH was slow to show an interest in funding research on women and AIDS—until it began to notice a rising incidence of pediatric AIDS. Current estimates of HIV transmission from mother to child (or fetus) vary widely from 12% to 65%.[57, 58] This alarming trend led to a research focus on pregnant women and issues of perinatal transmission. Highlighting maternal transmission was, after all, a logical outgrowth of the old understanding that women's health is equivalent to reproductive well-being. Although children with AIDS are clearly a pressing concern, this pediatric orientation blinded researchers to other important issues. As a result, epidemiologists answered questions about viral transmission of HIV through breast milk but not, for example, whether pregnancy accelerated the course of the disease in women.

The drug industry has been another obstacle to learning more about women and AIDS. Although in theory FDA has always permitted fertile women with life-threatening illnesses to participate in drug research, in practice fetal harm and liability concerns led to the widespread exclusion of "women of childbearing potential" from drug trials.[59] Yet before FDA approval of zidovudine (AZT), drug trials provided the only access to treatment for AIDS patients.

Still another reason for excluding women was cost. Including women in research and subsequent analysis of results by gender demanded larger study sizes and more sophisticated statistical techniques—both of which entailed greater expense. The call for women's inclusion in AIDS research comes at a time when policy makers are increasingly sensitive to criticism that AIDS research already commands too great a share of the NIH budget.

To reorient research priorities at NIH, grassroots organizing is critical. Although many women's organizations participated in the larger AIDS movement, the major AIDS activist groups tended to be more effective publicizing national funding priorities and access to experimental therapies for gay men, whom the disease affects in large numbers and who are better organized. Regional organizations devoted to women and AIDS have been so overwhelmed by the demand for direct services that they have had little time for public policy issues. In addition, these advocates have often lacked knowledge of the "insider politics" specific to the research community. Before the founding of the Society for the Advancement of Women's Health Research in 1990, no national advocacy organization focused exclusively on women's health research interests. Finally, the extraordinary battles over abortion politics have distracted women's health groups and policy makers from taking on important health issues such as women and AIDS.

To move an agenda within NIH, it is necessary to mobilize a scientific lobby and conduct professional meetings and conferences. It was not until late 1990, after the GAO report, that the first national meeting on women and AIDS occurred. This meeting finally led the National Institute of Allergy and Infectious Diseases (NIAID) to establish studies focusing on women, but not until a full decade after the disease was first observed in women. These new initiatives include

- The Women's Interagency HIV Study (WIHS), a large long-term study with a projected enrollment of 2,500 women, which is exploring the natural history of HIV infection in women
- The HIV Epidemiology Research Study (HERS), which is funded by CDC and which NIAID also supports; 1,200 women have been recruited into this study
- The Heterosexual AIDS Transmission Study (HATS), which examined the risk factors influencing heterosexual transmission of HIV to women and found that the risk was substantially increased for women who already had an STD
- Three clinical trials networks designed to identify effective therapies for men, women, and children with HIV infection and conduct sophisticated large-scale research studies[60]

Consequences of Women's Exclusion

The consequences of a male-centered definition of AIDS have been devastating to women with the disease. Physicians initially failed to diagnose the condition in women, which delayed treatment. Because insurance reimbursement and many social services were tied to the official AIDS definition—a definition that did not include gynecological conditions—women who were HIV positive but lacked other male-defined clinical symptoms were denied access to services and coverage. In fact it was not until January 1993 that CDC included cervical cancer in its AIDS definition.[61]

Women of childbearing potential—between ages 15 and 45—are a huge population. These women also are at greatest risk for contracting AIDS. The number of reported cases of American women with AIDS reached 58,000 as of December 31, 1994.[62] Worldwide, projections are frightening: the WHO's AIDS Program estimates that 14 million women will be infected with HIV by the year 2000 and that 4 million women will have died. (WHO's AIDS Program estimates come from a telephone interview with Dr. Paloma Cuchi, Regional Advisor for Self Information Systems and Special Projects, July 16, 1996.) AIDS advocates are hopeful that the various NIAID and CDC research studies are a sign that policy makers have recognized the crisis of HIV infection in women.

In both the United States and Africa, AIDS is increasingly spread through heterosexual contact. Repeated international surveys have documented that the public's understanding of the most common modes of AIDS transmission—sexual, intravenous, and perinatal—is high. However, the adoption of "safer sex" practices and other preventive strategies, such as condom use, reduction in the number of sexual partners, and elimination of needle-sharing among IDUs, has been less successful. To address this concern, the National Institute of Drug Abuse (NIDA) set up the Cooperative Agreement for AIDS Community-Based Outreach/Intervention Research Program, consisting of 21 sites across the United States plus one each in Puerto Rico and Rio de Janeiro, Brazil. This community-based program sends outreach workers into the field to recruit drug users who have not been in any kind of drug treatment for at least 30 days. The drug users are then exposed to a series of interventions regarding high-risk behaviors relating to sexual habits and drug use. Six to 9 months after acceptance into the program, they are evaluated to see if their behaviors have changed and, if so, to what extent. Preliminary results indicate some decrease in high-risk needle behaviors; however, researchers are finding that sexual conduct is much more difficult to change (interview by B. Jacobson with Helen Cesari, senior staff professional, NIDA, July 16, 1996). Other behavioral scientists also are exploring female-controlled methods, such as the female condom.

Because the mind-set that said "Women don't get AIDS" delayed the recognition of AIDS in women for a decade, results from the various research projects will not be available for several years. In the meantime, many women and children will die unnecessarily. The price women have paid for exclusion in the matter of AIDS—delayed diagnosis, treatment, and research, plus inadequate access to social services and insurance reimbursement—has been enormous. It is a price women have paid with their lives.

Conclusion

The AIDS story explains, with its demonstration of attitudinal blindness that kills, why we need this book: to ensure that women's health becomes a permanent priority for policy makers in the United States. Although the existence of the Office for Research on Women's Health at NIH and the Society for the Advancement of Women's Health Research gives cause for optimism, the danger of tokenism and marginalization is always possible given the history of the women's movement, which has taken two steps backward for every major leap forward. If, as one women's health advocate has proclaimed, the recent public and media attention to women's health research is analogous to the fall of the Berlin Wall—sudden and unexpected, but long overdue—we must be aware of the real danger of faddism. It is fun and trendy to devote an annual medical specialty conference to women's health. But it requires real substantive change to implement a women's health research agenda or restructure medical school curricula. While women's health remains a popular political issue, and before it loses its sheen, it is vital to institutionalize the needed research agenda so that it cannot be lost if public affection and sentiment switch course.

Advocates, of course, are not the only ones seeking to capitalize on the popularity of the women's health issue. Women's health has become an effective marketing tool for hospitals, the drug industry, and other players with nonexistent or negative track records on the issue. For example, Medical Economics Data, publisher of the *Physicians' Desk Reference*, the physician's bible of FDA-approved prescription drugs, released *The PDR Family Guide to Women's Health and Prescription Drugs* in 1994, a volume for women, not physicians, as part of the new interest in women's health. It is an open question whether the recent explosion of women's health clinics, centers, and programs is evidence of progress or if it is merely an attempt to take over the movement and change its direction, or both.

Women's Health Research: A Medical and Policy Primer represents an effort on the part of women's health advocates to define a research and policy agenda for the future. The book creates a vision of a research community composed of investigators and institutions that take women's health research needs seriously. It calls for studies to answer those needs as carefully and rapidly as possible within the confines of quality scientific inquiry. It challenges researchers in women's health to think expansively, to use multiple insights derived from many disciplines, and to move forward to a base of knowledge rather than our present condition of conjecture. It offers a women-centered definition of female health that will—in the end—improve the health, well-being, and productivity of all women in the United States and throughout the world.

Endnotes

[1] U.S. General Accounting Office, National Institutes of Health: *Problems in Implementing Policy on Women in Study Populations*. Statement of Mark V. Nadel, Associate Director of National and Public Health Issues, Human Resources Division, before the Subcommittee on Health and the Environment, Committee on Energy and Commerce, U.S. House of Representatives (GAO/T-HRD-90-80), June 18, 1990

[2]U.S. Congress, House of Representatives: Appropriations Act. H.R. 5677. 103rd Congress, 2nd session, 1992

[3]Steering Committee of the Physicians Health Study Research Group: Final report on the aspirin component of the on-going physicians health study. *New England Journal of Medicine* 321:129–135, 1989

[4]Blumenthal SJ, Barry P, Hamilton J, et al: *Forging a Women's Health Research Agenda.* Washington, DC, National Women's Health Resource Center. October 1991

[5]Wenger NK, Speroff L, Packard B: Cardiovascular health and disease in women. *New England Journal of Medicine* 329:247–256, 1993

[6]National Institutes of Health: *Opportunities for Research on Women's Health,* Part 1. Hunt Valley, MD, September 4–6, 1991 (hereafter called Hunt Valley, Part 1 or Part 2)

[7]Manson JE, et al: A prospective study of aspirin use and primary prevention of cardiovascular disease in women. *Journal of the American Medical Association* 266:521–527, 1991

[8]Lilienfeld AM, Lilienfeld DE: *Foundations of Epidemiology.* New York, Oxford University Press, 1980

[9]Appel LA, Bush T: Preventing heart disease in women. *Journal of the American Medical Association* 266:565–566, 1991

[10]"U.S. Plan Aspirin Study of Women 1991." *The New York Times,* July 30, 1991 (as of July 15, 1996, no results are available, according to Paula Williams, Information Specialist, NIHLB)

[11]Annual Report of the Society for the Advancement of Women's Health Research. Washington, DC, 1991

[12]U.S. Bureau of the Census: *U.S. Population Estimates by Age, Sex, and Race: 1993 to 2050.* New York, Census Bureau User Service (phone call, April 11, 1995, 212-264-4730)

[13]Pharmaceutical Manufacturers Association: 1992 Survey: 91 medicines in testing; three approved this past year, in *Development: AIDS Medicines, Drugs, and Vaccines.* 1992, p 8

[14]U.S. General Accounting Office: *Women's Health: FDA Needs to Ensure More Study of Gender Differences in Prescription Drug Testing.* Report to Congressional Requesters (GAO/HRD-93-17), October 1992

[15]Food and Drug Administration: Guideline for the study and evaluation of gender differences in the clinical evaluation of drugs. *Federal Register* 58(139), July 22, 1993

[16]Guralnik JM, LaCroix AZ: Assessing physical function in older populations, in *The Epidemiologic Study of the Elderly.* Edited by Wallace RB, Woolson RF. New York, Oxford University Press, 1992

[17]Hunt Valley, Part 2

[18]Austin L, Jacobson B: Managing incontinence can save dignity and cut costs. *Provider* 12(7):44, 1986

[19]Love S: *Dr. Susan Love's Breast Book.* Reading, MA, Addison Wesley, 1990

[20]Johnson JA: *Breast Cancer* (93-15 SPR). Congressional Research Service, The Library of Congress, May 25, 1993

[21]Ibid.

[22]Haseltine F, Hammond CB: Introduction, in *Menopause: Evaluation, Treatment, and Health Concerns*, Vol 320. Edited by Hammond CB, Haseltine FP, Schiff I. New York, Alan R Liss, 1989, pp xi–xxii

[23]Blumenthal SJ, Johnson T: *Facts and Research Needs*. Paper compiled for the Society for the Advancement of Women's Health Research, 1992 (hereafter called Facts)

[24]Beyene Y: *From Menarche to Menopause: Reproductive Lives of Peasant Women in Two Cultures*. New York, State University of New York Press, 1989

[25]National Osteoporosis Foundation: *Boning up on Osteoporosis: A Guide to Prevention and Treatment*, 1989

[26]Hunt Valley, Part 1

[27]Family Violence Prevention Fund

[28]Hunt Valley, Part 1

[29]American Medical Association Council on Ethical and Judicial Affairs: Gender disparities in clinical decision making. *Journal of the American Medical Association* 266:559–562, 1991

[30]Hunt Valley, Part 1

[31]Ibid.

[32]Ibid.

[33]Altman LK: "AIDS cases from sex on rise for women." *New York Times*, July 23, 1993

[34]"AIDS risk held twice as high in women." *New York Times*, November 11, 1994

[35]Petchesky RP: *Abortion and Woman's Choice: The State, Sexuality, and Reproductive Freedom*. Boston, MA, Northeastern University Press, 1985

[36]Ibid.

[37]Krieger N, Fee E: Man-made medicine and women's health: the biopolitics of sex/gender and race/ethnicity. *International Journal of Health Services* 24:265–283, 1994

[38]Hunt Valley, Part 1

[39]Johnson T: Health research that excludes women is bad science. *The Chronicle of Higher Education* B1-2, October 14, 1992

[40]Hunt Valley, Part 1

[41]U.S. Congress, Senate: National Institutes of Health Revitalization Act. S.1. 103rd Congress, 1st Session, 1993

[42]Mastroianni AC, Faden R, Federman D (eds): *Women and Health Research: Ethical and Legal Issues of Including Women in Clinical Studies*, Vol 1. Washington, DC, National Academy Press, 1994

[43]Halsey NA: Increased mortality after high titer measles: too much of a good thing. *Pediatric Infectious Disease Journal* 12:462–465, 1993

[44]Hunt Valley, Part 1

[45]Johnson T, op. cit.

[46]Weiss K: Vaginal cancer: an iatrogenic disease, in *Women and Health: The Politics of Sex in Medicine*. Edited by Fee E. New York, Baywood, 1983, pp 59–75

[47]Persaud TVN: *Problems of Birth Defects: From Hippocrates to Thalidomide and After*. Baltimore, MD, University Park Press, 1977

[48]Hunt Valley, Part 1

[49]Healy B: A celebration and new resolve. *Journal of Women's Health* 1(1): xvii, Spring 1992

[50]Treichler PA: AIDS, gender and biomedical discourse: current contests for meaning, in *AIDS: The Burdens of History*. Edited by Fee E, Fox DM. Berkeley, CA, University of California Press, 1988, pp 90–266

[51]ACT UP/NY Women & AIDS Book Group: *Women, AIDS & Activism*. Boston, MA, South End Press, 1990 (hereafter called ACT UP/NY)

[52]De Bruyn M: Women and AIDS in developing countries. *Social Science and Medicine* 34:249–262, 1992

[53]National Institute of Allergy and Infectious Diseases (NIAID) press release, February 1995

[54]Kline A, Kline E, Oken E: Minority women and sexual choice in the age of AIDS. *Social Science and Medicine* 34:447–457, 1992

[55]Schiller NG: What's wrong with this picture? The hegemonic construction of culture in AIDS research in the United States. *Medical Anthropology Quarterly* 6:237–254, 1992

[56]ACT UP/NY, 1990

[57]DeBruyn M, op. cit.

[58]Ryder RW, Behets F: Reasons for the wide variation in reported rates of mother-to-child transmission of HIV-1. *AIDS* 8:1495–1497, 1994

[59]U.S. Department of Health, Education and Welfare (HEW), Public Health Service (PHS), Food and Drug Administration (FDA): *General Considerations for the Clinical Evaluation of Drugs* (HEW/FDA-77-3040), 1977

[60]NIAID, op. cit. 1995

[61]Skinner T, Centers for Disease Control and Prevention spokesperson. Interview, August 9, 1993

[62]NIAID, op. cit. 1995

2

Women's Health Research: A Historical Perspective

Tracy L. Johnson, M.A.
Elizabeth Fee, Ph.D.

Within the past half decade, the research community has witnessed a remarkable policy reversal with respect to women's participation in clinical research. Until recently, federal regulations and guidelines pertaining to human subjects in research often limited the participation of women—especially pregnant women and, more broadly, "women of childbearing potential." Many of these policies dated from the 1970s and derived from a complex interplay of historical events and perceptions, including assumptions about female vulnerability, ethical and legal (particularly, *liability*) concerns, and a presumption that research risk often outweighs benefits. They were sustained by a scientific community that believed gender differences are rare and, when they exist, are negligible.[1]

Yet in a relatively recent flurry of activity, a number of federal agencies have issued revised policies that effectively shift women's participation in clinical research from a policy of *exclusion* to one of *inclusion*. The impetus for this policy shift is credited to the publication of a General Accounting Office (GAO) investigation in 1990, which revealed that the National Institutes of Health (NIH) had made "little progress" toward implementing its 1986 policy encouraging the inclusion of women as subjects in clinical research.[2] Subsequent press coverage—in both medical and popular journals—drew attention to several large-scale clinical trials with all-male study populations, for example, the Physicians Health Study[3] and Multiple Risk Factor Intervention Trials (MR. FIT).[4] These revelations resonated with women policy makers and the public, who became concerned about gaps in scientific knowledge as a result of "protective" policies.[5]

Reeling from the outcry created by the GAO report, NIH quickly issued a strengthened policy titled *Special Instructions for Inclusion of Women and Minorities in Clinical Research Studies*, which now appears in all of the *NIH Guide Request for Proposal Announcements* (RFAs). The policy requires "special attention to the inclusion of women and minorities in study populations" and "a specific justification" for exclusions or inadequate representation.[6] Moreover, a 1990 *NIH Policy Notice* stated that the inclusion of women in study populations will be considered a matter of scientific and technical merit in peer review.[7] NIH also created a new Office for Research on Women's Health (ORWH) to coordinate women's health activities and to ensure that NIH would adequately address women's health research concerns in the future.[8]

Seemingly overnight, women's health became a national priority. NIH launched a multimillion dollar Women's Health Initiative studying the prevention of disease in older women. Numerous medical and scientific associations—among them, the American College of Cardiology, American College of Epidemiology, and the Institute of Medicine (IOM)—dedicated annual conferences to women's health after the first was convened by the Society for the Advancement of Women's Health Research. NIH and other federal policies regulating women's participation in research were reevaluated and revised. In 1994, the U.S. Food and Drug Administration (FDA) issued new guidelines, and President Clinton signed the NIH Revitalization Act into law—both of which explicitly addressed the question of women's participation in clinical research.

Historical Context

To make projections about where the women's health research movement is headed, it is instructive to examine where it has been. This chapter outlines key legislative and regulatory developments in past re-search policy, describes their social and political influences, and con-cludes with directions for future policy development.

Food and Drug Act of 1906

At the turn of the 20th century, the practice of medicine and research was different from the way it is now. Allopathic medical physicians were not yet hospital-based but rather private practitioners in direct compe-tition with other healers: homeopaths, osteopaths, naturalists, midwives, and so forth. Many practitioners and healers competed on the basis of the contents of their "little black bag," peddling a whole spectrum of nostrums, tonics, and patent medicines.[9] Research on these sub-stances was not required. Moreover, the scientific investigation of the day was highly variable and reserved for the socially undesirable—prisoners, poor people, mentally ill persons, and elderly individuals.[10]

Practitioners jealously guarded this laissez-faire, free-market ap-proach to medicine and research. They did this so intensely that the first, modest attempt at federal regulation in the form of the Food and Drug Act of 1906—which prohibited false and misleading statements on medicine labels—was criticized by opponents as "unconstitutional, unenforceable and manifestly absurd."[11]

Manufacturers of patent medicines targeted women, especially for problems "peculiar to her sex." Before the 1906 regulations, for example, the label of the extraordinarily popular Lydia Pinkham's Vegetable Com-pound indicated that it was "A sure cure for prolapsus uteri, of falling of the womb and all female weaknesses including irregular and painful menstruation, inflammation and ulceration of the womb and for all weakness of the generative organs of either sex."[12]

After 1906, the label read: "Recommended as a vegetable tonic in conditions for which this preparation is adapted."[13]

Despite such labeling changes, the 1906 Act did not ensure against toxicity; it merely monitored drugs' strength and purity.[14] Two women physicians, Palmer and Greenberg, wrote in 1936 about the implicit public health concerns, particularly the exploitation of women. They cited, for instance, a drug trade newsletter that revealed that 92 differ-ent douche powders were on the market. In addition, household prod-ucts such as Lysol were recommended by manufacturers for feminine hygiene. According to Palmer and Greenberg, advertisements sought to exploit women's modesty by suggesting that "some problems are so intimate that it is embarrassing to talk them over with doctor." They criticized the 1906 regulation for its failure to require safety testing and to regulate drug advertising.[15]

Food, Drug and Cosmetic Act of 1938

Despite mounting public pressure, several attempts at reform in the early and mid-1930s failed. Then tragedy struck. Elixir Sulfonamide, a popular prescription drug, was converted into liquid form for children. Although the drug was tested for appearance, scent, and taste, it was not checked for toxicity. It caused severe kidney damage and 107 deaths. This episode provided the impetus for 1938 Food, Drug and Cosmetic Act requiring manufacturers to prove drug *safety* in advance of market release.[16] Unfortunately, this pattern of tragedy/scandal and *then* reform recurs repeatedly in the evolution of research regulation.

Nuremberg Code

Public concern and sensitivity to ethical issues in research were greatly strengthened by the 1945–1946 Nuremberg War Crime Trials, which revealed Nazi atrocities in human experimentation perpetrated on Jews and "undesirables." Nazi medical officials, for example, defended deplorable research practices such as the submersion of Dachau concentration camp prisoners in freezing water to measure exposure thresholds to cold temperatures. At Nuremberg, Nazi medical leader Dr. Karl Brandt testified that

> For the doctor would be at that juncture a mere instrument, like an officer on active service, for instance, who on receipt of an order puts a detachment of three or five of his men in a position where they must inevitably perish. The situation [human experimentation], when considered in relation to our circumstances in Germany during the war, is in principle the same.[17]

Also exposed at Nuremberg were several instances of questionable Allied research practices, including a United States program that involved malaria experiments on 800 Illinois prisoners.[18] To guard against future unethical research programs and practices, the trials gave rise to the Nuremberg Code, the first international policy of informed consent. Specifically, the code required that research subjects have the "legal capacity," "free power of choice," "sufficient knowledge," and "sufficient comprehension" to consent to participate in research activities.[19]

Origins of Protectionism: The 1962 Amendments and the Federal Policy for the Protection of Human Subjects (45 CFR 46)

Amendments to the Food and Drug Act in 1962—institutionalizing a drug approval process resembling current standards—were inspired by thousands of thalidomide-induced birth defects in Europe during the 1950s. *Ignoring* animal research data that indicated adverse reproductive effects, manufacturers marketed and physicians prescribed thalidomide to pregnant women to "combat nausea." Later it was found to cause severe limb deformities and organ malformations in children exposed in utero.[20] The 1962 amendments required manufacturers to demonstrate drug *efficacy* as well as drug safety, demanded that product advertising clearly indicate associated *risks* as well as benefits, and compelled the FDA to collect adverse reaction reports.[21]

In the 1960s and 1970s, diethylstilbestrol (DES) and the Dalkon Shield provided two additional examples of an unsafe drug product and a poorly designed device that were marketed without adequate testing, causing injury, reproductive harm, and even death.

Before its use in humans, DES had been used as a feed additive for cattle and was known to cause reproductive harm. Yet, incredibly, DES was not evaluated for teratogenic effects, nor were "dose-ranging" studies—to test safety and efficacy—conducted.[22] Commonly prescribed to pregnant women during the 1940s, 1950s, and 1960s to prevent miscarriages, DES has been associated with rare cancers of the vagina, infertility, and the abnormal development of reproductive organs in male as well as female children exposed in utero. Third-generation effects also have been observed.[23] A "classic example of teratogenic liability on a grand scale," the DES tragedy resulted in numerous legal suits, many of which were successful.[24]

Similarly, the intrauterine device (IUD) marketed under the name Dalkon Shield—which caused infection, hemorrhage, reproductive harm, and sometimes death—also sparked several large lawsuits. The manufacturer ultimately withdrew the product 4 years after its market release. Congressional hearings that revealed exaggerated manufacturer claims, poor research methodology, and selective presentation of results served as the impetus for this withdrawal.[25]

The thalidomide, DES, and Dalkon Shield disasters—and, particularly, the growing threat of liability—resulted in the pharmaceutical industry's adoption of increasingly conservative postures with respect to the participation of premenopausal women in clinical drug trials. In addition, revelations of the Tuskegee Study, an observational investigation involving 400 rural African American men whose syphilis remained untreated for 35 years, well after antibiotic treatment was widely available, served to solidify a protectionist sentiment, which was ultimately reflected in public policy.[26] More than 20 years after publication of the *New York Times* article that broke the Tuskegee story, the study continues to inform the discourse surrounding the ethics of human research, particularly with respect to the recruitment and retention of racial and ethnic minorities in clinical research.[27]

The Federal Policy for the Protection of Human Subjects (45 CFR 46) was announced in 1974 in response to concerns of research abuse. Significantly, regulatory language regarding "equitable subject selection" did not aim to guarantee equal *access* to studies, but rather to prevent a scenario in which one group (e.g., public patients) was required to bear the risk of research for the benefit of another (e.g., private patients).[28] Given the history of exploitation in research, it is understandable that federal policy focused on research risk rather than potential benefits. However, the emphasis on protecting *vulnerable* populations, including pregnant women, from research abuse has had consequences that policy makers may not have intended.

Indeed, portions of 45 CFR 46 that are still in effect strike the modern reader as paternalistic or even bizarre. For instance, one curious section reads:

> When some or all of the subjects are likely to be vulnerable to coercion or undue influence, such as children, prisoners, *pregnant*

women, mentally disabled persons, and economically or education-ally disadvantaged persons, additional safeguards have been included in the study to protect the rights and welfare of these subjects.[29] (emphasis added)

Contemporary critics of the policy have questioned what makes pregnant women especially "vulnerable to coercion" or "undue influence." Some also have asked why there was no feminist outcry. Here it is instructive to examine the context. The birth of the women's health movement occurred in the early 1970s, which adopted a critical orientation toward medicine. After the thalidomide, DES, and Dalkon Shield disasters, some women's health advocates concluded that federal policy, being overbroad and paternalistic, at least protected women from serving as guinea pigs in ill-conceived research projects.[30] Indeed, women's organizations of the 1970s, like Palmer and Greenberg in 1936, were more likely to frame the issue of women's health research as inappropriate *inclusion* and *exploitation* rather than exclusion. Focusing on reports that women received DES without their knowledge as a part of an experimental protocol, these early women's health activists supported improved informed consent procedures and other protective measures for women as research participants and consumers.[31]

1977 FDA Guidelines

In 1977, the FDA issued a guideline limiting the participation of women of "childbearing potential"—broadly defined—in drug research. The guideline permitted women's inclusion in clinical drug testing only after animal reproduction studies and the early Phase 1 and 2 (safety and efficacy) tests.[32] However, because manufacturers were not required to conduct animal reproduction studies, and because liability concerns were pervasive, women were commonly excluded from the later stages of research.[33] Although exceptions were made to include women with life-threatening conditions, researchers, for example, invoked "FDA restrictions" to exclude women with acquired immunodeficiency syndrome (AIDS) from drug trials or to allow their inclusion only after sterilization. A 1992 GAO survey of recently approved drugs found that, although some women were included in most studies, "for more than 60 percent of the drugs, the representation of women in the test population was less than the representation of women in the population with the corresponding disease."[34]

Considerable asymmetry existed in federal requirements for research affecting male versus female reproductive potential. According to FDA guidelines, even research that has resulted in reproductive harm in male animals could go forward depending "upon the nature of the abnormalities, the dosage at which they occurred, the disease being treated, the importance of the drug, and the duration of drug administration."[35] In contrast to this nuanced risk-benefit analysis, FDA's sweeping definition of "women of childbearing potential" virtually excluded all menstruating women from early testing of drug therapies.[36] Critics of these 1977 guidelines have suggested that the policy is more a reflection of gender stereotypes—female susceptibility and male invulnerability—than of sound scientific considerations.[37]

1993 FDA Guidelines

In response to recent policy changes at NIH and in an attempt to head off congressional action,[38] the FDA reversed its policy in 1993, noting that "fetal protection can be achieved by measures short of excluding women from early trials."[39] It issued a new *Guideline for the Study and Evaluation of Gender Differences in the Clinical Evaluation of Drugs* (1993), which effectively rescinded the 1977 guidelines. In doing so, the FDA acknowledged that the 1977 policy "had resulted in the exclusion of most women capable of becoming pregnant in the earliest phases of clinical trials."[40] The 1993 policy strongly encouraged the inclusion of "representatives of both genders" in drug trials but stopped short of *requiring* women's participation. The guideline also encouraged gender analysis, increased the study of pharmacokinetics, supported contraceptive use by female research participants, and strengthened informed consent procedures.[41]

1993 NIH Revitalization Act

In June 1993, President Clinton signed into law the NIH Revitalization Act, which contained a provision called *Subtitle B—Clinical Research*

Equity Regarding Women and Minorities. Subtitle B *requires* the inclusion of women—in sufficient numbers to ensure "a valid analysis"—in most clinical *trials*. Because this section seems to imply the need for increased sample sizes and therefore cost, this provision stirred controversy and debate within the scientific community.[42]

The NIH Revitalization Act was the reauthorizing legislation for the entire NIH. President Bush had vetoed the bill in 1992 because of provisions to lift the federal moratorium on fetal research *and* because the administration deemed it "not necessary to increase support for research directed at women's health needs."[43] An emergency resolution was secured to fund NIH until the following year. Confident that recently elected President Clinton would be supportive, the first bill the Senate introduced in January 1993 was this NIH legislation. As predicted, Congress passed the bill promptly.

The Congressional Caucus for Women's Issues helped draft Subtitle B in an attempt to close what it viewed as potential "loopholes" in current NIH policy with respect to women's participation in research activities (Susan Wood, Congressional Caucus of Women's Issues, personal communication, April 1993). Unlike the NIH policy, the act is legally binding, and it calls for U.S. Department of Health and Human Services (DHHS) guidelines to ensure the adequate representation of women in NIH-funded clinical research. The act differs from NIH policy in at least two respects. First, whereas NIH policy allows that unreasonable expense might be an acceptable rationale for women's exclusion from certain clinical trials, the act explicitly disqualifies cost considerations.[44] Second, NIH policy does not require that study designs provide statistical power to perform gender analysis except "whenever there are scientific reasons to anticipate differences between men and women."[45] For clinical *trials*, the act shifts the burden of proof, *requiring* a "valid analysis of whether the variables being studied in the trial affect women or members of minority groups." An exception applies only when "there is substantial scientific data demonstrating that there is no significant [gender] difference."[46] If the requisite scientific data exist, women must be counted among the study population, but the sample as a whole can be considered homogeneous with respect to gender. Therefore, in this case at least, including women will not require large increases in sample size.[47]

From Protectionism to Access

A number of factors have influenced these rather remarkable policy reversals at FDA and NIH. AIDS activism in the 1980s brought the first real challenge to protectionist policies.[48] In May 1987, the FDA responded to pressure from AIDS activists and issued regulations expanding access to experimental drugs used to treat serious and life-threatening illnesses.[49] Activists also succeeded in increasing federal appropriations for AIDS research. It is significant that researchers and policy makers, who once considered research as a dangerous project from which vulnerable groups needed protection, changed their conception to see scientific investigation as promoting the public good.

Policy developments at NIH and FDA reflect an ongoing philosophical reorientation that is occurring within ethics and law—a shift away from paternalistic physician practices and policies and toward greater patient autonomy. Concepts of joint decision making in clinical care and informed consent in research have now gained widespread recognition. In short, the rights of patients and research subjects—particularly women—have come sharply into focus. For example, the preamble to the newer (1993) FDA policy cites the Johnson Controls case as providing legal precedent to affirm women's right to make autonomous decisions about their own bodies:

> The FDA takes serious note of the [Supreme] Court's position on a woman's right to participate in decisions about fetal risk and believes it is appropriate to consider the Court's opinion in developing policy on the inclusion of women in clinical trials.[50]

In addition, the possibility of liability claims arising from women's exclusion was influential in changing attitudes.

Women AIDS activists were among the first to observe the parallels between the women's health and AIDS movements and sought to galvanize feminist activism.[51] Even after the FDA liberalized its policy in 1987, women with AIDS still faced exclusion from many clinical drug trials because of their reproductive potential.[52] The women's health community took careful note of the success of AIDS activists in reorienting financial and scientific resources to address AIDS research needs more effectively. AIDS activism provided women with a language and a political strategy with which to pursue a women's health research agenda.[53]

In addition, changing demographics provided the necessary critical mass. Maturing women of the baby-boom generation became increasingly concerned about the lack of attention to their health and well-being. Dramatic increases in the number of women enrolling in medical school during the 1970s[54] provided a vocal minority of medical professionals in the subsequent decade who questioned current priorities and policies in women's health research. In particular, they criticized governmental policies (e.g., 1977 FDA guidelines) that excluded women from medical research because of their reproductive potential.[55] Women in medicine began to link the lack of national focus on women's health to such "protective" policies.

Many women and women's groups played significant roles in mounting political pressure. Among them were women in Congress who questioned funding priorities; women in the media, especially science writers, who kept the issue before the public eye; women's organizations, such as the Society for the Advancement of Women's Health Research, the Breast Cancer Coalition, the Boston Women's Health Book Collective, the National Black Women's Health Project, and the National Women's Health Network; and baby boomers, who flexed their new-found economic and political muscle.

The new federal policies were not without critics, especially within the scientific community. In addition to raising concerns of unintended pregnancy, fetal harm, and liability, investigators pointed to practical considerations that made women's participation in research more time-consuming or costly. They charged that women were more difficult to recruit into studies and that their inclusion added complexity by introducing a new variable—the menstrual cycle—for which researchers must control. Claiming that gender differences are rare and usually small, some researchers defended all-male study populations as cost-effective, maintaining that results can normally be generalized to women. In contrast, statistically valid gender analysis demands increased sample sizes that can become unwieldy and expensive.[56]

However, NIH officials and other researchers who had defended women's exclusion from clinical research were often perceived as arrogant and dismissive. Their arguments also revealed the androcentric assumption that it is possible to generalize across gender, as well as the *inconsistent* assumption that the inclusion of women increases the variability within a sample (the "variance"). Countering this misperception, a recent IOM report notes: "Person-years of follow-up are person-years of follow-up whether they are female or male years, *unless* the researchers have plausible hypotheses of gender differences in response."[57] Moreover, the likelihood and significance of gender difference are matters of debate.

Because the NIH Revitalization Act requires larger samples only when gender differences are either anticipated or unknown, women's health advocates have argued that the extra expense in these cases is justified. They admit that the inclusion of women will have other implications for costs and design. Researchers will have to deal with unique recruitment issues, which may include child care and transportation. Investigators also will need to conceptualize and explore gender-based hypotheses, which may entail the collection of additional variables. Advocates do not deny that such considerations may add to current research costs, but rather question the implicit assumption that the costs associated with an all-male sample are appropriate, whereas the additional expense of including women is excessive.[58]

IOM Recommendations

Even with passage of the NIH Revitalization Act, the issue of women's participation in clinical research is not settled. Final word may depend on future regulations from DHHS that will control the operation of the act. As of early 1996, no regulations had been issued (personal communication from Barbara Allen, DHHS Office on Women's Health, February 1996). Thus, the IOM committee proposes weighing the cost of increasing sample sizes against the likely scientific benefit.

However, it is not clear that an overly rigid, "exceptionless" regulation reflects legislative intent. The NIH Revitalization Act clearly charges the Secretary of DHHS with the responsibility of establishing guidelines regarding "the circumstances under which the inclusion of women and minorities as subjects in projects of clinical research is inappropriate for purpose of subsection (b)."[59]

Moreover, the extent to which researchers can recognize *in advance* the potential for gender differences remains controversial. The recent experience of researchers at Johns Hopkins University raises doubts about this "crystal ball" approach. Investigators followed up children who received a new high-titer measles vaccination in Haiti and discovered that mortality rates among children differed significantly by sex—with girls experiencing higher mortality. The authors noted that there was "no evidence of selection bias or preferential health care by sex" and that the "biological basis for this [gendered] effect on mortality has not been determined."[60] Hence, the Congressional Caucus for Women's Issues and others have argued that the dearth of scientific literature on gender-mediated effects serves to hamper the ability to "anticipate" such differences (personal communication from S. Wood, May 1993).

Conclusion

Although recent events have focused attention on women's participation in clinical trials, one must not lose sight of the fact that the history of research on women is one of inappropriate *inclusion* as well as of exclusion. Responding to a history of abuse in drug testing and contraceptive research—all too often on poor women and women of color in the United States and abroad—some feminists have decried all experimentation on women. The observation that women have served as objects but not subjects of science is not new. The tendency of male "intellectuals" to make women objects prompted Virginia Woolf to comment: "Have you any notion how many books are written about women in the course of one year? Have you any notion how many are written by men? Are you aware that you are, perhaps the most discussed animal in the universe?"[61]

Cross-culturally, dominant social groups generally frame questions and conduct experiments, whereas less dominant or socially undesirable groups—poor people, mentally ill persons, and elderly individuals, as well as prisoners, racial and ethnic minorities, and women—are relegated to study participants or play no role at all.

Recognizing this, we can argue that we need ethical and responsible human research before drugs and treatments are incorporated into general medical practice. Thus, as the IOM committee writes, "in designing recruitment and consent procedures, investigators must [respond] to the concerns and needs of communities that have a history of exploitation or abuse in previous clinical studies."[62] Federal guidelines that ensure access to research while providing appropriate protection are necessary to curtail the most flagrant abuses but are merely one step toward the larger goal of a women-centered research agenda. We also must look to structural issues—how is research funded, who sets priorities, and what is the nature of the power structure that makes research decisions. Beyond mere inclusion and "numerical parity" for women, we need efforts to incorporate women and women's perspectives at every level of federally funded research, from policy, to peer review, to design and practice. A move away from the case-by-case review of research in favor of looking at the research agenda as a whole, as suggested by IOM, is perhaps premature until mechanisms for accountability are securely in place. For now, we need the mandatory inclusion of women in studies to ensure that research on women becomes and remains a reality.

Endnotes

[1]Mastroianni AC, Faden R, Federman D (eds): *Women and Health Research: Ethical and Legal Issues of Including Women in Clinical Studies*, Vol 1. Washington, DC, National Academy Press, 1994

[2]U.S. General Accounting Office, National Institutes of Health: *Problems in Implementing Policy on Women in Study Populations*. Statement of Mark V. Nadel, Associate Director of National and Public Health Issues, Human Resources Division, before the Subcommittee on Health and the Environment, Committee on Energy and Commerce, U.S. House of Representatives (GAO/T-HRD-90-80), June 18, 1990

[3]Steering Committee of the Physicians Health Study Research Group: Final report on the aspirin component of the on-going physicians health study. *New England Journal of Medicine* 321:129–135, 1989

[4]Blumenthal SJ, Barry P, Hamilton J, et al: *Forging a Women's Health Research Agenda: Clinical Pharmacy Panel Report*. Washington, DC, National Women's Health Resource Center, October 1991

[5]Johnson T, Fee E: *Women's Participation in Clinical Research: From Protectionism to Access*. Commissioned paper for the Committee on the Ethical and Legal Issues Relating to the Inclusion of Women in Clinical Studies, Institute of Medicine, Washington, DC, National Academy Press, 1994

[6]National Institutes of Health: *NIH Guide for Grants and Contracts*. 22(5):3, February 5, 1993

[7]National Institutes of Health (NIH) and Alcohol, Drug Abuse, and Mental Health Administration (ADAMHA): NIH/ADAMHA Policy Concerning Inclusion of Women in Study Populations. *NIH Guide* 19(31):18–19, (P.T. 34, II; 1014002, 1014006), August 24, 1990

[8]National Institutes of Health, Division of Research Grants: *NIH/ADAMHA Tracking of Gender and Minority Representation in Clinical Research Studies* (Tech Notice No 214), March 27, 1992

[9]Starr P: *The Social Transformation of American Medicine: The Rise of a Sovereign Profession and the Making of a Vast Industry*. New York, Basic Books, 1982

[10]National Commission for the Protection of Human Subjects of Biomedical and Behavioral Research: *The Belmont Report: Ethical Principles and Guidelines for the Protection of Human Subjects of Research*, April 18, 1979

[11]Young JH: *Pure Food: Securing the Federal Food and Drugs Act of 1906*. Princeton, NJ, Princeton University Press, 1989

[12]Palmer RL, Greenberg SK: *Facts and Fraud in Woman's Hygiene: A Medical Guide Against Misleading Claims and Dangerous Products*. New York, Vanguard Press, 1936

[13]Ibid.

[14]Young JH, op. cit.

[15]Palmer RL, Greenberg SK, op. cit.

[16]Young JH: *The Early Years of Federal Food and Drug Control*. Madison, WI, American Institute of the History of Pharmacy with the cooperation of the American Pharmaceutical Association, 1982

[17]Fletcher JC: Evolution of informed consent, in *Research Ethics: Progress in Clinical and Biomedical Research*. Edited by Bergt K, Tranoy KE. New York, Alan R Liss, 1983, pp 187–228

[18]Ibid.

[19]Gallant PM, Force R: *Legal and Ethical Issues in Human Research and Treatment*. New York, SP Medical & Scientific Books, 1978

[20]Persaud TVN: *Problems of Birth Defects: From Hippocrates to Thalidomide and After*. Baltimore, MD, University Park Press, 1977

[21]Food and Drug Administration (FDA): *Evolution of U.S. Drug Law: From Test Tube to Patient: New Drug Development in the United States* (HFI-40), 1988, Revised March 1990

[22]Bowles LE: The disfranchisement of fertile women in clinical trials: the legal ramifications of and solutions for rectifying the knowledge gaps. *Vanderbilt Law Review* 45(4):877–920, 1992

[23]Brody JE: "Personal health: adult years bring new afflictions for DES 'babies'." *New York Times*, February 10, 1993

[24]Bowles LE, op. cit., pp 907–916

[25]Corea G: *The Hidden Malpractice: How American Medicine Treats Women as Patients and Professionals*. New York, William Morrow, 1977

[26]Jones JH: *Bad Blood: The Tuskegee Syphilis Experiment*. New York, Free Press, 1981

[27]Johnson T, Fee E, op. cit.

[28]U.S. Department of Health and Human Services (DHHS): *Federal Policy for the Protection of Human Subjects* (Title 45 Code of Federal Regulations Part 46, pp 101–124, Subpart A [FR Doc. 91–14262]), Revised June 18, 1991

[29]Ibid.

[30]The Boston Women's Health Book Collective: *Our Bodies, Ourselves*. New York, Simon & Schuster, 1973

[31]Weiss K: Vaginal cancer: an iatrogenic disease, in *Women and Health: The Politics of Sex in Medicine*. Edited by Fee E. New York, Baywood, 1983, pp 59–75

[32]U.S. Department of Health, Education and Welfare (HEW), Public Health Service (PHS), Food and Drug Administration (FDA): *General Considerations for the Clinical Evaluation of Drugs* (HEW/FDA-77-3040), 1977

[33]Kinney EL, et.al: Underrepresentation of women in new drug trials: ramifications and remedies. *Annals of Internal Medicine* 95:495–499, 1981

[34]U.S. General Accounting Office: *Women's Health: FDA Needs to Ensure More Study of Gender Differences in Prescription Drug Testing* (Report to Congressional Requesters [GAO/HRD-93-17]), October 1992

[35]U.S. Dept. HEW, PHS, FDA, op. cit., p 11

[36]U.S. Dept. HEW, PHS, FDA, op. cit., p 12

[37]Kinney EL, et al, op. cit.

[38]U.S. House of Representatives: Pharmaceutical Interactions Safety Act (Discussion Draft), 1993

[39]U.S. Department of Health and Human Services, Public Health Service, Food and Drug Administration: *FDA Talk Paper: FDA Plans Policy Change on Women in Clinical Trials*, April 5, 1993

[40]Ibid.

[41]Guideline for the study and evaluation of gender differences in the clinical evaluation of drugs. *Federal Register* 58(139):39406–39416, July 22, 1993

[42]Wittes BW, Wittes JW: "Group therapy: research by quota." *The New Republic*, April 6, 1993, pp 15–16

[43]Johnson T: Health research that excludes women is bad science. *Chronicle of Higher Education*, October 14, 1992

[44]U.S. Congress, Senate: National Institutes of Health Revitalization Act. S.1. 103rd Congress, 1st session, 1993

[45]U.S. Department of Health and Human Services, Public Health Service, National Institutes of Health: *NIH Instruction and Information Memorandum:32* (OER 90-5), December 11, 1990

[46]U.S. Congress, Senate, op. cit.

[47]Johnson T, Fee E, op. cit.

[48]Rothman DJ, Edgar H: Scientific rigor and medical realities: placebo trials in cancer and AIDS research, in *AIDS: The Making of a Chronic Disease.* Edited by Fee E, Fox DM. Berkeley, CA, University of California Press, 1992, pp 194–206

[49]Rothman DJ, Edgar H: New rules for new drugs: the challenge of AIDS to the regulatory process. *Milbank Quarterly Supplement* 68(1):111–142, 1990

[50]Federal Register, op. cit., pp 39406–39416

[51]ACT UP/NY Women & AIDS Book Group: *Women, Aids & Activism.* Boston, MA, South End Press, 1990

[52]American Civil Liberties Union: *AIDS and Civil Liberties Project: Testimony on the Discrimination in Access to Clinical Trials of AIDS Drugs.* Before the Human Resources and Intergovernmental Relations Subcommittee of the Committee on Government Operations, April 28, 1988

[53]Johnson T, Fee E, op. cit.

[54]American Medical Association (AMA): *Women in Medicine in America: In the Mainstream.* Chicago, IL, AMA, 1991

[55]American Civil Liberties Union, op. cit.

[56]Wittes BW, Wittes JW, op. cit., pp 15–16

[57]Mastroianni AC, Faden R, Federman D, op. cit., p 6

[58]Johnson T, op. cit.

[59]U.S. Congress, Senate, op. cit.

[60]Halsey NA: Increased mortality after high titer measles vaccines: too much of a good thing. *Pediatric Infectious Disease Journal* 12:462–465, 1993

[61]Woolf V: *A Room of One's Own.* New York, Harcourt, Brace & World, 1929

[62]Mastroianni AC, Faden R, Federman D, op. cit., p 19

Part 2

What We Know

3

How Female and Male Biology Differ

Estelle Ramey, Ph.D.

Considering the discouraging statistics regarding the excess illness experienced by women, noted in Chapter 1, one would think that Shakespeare was right when he wrote, "Frailty, thy name is woman." This belief has been repeatedly underlined by everyone from the Apostle Paul to Freud to early 20th century gynecologists such as Drs. Horatio Storer and Charles Meigs. Storer's contribution came in this statement: "It was the Almighty who, in creating the female sex, had taken the uterus and built a woman around it." Meigs's widely used obstetrical textbook declared, "A woman has a head too small for intellect but just big enough for love." Later in the century, male gynecologists continued their insistence on woman as womb, claiming that too much female thinking takes vital energy from the uterus and overheats small brains, leading to sterility and madness; that raging female hormones make women unfit for responsible jobs, thereby putting child rearing in the irresponsible job category; and that successful women are endocrine freaks with hair on their chests but none on their heads, the result of an excess of the male hormone testosterone. This image has not faded completely even now, with women viewed as aging less attractively than men, so that the common perception is that men mature while

47

women rot—this, despite insurance statistics showing that, for every 100,000 people, 803 men die to 447 women.[1]

Nothing could be further from the truth than the doctrine of "frail womanhood." Women have a terrific biological advantage over men. Understanding female biology is therefore vital—to find ways of using women's biological strengths to counteract their excess illness and allow them to live to a vital old age, and to see what we can learn from female biology that may permit the modification of male biochemistry at critical sites, such as the cardiovascular system, to reduce early male death. It is time to look for answers to this basic question: why does the female of every mammalian species, including our own, resist stress better than the male, perform better than the male when it comes to chronic physical demands, and outlive the male even when lifestyles are the same? We need to answer these questions from three perspectives—cellular, for the basic scientist; whole organism, for researchers and clinicians; and societal, for those who study how human behavior affects the way we live.

The Immune System

Women throughout their life span respond more vigorously to infections and other conditions requiring activation of the immune system. This is because the X chromosome carries a gene complex governing immunoresponsiveness and a double dose of Xs augments this capacity. In addition, estrogens act on the liver to produce more immune globulins, proteins that make antibodies to fight disease. Men do not have this advantage. Although women benefit from their lusty immune systems with a strong reaction to viral and bacterial invaders and, possibly, to some cancer-causing viruses, the very robustness of immune systems probably accounts for a greater incidence of autoimmune diseases, such as multiple sclerosis, lupus erythematosus, and rheumatoid arthritis. Female cardiac transplant patients reject organs more frequently and earlier than male patients. In addition, male transplant patients who receive female bone marrow experience more graft versus host disease.[2]

Pregnancy reduces female immune responsiveness. For example, pregnancy is associated with spontaneous remission of rheumatoid arthritis, which is four times more frequent in women than men. Pregnant renal transplant patients can have their dosage of immunosuppressant drugs reduced or eliminated until delivery, when it must immediately be re-administered at full strength. Research is needed to assess the effect of hormone replacement therapy on both the transplanted tissue and the autoimmune disease itself in nonpregnant patients.[3]

Conception to Puberty

The female advantage starts in utero. The Y (male) chromosome is smaller and lighter than the larger, heavier, and somewhat lethargic X (female) chromosome. In addition, the sperm carrying the Y chromosome are Olympic speed swimmers, producing 130 to 150 male conceptions for every 100 females. But by the time the fetus emerges from the womb, the ratio falls dramatically—to 106 boys born for every 100 girls.

There are good biological reasons for this. From the moment of conception the two X chromosomes of the female give her better genetic backup systems than the male XY configuration. The Y chromosome apparently contributes only maleness and seems to have no other genes that can match those on the X chromosome for traits such as blood clotting and a peppier immune system. That is why a sex-linked disease such as hemophilia is overwhelmingly (85%) male. Each X chromosome has a gene for clotting. The boy who receives an abnormal gene for blood clotting on the X chromosome from his mother does not have a chance to neutralize this trait because he lacks a second X chromosome; he has only a Y chromosome that carries no blood clotting gene. If there is an error on a girl's X chromosome, her other X can override it, but males get no second chance. This makes male fetuses much more vulnerable to inborn errors of metabolism, producing a significantly higher death rate in utero. Male fragility persists after birth. In the first week of life, 30% more male than female babies die from congenital disorders. In fact, about 75% of all genetically mandated abnormalities have a higher incidence in boys than girls. All learning disabilities, for example, are seen more in boys than girls.[4]

Testosterone

For the first 6 weeks after conception, all fetuses are developing females despite their genetic differences. At 6 weeks the Y chromosome comes into play, mandating the first secretion of testosterone, which causes the male sex organs to begin maturing and alters brain development and enzymatic patterns in other organs such as the liver. At this crucial changeover time, there is a high incidence of abnormalities.

Testosterone slightly inhibits the growth of the left side of the cerebral cortex, whereas the right side grows more rapidly. This may account for better spatial ability in men but at a cost to verbal facility and digital dexterity, which are better in girls. Testosterone also produces a slower rate of overall maturation of the male brain. Females develop both sides of the brain more equally and establish a more extensive interconnection between the two sides. Later in life this allows women to tolerate brain damage better. For example, if a stroke impairs one area of the brain, a woman is more likely to recruit other areas to take over the job of the injured region. Thus, women tend to recover better from strokes than similarly afflicted men. It also has been suggested that this bilateral symmetry in women's brains enables them to do more than one job at a time more comfortably than men. No mother or home manager could survive without this typical female versatility.[5]

Puberty to Menopause

At puberty, women get another biological boost from the sex hormones, the estrogens and progestins. They protect the heart and blood vessels from rapid aging, whereas the male hormones accelerate the aging of these tissues, making men more susceptible to fatal heart disease. Animal research in our laboratory has shown that male sex and testosterone treatment increased sudden death in mice; that, in rodents bred to study arterial blood clots (thrombosis), maleness itself is significantly deleterious; and that testosterone dramatically increased thrombosis in animal models of both sexes. However, when estradiol, the most potent naturally occurring estrogen in humans, was administered subcutaneously to these animals, thrombosis was significantly reduced. The data indicate that estradiol may have a beneficial anticlotting effect on the elements of the blood but not necessarily on the vascular wall itself. However, there is no conclusive evidence yet in humans that male sex per se is a risk factor for the development of thrombosis, although plaque formation in the coronary arteries and consequent plaque rupture are greater in men than in postmenopausal women, even though the incidence of heart disease in women jumps sharply after menopause.[6] More research is needed to determine what protects women's coronary arteries from excessive plaque formation even after menopause.

Testosterone produces big muscles and taller stature, but estrogens give women a much superior ability to resist stress and a greater capacity for long-term energy expenditure. Estrogens are protective in at least two ways. They act on the liver to produce more high-density lipoprotein (HDL), the so-called good cholesterol that removes cholesterol from the bloodstream and thus protects against its damaging buildup in blood vessels. Estrogen therefore has a favorable effect on blood lipids (fats), allowing women during the childbearing years to provide the fetus with sugar (glucose) from fatty acids circulating in the bloodstream. Estrogen's beneficence vis-à-vis blood lipids is the basis for estrogen replacement therapy (ERT) after menopause. Estrogens also regulate the manufacture of prostaglandins, hormones that protect women from forming fatal blood clots or experiencing coronary artery damage. Thus, women develop heart disease some 10 to 15 years after men.

Although conventional and media wisdom in the 1980s blamed the stress of earning a living and competing in the real world for male cardiac vulnerability and predicted similar increased illness and death for women after large numbers of them entered the labor force, this did not happen. In fact, a study by the Metropolitan Life Insurance Company of men and women listed in *Who's Who in America* found that these hardest running and most competitive people in the country outlived a matched group of less successful colleagues by 29%.[7]

Science gives estrogen credit for protecting women from heart disease for valid reasons. One is that laboratory animals show the same female cardiac strength and male cardiac weakness as the human species and they do not go to work. The killer stress apparently is not hard work, competition, or lack of time for recreation; it is an internalized perception that one lacks control over one's fate in a culture that rates such control at the top of the value scale. In fact, a sense of helplessness and a perception that rewards and punishments have no relation to effort have been shown to produce fatal cardiovascular damage even in laboratory rats, especially in males. The longevity of Supreme Court justices and symphony orchestra conductors, who have quintessential control over events, is legendary.[8]

The second reason comes from research on estrogen's effects in different groups of women. For example, one study of large numbers of women who had their ovaries removed in their 20s and did not receive hormonal replacement found that these women developed heart disease about 15 years before women with intact ovaries or women who took ERT after ovarian removal.[9] Observational studies suggest that the risk of coronary heart disease among healthy postmenopausal women taking oral estrogen is reduced by approximately 50%, with an even greater benefit of protection from a second heart attack for women who already have coronary heart disease (CHD).[10] Although many postmenopausal women are using combined hormone replacement therapy (HRT), with progestin added to estrogen to protect against endometrial cancer, recent evidence from the Postmenopausal Estrogen/Progestin Interventions (PEPI) Trial, a large controlled, double-blind study of 875 women, indicates that progestin—depending on the kind of synthetic preparation used—reduces but does not eliminate the favorable effect that estrogen has on blood lipids.[11] (See Chapter 7 for a full discussion of the PEPI study.) In addition, recent observational data suggest that there are benefits from adding progestin to estrogen, particularly on women's lipid levels and anticoagulation tendencies.[12] Definitive answers to the risks and benefits from HRT for perimenopausal women must await the dawn of the new century, when the results of the Women's Health Initiative, which is studying this question in a much larger cohort of older women, are due. If estrogen is so beneficial to cardiovascular health, we need research to find a nonfeminizing estrogen for men.

How Hormones Affect Females and Males

Biology dictates that the primary role for both females and males is to reproduce themselves to ensure the survival of the species. Historically, both sexes had to live only long enough to bear children. Nature en-dowed the human male with the strongest sex drive of all animals and powered the male brain with the hormone testosterone, which dictated that inseminating the female was the male's primary function. When our species was being established as a unique development in evolution because of our greater brains and more skillful hands, life expectancy for both sexes was only about 18 years. Species survival therefore depended on a constant and urgent sex drive in young males, a high rate of sperm production, and, to ward off danger, a vigorous, rapidly responding mus-culature, endurance, and speed.

Females, however, needed large amounts of estrogen and progestin to sustain ovulation, fertilization, implantation, gestation, and delivery. Because the human fetus is extremely vulnerable to environmental threats, the pregnant woman required more protection than the male. The male, in fact, had to provide this protection for the pregnant fe-male and their vulnerable offspring. Testosterone was the key to fulfill-ing this need because it produces more of the stress hormones—adrenaline and cortisone—in the male. These stress hormones prime the cardiovascular system for fight or flight. Males therefore respond to danger with explosive muscular activity, a sudden rise in blood pres-sure, a strong heartbeat, and greatly increased cardiac output to bring blood to the muscles and provide them with the large amount of oxy-gen and nutrients they need to function under stress. In addition, be-cause these early males were at high risk of injury as they fought off large animals and other males, the stress hormones also shorten bleed-ing time by increasing the rate of blood clotting at the site of damage to blood vessels.

In short, testosterone mandated a brief, lusty, athletic life in early males. But testosterone is not a benign hormone. The high blood pres-sure it provokes causes damage to blood vessels and makes the liver produce low-density lipoprotein (LDL). LDL is known as the "bad" cho-lesterol because it can be oxidized by free radicals, and oxidized LDL damages blood vessels. In fact, LDL with a free radical acts like a loose cannon in the bloodstream. Early males did not have to worry about this because they did not live long enough to experience such damage. But the stress response takes an enormous toll on modern males. Whereas early man was able to counteract elevated blood pressure by vigorous muscle work, in our high-technology society, most stresses and dangers are not appropriately met by running or fighting. Instead, they are internalized, contributing to high rates of hypertension and cardiovascular disease.[13]

In the laboratory, we have shown that when we inhibit testosterone secretion in young male rats and other animals, their life span markedly increases despite stressful conditions.[14] But this also produces impotence and an overall reduction in vigor so that testosterone inhibition is not the treatment of choice for increasing male life expectancy.

Meanwhile, nature has been much kinder to females. The female hormones act to protect the heart and blood vessels. For example, the pregnant woman develops a markedly expanded blood volume to provide the fetus with an elevated circulation. If a woman's blood vessels were as rigid as male vessels, this expanded blood volume would cause her blood pressure to rise to levels dangerous for the fetus. But the substantial amount of estrogen a pregnant woman secretes makes her blood vessels more elastic. It also makes them less vulnerable to elevated blood pressure caused by stress even if she never gets pregnant. Recent research has shown that the more babies a woman has delivered, the greater is the diameter of her blood vessels, with the added advantage of fewer damage sites. The fact that estrogen stimulates the liver to produce more of the beneficial HDL means a woman is protected from atherosclerosis.[15]

Posture

Because we developed from four-legged animals, the human spinal column is designed for walking on all fours. The move to an upright position created backache. It also readjusted the position of the pelvis and reshaped the birth canal, making delivery more difficult for human females. Thus, natural selection favored women who produced small babies. In general, all normal infants are born less mature than any other species and require years of protection. Because the birth canal is inappropriate for a baby, delivery can damage it as well as the infant. Pregnancy further complicates matters for females because the heavy weight of the fetus pressing on the veins in the legs causes varicose veins.

The Mature Adult

Mother Nature releases her wrath on women at maturity. No longer needed biologically once fertility is lost, women become expendable. After menopause, women are relatively deficient in estrogen and more like the male regarding the secretion of sex hormones. Thus, damage to their cardiovascular system accelerates, and heart disease becomes their leading cause of death. Replacement of female hormones serves to protect the aging woman's heart and blood vessels, although the final word on the correct combination of hormones and dosages awaits completion of current research. Additional research to explain and then counteract women's higher death rate after myocardial infarction and poorer response to traditional treatments for heart attacks is needed, as well as uncovering new treatment methods (see Chapter 7). In addition, future research should focus on younger women to discover better ways of preventing cardiovascular disease and osteoporosis. We need sociological research to learn the true negative health effects of poverty and hunger among older Americans—most of whom are women—and how to counteract them. According to a 1993 report from the Urban Institute, between 2.5 and 4.9 million elderly Americans experience hunger and "food insecurity." The report defines "food insecurity" as having to decide between buying food and medicine or between paying the utility bill and having enough to eat.[16] On the plus side, women who work outside the home seem to enjoy a health advantage, possibly because a paycheck gives them not only a higher income but also greater control over their lives.

Men also experience a decrease in testosterone production and loss of sexuality with advancing age. Recent behavioral changes among white middle- and upper-class men indicate that they have become more health conscious. Their rate of smoking has dropped from 60% to 30%, and many are eating less meat, more fish, more complex carbohydrates, and less protein. They are exercising more, moving away from previous ideals of exemplary masculinity, which included a lack of emotional expression and a belief that it was good to endure fatigue and pain. They are seeking more medical care to control hypertension and other risk factors. But these well-educated and well-heeled males represent only a blip on the health radar screen—because blue collar, African American, and Hispanic males have made relatively fewer lifestyle changes.

How Lifestyle Affects Female Biology

At a conference on aging in 1982, Dr. Palmore, of Duke University, concluded that "about half of the greater longevity of women is due to genetic difference and about half to difference in life style."[17] Lifestyle variations also affect males, exaggerating their vulnerability. From childhood, boys are encouraged to take life-threatening risks and to use guns and other weapons to prove their masculinity. Thus, murder, accidents, and suicide are a major cause of death among men throughout the life span, three times the rate in women. Women do attempt suicide more often than men but use revocable forms of self-destruction—such as pills—and often call for help. Men, because they tend to use guns to kill themselves, are usually more successful than women. We need behavioral research on how to reduce violent male behavior, not only to protect women victims of it, but also to protect men from their own life-threatening behavior.

Smoking

Women who smoke throw away many of their biological aces. Lung cancer is now the leading cause of cancer death among women, surpassing breast cancer fatalities, largely because women started smoking in large numbers right after World War II, and the lethal effects of smoking are now taking their toll. Smoking accounts for about 30% of all cancer deaths and about 25% of all deaths from heart disease.[18] For women, smoking has been a disaster, removing the inherent advantage nature provides. Between 1960 and 1962 and 1990 and 1992, for example, death rates from lung cancer in women rose 438%; there also was a 67% increase in female mortality from cancer of the larynx.[19] But even women who smoke maintain some advantage. The Framingham study and other reports show that for matched smokers and nonsmokers, women survive better than men.[20] Because women find it harder to stop smoking than men do, we urgently need research on preventing teenage smoking in girls and finding more effective techniques to help women stop smoking.

Bone Mass and Strength

Osteoporosis is a major cause of disability for older women, who are far more vulnerable to this condition than are men. This is because women have smaller bones and they lose about 50% of their cancellous bone and 30% of their cortical bone over their lifetimes, compared with 30% and 20%, respectively, among men. In addition, the drop in estrogen after menopause accelerates bone loss. But bone loss does not occur overnight with the cessation of menstruation. From their late 20s and early 30s, women show some bone loss. Asian women have the most rapid loss, white women have less rapid loss, and African American women have the least rapid loss.[21]

Genes play a major role in determining how dense a person's bones become, which is why a family history (a mother or sister with osteoporosis) increases one's risk, but genes are not the whole story. Bone loss can be mitigated by two things pre- and postmenopausally—regular weight-bearing exercise and a high-calcium intake, either from milk products or calcium supplements up to about 1,500 milligrams daily. Red meat should be consumed in limited quantities because as the body metabolizes it, calcium loss increases. Estrogen supplementation after menopause amplifies the effect of both exercise and calcium consumption. Regular exercise provides muscle and, in the case of aerobic exercise, cardiovascular conditioning, as well as an outlet for emotionally induced body changes. Women have known this intuitively for years as they have stormed through housecleaning as a release from anxiety and tension. But there are better forms of exercise. As women age they should engage in the safest of these—brisk walking, stretching and flexing, and swimming. Women's joints are especially vulnerable to damage, and many exercise regimens increase the aging process in the joints. For older women, exercises done in water are the most protective, even for arthritic joints.

Diet

Women, even those who are lean, have a higher percentage of fat in their bodies than men. This fat gives them a larger reserve energy for endurance demands, which is why female athletes are less dependent on carbohydrate loading for distance events. The fat layer makes a woman's slightly lower body temperature more stable than a man's. Women also retain water and salts better and do not need as much fluid during exercise as men. They rely less on sweating to dissipate heat but have a more efficient distribution of sweat glands. A woman who keeps her salt intake down and drinks six to eight glasses of water daily maintains vascular and bowel function at optimal levels. Dietary fiber also contributes to better bowel function and may protect against colon cancer, a major killer of women. Current recommendations from the new Food Pyramid of the U.S. Department of Agriculture (USDA) call for 6 to 11 servings from grains daily—mainly breads, cereals, rice, and pasta.

Dietary fat intake, typically 40% or more of calories in American diets, is much too high. Current recommendations are that 30% or less of calories should come from fat, and no more than 10% from saturated fat. But some fat is critical for health. It is possible to be too thin, and there is some evidence that the older woman is healthier at a slightly heavier weight than in her leanest years. Extra pounds may also slow the development of osteoporosis because of the greater weight on the bones.

But overweight and obesity represent a serious threat for many diseases in women and may be related to breast and colon cancer. Obesity also is a risk factor for heart disease, high blood pressure, non-insulin-dependent diabetes, and cancers of the cervix, endometrium, uterus, ovaries, gallbladder, and biliary passages. Obesity is a widespread problem; the Framingham study found that 70% of women older than 40 are overweight or obese.[22] Americans, despite all the media attention to nutrition and exercise, are getting fatter. Dramatic increases in overweight persons have occurred in the past decade in both sexes and all races, making it unlikely that we will reach the goals of Healthy People 2000—namely, to reduce the prevalence of overweight persons to no more than 20% of the United States population.[23] However, severe diets that provide fewer than 1,000 calories a day can be damaging. Repair and growth of tissues occur constantly and require calories.

Americans tend to consume too much protein so that even active women do not have to increase their protein intake. Fish protein seems to be the best kind of animal protein in terms of conserving calcium and protecting blood vessels. As far as carbohydrates go, despite bad press, sugar in moderation is not damaging, except to teeth. However, the best sources of carbohydrates are beans, pasta, and rice, particularly in the light of data that show how they benefit the body. Pasta, for example, does not produce an elevation in blood sugar in the same way that a potato does. As a result, the pancreas does not make more insulin, and the body deposits less fat. Furthermore, these complex carbohydrates seem to suppress the appetite centers in the brain because they release certain brain hormones that give us a sense of satiety. A high-protein meal is not nearly as efficient in controlling appetite.

Antioxidant vitamins such as vitamins C, E, and beta-carotene have recently been recommended as a way of preventing or slowing damage from free radicals by protecting cell membranes from oxidation. Carrots, cabbage, brussels sprouts, and broccoli contain large amounts of beta-carotene. But dosage is important. At a recent meeting sponsored by the U.S. Food and Drug Administration (FDA) on antioxidant vitamins and cancer and cardiovascular disease—cosponsored by the Federal Trade Commission (FTC), the Department of Health and Human Services (DHHS), the National Institutes of Health (NIH), the American Cancer Society, the Congressional Research Staff, the Institute of Medicine of the National Academy of Sciences, and the American Medical Association—the expert participants agreed unanimously that "vitamins C, E, and beta-carotene are mischaracterized by describing them solely as 'antioxidant' (fighters against harmful free radicals), since they are in fact redox agents, antioxidant in some circumstances (often so in the physiologic quantities found in food), and prooxidant (producing billions of harmful free radicals) in other circumstances (often in the pharmacologic quantities found in supplements). Vitamin C is a special case since, in the presence of iron, it is violently prooxidant, and, for genetic reasons, about 10% of American whites and 30% of American blacks have high blood iron" (letter dated November 3, 1993, from conference participant Victor Herbert, M.D., J.D., to the FDA and FTC, outlining points of consensus achieved by the conference, private communication to

B. Jacobson). Additional research is sorely needed to sort out the dosages, risks, and benefits of these vitamins.

One recent study[24] of 30,000 male smokers in Finland found that vitamin E had no effect on the development of lung cancer and that beta-carotene showed a "slight but statistically significant increase in risk for the disease." In addition, vitamin E had no apparent effect on total mortality, although it seemed to protect study participants from thrombotic strokes while making them more prone to hemorrhagic strokes. The beta-carotene group in the study had an 8% higher overall mortality than those in the vitamin E and the no supplement groups.[25] It is wise to get needed vitamins from food by following the current recommendations from the USDA to consume three to five servings of vegetables and two to four servings of fruit every day.

Some fruits and vegetables contain both carcinogens and antioxidants, and some vegetables are higher in mutagens than others. These include beets, spinach, celery, radishes, and alfalfa sprouts.[26] Many foods are touted as preservative-free in health food stores, but preservatives are necessary to retard oxidation, and their use, along with widespread refrigeration, probably accounts for the steep drop in stomach cancer in developed countries. In addition, cooking methods affect food value. High heat and charcoal broiling may encourage the formation of carcinogens. Fats are particularly suspect, and rancid fats have been implicated in colon and breast cancer. Unsaturated fats in particular are easily oxidized on standing or cooking and can form carcinogens. This suggests that refrigerating oils, and cooking on low heat or with a microwave, may be of some use in decreasing the amount of carcinogens in the diet.

Women are more susceptible than men to alcohol-induced liver disease. One reason is their smaller size; another is that they have more fat and less water in their bodies, which produces a higher blood-alcohol level because there is less fluid in which the alcohol can be distributed. In addition, women have fewer of the enzymes that break down alcohol in the stomach so that more alcohol ends up in the bloodstream. Women also are more susceptible to alcohol just before menstruation, when oxidation of alcohol is slowest. This is why the USDA recommends only one drink daily (either 12 ounces of beer, 5 ounces of wine, or 1.5 ounces of distilled spirits) for women, although it allows two drinks for men. Pregnant and lactating women should not drink any alcohol because a safe dose for the fetus has not been determined. On the plus side, a number of studies have shown that moderate drinking (from three drinks a week to one or two daily) is associated with a high HDL and a reduced frequency of heart disease.[27]

Endnotes

[1]Ramey ER: How to use the natural biologic strengths of women to live to 100, in *Women: A Developmental Perspective*. Washington, DC, U.S. Government Printing Office, 1983

[2]Ramwell PW, Ramey ER: Cardiovascular sexual dimorphism, in *Sex Steroids and the Cardiovascular System*. New York, Springer-Verlag, 1992

[3]Ibid.

[4]Ibid.

[5]Ibid.

[6]Ibid.

[7]Ramey ER: Lecture at Amherst College, 1992

[8]Ibid.

[9]Ramey ER, op. cit., 1983

[10]Wenger NK, Speroff L, Packard B: Cardiovascular health and disease in women. *New England Journal of Medicine* 329:247–256, 1993

[11]The Writing Group for the PEPI Trial: Effects of estrogen or estrogen/progestin regimens on heart disease risk factors in postmenopausal women. *Journal of the American Medical Association* 273:199–203, 1995

[12]Ibid.

[13]Ramey ER, op. cit., 1992

[14]Ibid.

[15]Ibid.

[16]Whitmire R: "Report: elderly suffer dramatically from hunger." *The Burlington Free Press*, Burlington, VT, November 15, 1993

[17]Ramey ER, op. cit., 1983

[18]Ibid.

[19]American Cancer Society: *Cancer Facts & Figures—1996*. Atlanta, GA, American Cancer Society, 1996

[20]Ramey ER, op. cit., 1983

[21]Riggs BL, Melton LJ: The prevention and treatment of osteoporosis. *New England Journal of Medicine* 327:620–627, 1992

[22]Simopoulos AS, Herbert V, Jacobson B: *Genetic Nutrition: Designing a Diet Based on Your Family Medical History*. New York, Macmillan, 1993

[23]Kuczmarski RJ, Flegal KM, Campbell SM, et al: Increasing prevalence of overweight among U.S. adults. *Journal of the American Medical Association* 272:205–211, 1994

[24]Second thought about antioxidants. *Harvard Health Letter* 20(4):4–6, February 1995
[25]Ibid.
[26]Ramey ER, op. cit., 1983
[27]Simopoulos AS, Herbert V, Jacobson B, op. cit.

4

How One Gender Difference Affects Society

Esta Soler
Marya Grambs, M.S.

I n Chapter 3, we pointed out some of the attributes men possess because of the male hormone testosterone, specifically, a large and powerful musculature, great speed and endurance, the strongest sex drive known among mammals, and high stress levels thanks to testosterone's production of adrenaline and cortisone. In primitive times, males used these characteristics to advantage, inseminating females to ensure species survival, hunting large animals for food, fighting marauders—animal and human—and covering substantial distances in their nomadic existence. Now, with the need for such dramatic responses eliminated by elements of our technological society—from supermarkets to automobiles to overpopulation—these male characteristics are either turned inward, producing high blood pressure, elevated stress levels, and cardiovascular disease, or turned against other men, and, most strikingly, against women and children.

Perhaps the clearest view of this latter tendency is contained in the following excerpt:

> Betty was in an abusive marriage for 6 years. One day, her husband tried to hit her in the face when she was holding their 3-year-old daughter. "When I moved my head, he accidentally hit the baby and

broke her nose. The blood was everywhere. It splattered all over the windshield of the car. That's when I decided I was leaving and getting away for good," she recalls.

The day she and her daughter moved into their own apartment still resonates in Betty's memory. "We walked through the door, and my daughter turned around and said, 'This is a woman's house. No man allowed.' This came from a 4-year-old," says Betty. "That's something I'll never forget."[1]

Although women's genetic makeup may protect them against stress, immune attack, and cardiovascular disease, unfortunately neither their genes, their health care providers, nor their communities offer them virtually *any* protection from the harm caused by the epidemic of domestic violence, which has become an American public health crisis of unparalleled magnitude. In 1993, almost 4 million American women reported being physically abused by their husbands or boyfriends. Almost half (42%) of all women murdered in this country are killed by their husbands or partners.[2]

Although many women may never call a law enforcement officer for help, almost every woman in America does visit a physician's office or clinic setting at some point in her life. Whether for pregnancy-related services, gynecological checkups, or basic medical care, most women interact with health care providers. Women who are battered by their partners may have the most contact of all. At least 1.5 million women seek medical care for abuse-related injuries each year, with abused women representing one-third of all emergency department trauma visits.[3] This gives the health care sector an unparalleled opportunity to make a difference in the struggle against domestic violence.

Unfortunately, although medical caregivers treat the physical problems women experience as a result of battering, they rarely address the underlying cause of those injuries. For the most part, abused women return to the dangerous situation that produced the damage in the first place. They have clearly not been served well by the public health system.

In 1985, the U.S. surgeon general identified family violence as a priority public health issue.[4] Now, little has changed; in 1994, the U.S. secretary of health and human services called on Americans to recognize the terrible toll of domestic violence, naming it "domestic terrorism."

One of the most tragic health-related aspects of domestic violence occurs when women are pregnant. One in five teenagers and one in six adult women report being abused while pregnant; this makes it more likely that these women will deliver low-birthweight babies than those who are not battered.[5] Evidence is mounting that domestic violence is starting at earlier and earlier ages among teens. Experts believe that it may now be double the 16.8% rate reported among college students a decade ago.[6]

Poor girls in inner-city communities may be at even higher risk. An article in *The Wall Street Journal* commented that

> domestic violence may well prove to be the most troubling issue facing poor, urban minority communities for a long time to come. . . . The atmosphere in a neighborhood like this one [Brooklyn's Bedford-Stuyvesant] fosters a very vicious form of domestic violence. . . an atmosphere in which young men are "taught" by their fathers, if they have one, and older brothers to refer to women as "ho's" ["whores"] who need abuse; where physical violence is a common means of ending verbal disputes; and where women are mistrusted and detested.[7]

The article went on to say that "extreme distrust of women, and belief in physical violence as the solution to familial disputes, is commonplace among all too many inner-city young men." The author of this story had grown up in this inner-city neighborhood; all five of his sisters had been battered by their male partners.

Domestic violence damages more than the physical health of its adult women victims. It can have a devastating effect on women's *mental* health. Research documents that two-thirds of hospitalized female psychiatric patients were physically abused as adults.[8] This violence also often leads to depression and even suicide.[9]

Adult and teenage women are not the only victims. When battered women are mothers, their children are often harmed as well, in several ways. First, there is an extraordinarily high incidence of child abuse in families experiencing domestic violence: three-quarters of abused women report that their children also are abused.[10] The rate of child abuse is 15 times greater in families if family violence is present than if it is not.[11] The problem is escalating; there were 2.9 million reports of child abuse and neglect in the United States in 1992 compared with 1.2 million 10 years earlier. More than three children die every day in America from abuse, with 85% of them younger than 5 years.[12]

Second, domestic violence teaches children that violent behavior is acceptable. Men who grew up in violent homes, for example, are three times more likely to abuse their own wives, with the sons of the most violent parents 1,000 times more likely to become wife beaters.[13] The effects of violence show up even earlier; according to one study, violent juvenile delinquents come from homes in which domestic violence occurs four times more often than in the homes of nonviolent juveniles. All the children studied were younger than 12 years and were seriously disturbed, requiring admission to an inpatient child psychiatry ward in New York. But the difference between these violent and nonviolent disturbed youngsters was that the violent children came from violent homes, where, usually, the father seriously abused the mother.[14]

Finally, witnessing domestic violence is itself a form of child abuse because it can cause severe trauma to the child. Growing up in a home in which violence breaks out unpredictably, anger is frequently explosive, parental behavior is inconsistent, children must take care of parents, and terror is a frequent experience can produce long-lasting effects on children. According to several studies, many of the children of battered women have reduced self-esteem and social competence, as well as increased aggression, behavior problems, anxiety, and other symptoms of high distress or maladjustment.[15]

The Institutional Toll of Violence

Domestic violence has an enormous impact, not only on the lives of millions of women and children, but also on our health care system. Domestic violence causes a high level of injury to American women, accounting for three times as many emergency department visits as car crashes and muggings combined.[16] The issue can be viewed not only as an acute care problem, but also as a chronic health problem because, in most cases, the violence occurs repeatedly and often escalates. One study showed that approximately one in five abused women seen by physicians had sought medical attention for injuries from abuse *11 times* before.[17] This means that when a health care provider comes in contact with an abused woman, that provider has an important opportunity to stop the cycle of violence, prevent the woman from receiving further injury, and free up the health care system from the continual and repetitious treatment of injuries stemming from the same cause.

Why the Epidemic Continues Unchecked

One of the fundamental reasons that domestic violence continues at such epidemic levels involves the subtle but pervasive ways that American society accepts and condones disrespect for women and violence against them. Throughout the media—in advertising, radio, television, and literature—abuse of women is often presented as funny, and much of the humor portrays women as stupid and ridiculous, sometimes even in need of physical control. Becoming the butt of jokes, women are demeaned, and violence against them is mocked. For example, in the mid-1980s, a friend working on Capitol Hill reported to us that a legislator was preparing to speak in Congress to support the Family Violence Services Act, which provided critical funding to battered women's shelters across the United States. A colleague took him aside and said, "I don't know why you're supporting this bill; all you're doing is taking the fun out of marriage." The colleague appeared to be serious.

On television and in the movies, the graphic depiction of horrifying acts of violence against women, and of women as victims of every type of assault, contributes to a climate that fails to take the abuse of women seriously. In fact, this constant barrage desensitizes society to violence in general and violence against women in particular.

The justice system has contributed to our cultural acceptance of violence against women in the way it has historically responded to domestic violence. Until recently, it was typical for police called to deal with an incident of abuse not to consider the problem significant, rarely arresting perpetrators. When battered women persevered and tried to press charges, district attorneys often refused to support their cases, and those lawsuits that made it to court were likely to be dismissed by judges. The general attitude was, "she provoked it"; "it's only a domestic dispute, not a matter for law enforcement or the justice system"; "it's a private, family problem, not our business"; or, "there's nothing wrong with a husband showing he's boss."

The cultural climate regarding abuse of women has improved some-what in the past two decades. Women have made gains in the work force, for example, and the justice system now pays attention to domes-tic violence complaints. Polls in the mid-1990s showed that 96% of Americans consider domestic violence a serious problem in society and that 94% believed that hitting a woman is always wrong.[18]

Despite these polls, the vast majority of Americans have covert at-titudes that implicitly condone violent behavior. The following story told by a friend is instructive:

> Ed is a liberal individual, progressive on social issues. He mentioned to a woman friend who is a domestic violence activist that he had just made a startling discovery: a man with whom he plays weekly tennis regularly beats his wife. Ed's woman friend asked him why he contin-ues to play tennis with that kind of person. "Because," Ed replied, "he's basically a nice guy." She responded, "No. If you know he beats his wife, he is not a nice guy. You should not play tennis with him, any more than you would play tennis with an anti-Semite or a racist."

The staggering number of abused women indicates that progress is not happening nearly fast enough. However, we do know from other social issues that what is learned can be unlearned. For example, smok-ing, which was the sine qua non of the 1940s, an absolute requirement for anyone wanting to appear sophisticated, has now become socially unacceptable, thanks to research pinpointing its health threat and an aggressive public education campaign. Therefore, we can assume that the broad cultural messages about male-female relationships can be changed as well, attitudes about what is acceptable behavior can be reframed, and children growing up with domestic violence can be taught new behav-iors. As we will see, health policy can play a pivotal role in modifying these attitudes.

The First Step Is Prevention

The issue of domestic violence is at a crucial turning point. Services have been created throughout society to respond to the epidemic of battering, many relevant laws have been improved, and the greater com-munity has, to a limited extent, become aware of the problem. What has not occurred, however, is a comprehensive commitment to prevent and reduce domestic violence within the health care community. We need a multipronged effort to stop the violence *before* it begins and research to discover the best ways to do this.

Such a health-based prevention program should include

- Public health education to increase awareness and create a cultural intolerance of domestic violence
- Routine screening of women for domestic violence in all health care settings, including those that care for pregnant teens and children
- Universal protocols to enable health care providers to identify and treat domestic violence
- Improved documentation by providers
- Domestic violence curricula established in all health and medical education programs
- Improved access to the health care system for victims by removing domestic violence as a preexisting condition for health insurance
- Improved data collection
- Activism in the elimination of guns

Changing Behavior and Attitudes

To be effective, prevention-based policies in the health system must educate health care providers and the public about this issue. This education should be done in a manner that counters the remaining cultural acceptance of violence and produces public outrage about, and a commitment to stop, violence against women. We have seen this happen with many health issues. In fact, every significant societal health problem, especially those that involve behavior, has required changing the way people think first and then they way they behave—whether it has been cigarette smoking, drunk driving, or high-risk sexual behavior.

For example, look at how health policy evolved on the question of cigarette smoking. The initial health policy response at the provider level was to treat lung cancer. Then, health educators and providers endeavored to convince smokers to stop because smoking turned out to be dangerous to health. Later, policy initiatives involved health education campaigns designed to stop people from starting by creating a cultural intolerance of smoking and by getting nonsmokers into the act by teaching them about the harmful consequences of secondhand smoke.

The effectiveness of such efforts can be seen in California, which has conducted a massive public education campaign against smoking that has saturated the media for the past several years, detailing the negative health effects of smoking and secondhand smoke. The campaign was financed by revenue obtained from an increase in the cigarette sales tax from 10 cents to 35 cents per pack passed in 1988. One-fifth of the revenues generated by this law, $100 million annually, went to tobacco-related public education. The combination of the increased cost of cigarettes and the education campaign resulted in a 15% drop in tobacco sales in California. Between 1987 and 1990, smoking prevalence declined from 26.3% to 21.2%.[19,20]

The issue of domestic violence is at a crossroads in the 1990s. Having first been identified as a policy issue in the United States in the 1970s, domestic violence was addressed initially by providing emergency shelter to victims. Then the justice system got involved, and efforts were made to improve the response of the criminal justice system and to hold batterers to the same legal standards as other violent criminals. In the ensuing years, public awareness has been raised, but a subtle acceptance of and a willingness to ignore domestic violence persist. The problem continues to flourish in part because of silence and because some sectors of society still view the issue as a private one.

It has only been recently—as the country has started to recognize the impact of domestic violence on women's health and on the health care system—that public officials have begun to develop new health policy and *prevention* efforts. We need public health education campaigns designed to encourage individuals to claim personal responsibility for stopping domestic violence, just as the individuals have taken responsibility for protecting the environment and stopping drunk driving, with slogans such as "friends don't let friends drive drunk" and a willingness to back up such statements with action. For example, if an individual knows someone—a family member, co-worker, or neighbor—who is being abused by, or who is abusing, his or her partner, the message should be do not ignore the abuse or turn your back. Offer the victim support and practical assistance, and assure her that it is not her fault. For the abuser, let him know that such behavior is unacceptable, that he must stop the abuse, and that he needs help. If you know children whose parents are in an abusive relationship, let them know that what is going on in their family is not right and that you are able and willing to help them. In this way, we can create a climate that communicates social sanctions against abuse while providing support to victims. However, it is extremely important not to intervene physically or verbally during a violent incident. In that case, a bystander or neighbor should call the police to take over because, clearly, a crime is being committed.

In 1993, the Family Violence Prevention Fund, a national domestic violence education and policy organization, conducted pioneering market research on public opinion about domestic violence to lay the groundwork for the first national public education campaign. Fund officials found that not only did a vast majority of the American public identify domestic violence as a serious problem, but also 34% had witnessed such abuse directly, more than the combined number of people who had seen a mugging or a robbery. Unlike a decade ago, most Americans were no longer buying the old excuses for abuse. The respondents were unwilling either to excuse *him* for his violent behavior ("he couldn't help it," "he was drinking") or to blame *her* for the violence ("she provoked it," "she deserved it"). In addition, the research indicated that most Americans felt helpless to do anything about this widespread problem. This implies that Americans are ready to get involved if only they are given some direction.

On the basis of that information, the fund launched a national public education campaign. Called "There's No Excuse for Domestic Violence," the fund's effort aims to reduce and prevent domestic violence by educating the public and creating a commitment to end the epidemic. The fund produced two radio public service announcements (PSAs), two television PSAs, and two print advertisements, in black-and-white and color versions for newspapers and magazines. One of these ads was done in several variations, showing white, African American, Asian American, and Latin American models. Bus shelter and billboard displays also were distributed. Sponsored by the Advertising Council and selected as its major public education initiative, the campaign, launched in June 1994, will continue for 10 years.

In one powerful scenario designed for radio and television, listeners or viewers hear the muffled violence of a fight in a nearby apartment. The message says, "If the noise coming from next door were loud music, you'd do something about it." Another television PSA shows a couple going to bed while they hear disturbing sounds from next door—a man yelling and a woman crying. The violent sounds escalate as the couple get into bed; they look at each other, worried and scared. Finally, the man leans over the bedside table and reaches not for the phone but for the light, which he turns off. The words flashing across the dark screen are, "Domestic violence. It is everyone's business."

The Advertising Council has arranged for millions of dollars of donated media space, enabling campaign messages to appear in national news magazines, on prime-time network television, in national and local newspapers, and on radio stations across the country. A national toll-free number, publicized on each PSA, provides free Action Kits to callers, suggesting specific local strategies that citizens can undertake to reduce and prevent domestic violence in their own communities. For example, in one Modesto, California, community, several women formed a "Neighborhood Watch" program—but with a different twist. Normally, such efforts are aimed at "stranger danger," stopping break-ins, theft, and muggings. In this case, domestic violence was added to the usual list of crimes. Neighbors were educated about the issue and told to call the police and notify their Neighborhood Watch coordinator whenever they heard screaming in the night. The next day, the coordinator and a friend of the victim visit, offering help and resources.

Other communities have organized a memorial march every time a battered woman is murdered; still others have enlisted all the businesses in a small town to post a sign in each establishment's window that says, "If you are in a scary or dangerous situation and need help, you may use our telephone to call Women's Emergency Services and/or the police. This is a safe haven. We are helping to create a community free of violence and abuse."

Saturating the media with prevention messages—even when the messages are unpleasant and intrusive—is an effective method for changing behavior. For example, a public service advertising campaign urging people, particularly men, to speak to their physicians about colon cancer—not an easy or comfortable subject—increased awareness about the issue from 11% to 29% after 6 months of advertising and up to 40% after 12 months. The number of people who spoke to their physicians about colon cancer increased by 43%, with the number of men increasing by 114%.[21]

Such a campaign against domestic violence should be implemented on a state-by-state basis. That this strategy can have a profound impact on health-related behavior has been demonstrated by the success of the California Health Department's antismoking campaign, illustrating the potentially positive role of public policy.

Editorial campaigns can be instrumental, too, in affecting public opinion. Such campaigns provide an important opportunity for health care providers to lend their names to outcries against domestic violence. Citizen efforts also can be extremely effective, as shown by the sharp reduction in drunk driving fatalities resulting from effective public education by Mothers Against Drunk Driving (MADD).

Routinely Asking About Abuse

Dr. Robert McAfee, president of the American Medical Association (AMA), described a patient who had come to his office every 3 months for a year, complaining of breast pain. The woman had a family history of breast cancer, so he ran several tests but never found any indication of cancer. Finally, the third time she came with the same complaint, he noticed bruises on her shoulder and ribs and asked if she bruised often. She replied, "Only on certain occasions." The woman proceeded to tell him about years of physical abuse at the hands of her husband, who was a respected businessman.[22]

Just as the general public has long ignored the problem of domestic violence and has failed to see it as a public health issue, the health care community has been guilty of the same blind spot. Although domestic violence victims come into regular contact with health professionals, physicians frequently treat only the injuries and fail to recognize abuse as the cause, identifying as few as 1 victim in 20.[23] Even when abuse is identified, health care professionals often provide inappropriate or even harmful treatment, such as not separating a victim from her abuser in the waiting or examining room, not documenting injuries, prescribing tranquilizers, or conveying the attitude that she deserved or provoked the abuse, was a "troublesome" patient, would not take responsibility for herself, or lived in an area in which such incidents were the norm.[24]

Many other reasons for failure to diagnose battering exist, including inadequate training, time constraints, and the victim's reticence. Physicians view discussing domestic violence with patients as opening a "Pandora's box" and express discomfort, fear of offending, powerlessness, and loss of control.[25] A 1993 Commonwealth Fund Harris Poll found that 92% of women who were physically abused did not discuss these incidents with their physicians.[26] However, whereas many battered women will not volunteer information about the true source of their injuries, they often will acknowledge the violence when the health care provider asks about it directly; uses a sensitive, nonjudgmental manner; and does this in a confidential setting.[27] But a great disparity exists between patient and provider perceptions: 90% of patients believe that physicians can help with physical and sexual abuse, although only 33% of physicians believe they can.[28] It should come as no surprise that battered women hold negative opinions of medical providers, rating health care personnel their least effective formal source of help.[29]

The escalating nature of domestic violence means that early identification and intervention can prevent further injuries; thus, it is critically important for health care professionals to inquire about abuse. Their questions might allow a woman to reveal the problem of violence to a non–family member for the first time. A question about abuse from a health care professional can break the victim's isolation, help her develop a safety plan, and increase her willingness to seek help. The provider who does not acknowledge the cause of the injury not only perpetuates the danger the patient is in, but also reinforces her sense of entrapment and helplessness, thereby contributing to her further victimization.[30]

Domestic violence can be identified fairly easily by the trained eye and ear. Indicators include certain patterns of injuries, fear or shame in the patient, certain psychosomatic complaints, and implausible explanations of injuries.[31] Health care workers should also become suspicious when the woman's husband or boyfriend cancels her medical appointment. Contrary to the fear of some providers, addressing domestic violence need not be overly time-consuming. One study found that as few as *three questions* asked by the provider in a private setting without the patient's partner present were effective in identifying the presence of domestic violence.[32] Ultimately, it is not difficult to distinguish a deliberately inflicted injury from an accidental one—if the health care worker *wants* to know. Providers can introduce the subject with a comment such as "Because violence is so common in many women's lives, I have begun to ask about it routinely. At any time, has your partner hit, kicked, or otherwise hurt or frightened you?" Questions about abuse also can be included in the medical history form given to new patients.

The provider should try to determine whether physical abuse has ever occurred, whether it has occurred within the preceding 12 months, and what was the frequency and severity of the abuse. The patient also should be asked directly if she is afraid of her partner and if she has support and options should she decide to leave. Providers should therefore have appropriate referral information available.

Because the health care setting presents such a valuable opportunity to detect abuse, in 1994 California enacted legislation that *requires* practitioners to screen for domestic violence, in the same manner that they routinely screen for alcohol and drug abuse, high-risk sexual behavior, and smoking. Some providers argue that this requirement alters their role from being medical caregivers to that of social workers, but such screening, as in other conditions, is part of the provider's responsibility to address the overall health of the patient.

Screening for domestic violence should take place during visits to adult health care providers' offices—primary care, family practice, obstetrics/gynecology, community clinics, and outpatient centers. It also is important for pediatricians to explore this issue with mothers of children with unexplained or unreasonably explained injuries because often, when there is child abuse in the family, the woman often also is abused. However, most health care providers who are trained to look for and recognize signs of child abuse do not know that they should be on the lookout for signs of domestic violence and, when they encounter an abused child, that they should ask if the mother is also being abused. It makes little sense to intervene in the abuse of the child and allow the father to continue to beat the mother. Therefore, routine screening for domestic violence should be instituted in all health care settings where children who might be abused are seen, including hospitals, offices of pediatricians and family practitioners, clinics, and child protective services. It also is vital that such screening be included in all teen pregnancy programs, as these patients are extremely vulnerable to abuse.

Ensuring That Providers Know What to Do

In January 1992, the Joint Commission on Accreditation of Healthcare Organizations (JCAHO) mandated new standards relating to the identification, evaluation, and care of adult victims of domestic violence. These standards require emergency departments and hospital-sponsored ambulatory care services to develop both written policies on domestic violence and a staff training plan. JCAHO's guidelines mark the first time hospital accreditation has been directly linked to compliance with domestic violence requirements for patient care, just as it has been coupled with compliance on other issues.

JCAHO is not the only health institution recognizing the importance of identifying and intervening to help victims of domestic violence. In September 1989, the U.S. Department of Health and Human Services released a report titled "Healthy People 2000," which recommended the development of baseline data on the number of emergency departments using domestic violence protocols and the dissemination of treatment protocols to at least 90% of hospital emergency departments. Many other professional health organizations have launched efforts to encourage their members to address domestic violence.

Despite these attempts, most hospitals do not have policies or protocols regarding domestic violence, and those that do exist are often inadequate. The Family Violence Prevention Fund surveyed almost 400 hospital emergency departments in California in 1994, assessing their capacity to respond to domestic violence victims seeking emergency care. We found that as few as one in five California hospitals appeared to be in compliance with the JCAHO standards; furthermore, only 23% of California physician directors reported that their emergency department had conducted an educational session on domestic violence for physicians.

Of the 57 protocols reviewed in this study, only 8 were adequate in addressing the dynamics and indicators of domestic violence and identifying appropriate interventions. Similarly, although one-fourth of the respondents reported they had domestic violence brochures, these brochures did not even mention spouse or partner abuse. The survey also discovered that physician directors and nurse managers believe that obstacles to identification and referral of patients lie in the patient's denial and failure to volunteer information, and not with the adequacy of the health care system's response.

This survey did find, however, that providers *want* the information; an overwhelming 88% of nurse managers said that they would use model policies and procedures on how to identify and refer battered adults, if they were available. It is clear that the tide of opinion about domestic violence is changing. In 1989 the American College of Obstetricians and Gynecologists joined with former Surgeon General C. Everett Koop to launch a public campaign aimed at helping physicians assist victims of domestic violence. In 1993, AMA launched a 3-year effort to improve physician identification and treatment of domestic violence and developed guidelines for primary care physicians.

These professional associations concluded that health care settings— including emergency departments, primary care offices, pediatricians, and obstetrics/gynecology services—need universal protocols accompanied by training. These protocols will show providers how to ask all their female patients direct and specific questions about abuse, including frequency, severity, and timing. For example, providers should

- Encourage their female patients to talk about problems related to domestic violence
- Listen nonjudgmentally
- Document the symptoms and injuries
- Assess the current danger
- Provide appropriate treatment, referral, and support
- Validate the woman's experience

The protocols also should include information about what to do in situations in which the woman denies abuse but the provider suspects it is occurring.

Record Keeping: Documenting the Violence

Domestic violence cases sometimes enter the criminal justice system, if the victim or the district attorney decides to press charges. For criminal charges to be brought against the perpetrator at some point after an injury, documentation of the injuries and other symptoms related to domestic violence is essential. This documentation provides evidence critical to prosecutors, enabling them to build a case even if the victim is too afraid to testify. Without documentation, a case cannot go forward. Thus, it is critical that all health care providers receive training about why it is important to record such information and how to do so correctly *and* legibly. A proper record can make it unnecessary for the practitioner to go to court to testify about the abuse, which saves time and money.

Institutionalizing the Response

Developing effective health policy about domestic violence entails more than incorporating screening mechanisms and implementing protocols. It is important to *institutionalize* the health care system's response so that institutions and practitioners have a heightened awareness of the issue and a built-in commitment to addressing it. To do this, there is no better time to start than now and no better place to start than with the schools that train health professionals. We must develop new curricula about battering, describing how the health care provider should intervene in domestic violence situations. Making these curricula an integral part of the professional school course work will confirm the importance of the issue, producing graduates who, as they start their clinical careers, can identify and treat victims of abuse. Medical, nursing, social work, mental health, and public health schools should incorporate curricula on domestic violence that includes information on

- Recognizing victims by identifying the types of injuries typically caused by physical abuse and the sort of behavior that indicates victimization
- Developing a multidisciplinary team approach to respond to victims' needs
- Learning how to feel comfortable asking the difficult questions necessary to diagnose abuse
- Learning how to respond to answers sympathetically and nonjudgmentally

- Developing appropriate interventions, treatment, and referral documentation

Increasing Access to Health Care: Preexisting Conditions

A woman was beaten up by her husband and shoved across the room. Later she sought life, health and mortgage disability insurance. She was denied all three, although she was only in her mid-20s. The letter from the insurance company said, "the decision is due to history of a domestic dispute." The company said this was for her own protection. However, a spokeswoman also said, "It wouldn't be prudent of us as a company to insure someone we knew was being abused any more than it would be to insure a diabetic not taking his or her medication.[33]

This insurance company was not alone. In fact, the policies of some of the nation's largest insurance companies have been to deny health insurance coverage to victims of domestic violence. This practice came to light in 1993 when a Pennsylvania woman was denied life, health, and disability insurance by State Farm Insurance Company and life insurance by First Colony Life Insurance because her medical records indicated an incident of domestic violence. Congressman Charles Schumer (D-New York) conducted a survey in 1994 and found that 8 of 16 underwriters refused to cover battered women.[34] Such a policy victimizes abused women twice—once for the original harm, and again when they are denied health insurance protection to which they are entitled. In essence, denial of medical coverage blames them for the abuse. It may, if they cannot pay for needed medical care out of pocket, subject them to additional negative health consequences.

Legislation has been developed to eliminate this unfair practice, and this is being pursued on a state-by-state basis. Pennsylvania, California, Washington, New Jersey, New York, Florida, Michigan, North Dakota, and Wisconsin have all introduced legislation that prohibits insurance companies from denying coverage to individuals based on incidents of domestic abuse. This coverage applies to life, health, disability, and homeowners insurance.

Should Reporting Be Mandatory?

In 1994, California enacted legislation that required health practitioners to report injuries caused by domestic violence to the police or a specified state agency, just as they are required to report incidents of child abuse. Although such mandatory reporting may sound appealing, it may cause more problems than it was intended to cure and, in fact, may represent a threat rather than a solution to the health and safety of abused women.

Proponents argue that mandatory reporting will enhance patient safety and care. However, there is a great likelihood that it will cause at least some abused women not to seek medical assistance. Many domestic violence victims believe that involving the police is not the best or safest response to their particular situation and will only place them and their children at greater risk.

Although some argue that mandatory reporting will increase provider awareness of domestic violence, we question whether this is the most effective way to do so. In addition, although such reporting is supposed to aid law enforcement, there is often no mechanism in the average police department for receiving and handling the information, raising questions regarding how the justice system will respond.

Ethical issues also arise. For example, reporting child abuse is mandatory because children are helpless to protect themselves, and the state must intervene to ensure their safety. With domestic violence, the patient is a competent adult. Such patients are already victimized and controlled by their abusers. Women victims may see mandatory reporting as yet another paternalistic approach that takes the decision-making power about their situation away from them. Then there is the matter of confidentiality; mandatory reporting not only breaches patient privacy but also alters the principle of informed consent.

Collecting Data About Violence

One of the biggest obstacles to an effective prevention program about domestic violence, especially within the health care system, is lack of data about the problem and its interrelationship to other health issues. Because domestic violence has not been considered a health problem in the past, little attention has been paid to documenting the issue and obtaining data.

This situation should be corrected. We need to develop data collection systems; health care providers and agencies in both the public and private sectors should collect the data for such systems. We need epidemiological studies by the U.S. Centers for Disease Control and Prevention (CDC) and the National Institutes of Health. The necessary data include

- The number of males and females killed each year in domestic violence situations, including mass murders, and number of homicides that have been preceded by domestic violence
- The number of domestic violence victims assaulted each year, and the number of women who leave violent relationships
- The number of suicides attempted and carried out by children, teens, women, and men as a result of domestic violence
- The number and rate of miscarriages, birth defects, and low-birthweight babies resulting from domestic violence
- The rate of relationship violence among teenagers
- The relationship between child abuse and wife abuse
- The rate of domestic violence among the homeless
- The rate of domestic violence in families of delinquents

The 1994 Violence Against Women Act approved by Congress allocated resources for research on domestic violence. In 1995, the U.S. Departments of Justice and Health and Human Services and CDC were investigating the most effective methods of carrying out this congressional mandate.

Too Many Guns

Guns turn a moment of anger or despair into death and often turn domestic violence into murder. Because domestic violence between adults tends to escalate in severity and frequency over time, the presence of a gun can transform a physical assault into a homicide in a split second. From 1976 to 1987, more than twice as many American women were killed with guns by their husbands or boyfriends than were murdered by strangers using *any* means.[35] More than 80% of women who are murdered each year are killed with a gun. A gun in the home makes it three times more likely that a family member or a friend will be killed.[36] The cost in human lives is immense, as is the price our health care system pays. An average gunshot wound costs $33,000 in medical care; the total cost to society of gun-related injuries is $4 billion annually.[37]

Yet the gun industry and its well-paid lobbyists are now marketing their guns to women, attempting to exploit women's fears by encouraging them to buy guns for self-protection. "Refuse to be a Victim," suggests one ad; another shows a woman and her daughter nervously approaching a car in a deserted parking garage, above the words, "Where we live, where we park, where we walk, with every step, American women must weigh their personal safety against the increasing odds of criminal attack." These ads have appeared in *Family Circle, Redbook,* and *Working Woman.*

Despite these advertising campaigns, most of the American population now favors a ban on handguns for the first time in history.[38] Moreover, violence in general, and domestic violence in particular, is becoming increasingly a public health issue.[39] These shifts in public opinion have created a unique opportunity to organize health care providers to take an active role against gun violence. Just as police chiefs from all over the nation helped push the 1993 crime bill through a wavering Congress by testifying that police officers were being killed by the huge proliferation of guns on the streets of America, so physicians and other health care providers—whose knowledge still commands public respect—can testify that guns make domestic violence a serious health issue that costs the nation 4 billion unnecessary dollars at a time when millions of Americans have no health care coverage.

Conclusion

After 20 years of efforts to address domestic violence, the United States is at a turning point as we begin to shift from an emergency and legal response to a preventive approach. Our health care system offers an enormous opportunity for prevention because victims of abuse seek help from the health system, affording providers an unparalleled chance to help women at the beginning or at various points in the cycle of violence and to break through the cloak of privacy, secrecy, and shame that often silences female victims. Because virtually everyone interfaces with the health system at some time, even abuse in women who do not initially seek help may be picked up by an alert physician, nurse, or other provider when the women come for another reason. In fact, health care providers are already seeing victims of domestic abuse; they just do not always know it, nor do they know what to do. That is why, in addition to an emergency-based criminal justice response, we have proposed a comprehensive prevention approach that will allow the health care system to fulfill its responsibility to help end this scourge that destroys the health of so many women.

Endnotes

[1] Briggs J, Davis M: The brutal truth: putting domestic violence on the black agenda. *Emerge*, September 1994, pp 50–58

[2] Harris L: *The First Comprehensive National Health Survey of American Women.* Analysis by the Center for the Study and Prevention of Violence, Institute of Behavioral Science, University of Colorado. The data used to calculate this percentage came from the FBI's 1988–1989 Uniform Crime Reports (UCR), New York, Commonwealth Fund, 1993

[3] McLeer S, Anwar R: A study of battered women presenting in an emergency department. *American Journal of Public Health* 79(1):65–66, 1989

[4] Koop E: *Surgeon General's Workshop on Violence and Public Health Report: Source Book.* Atlanta, GA, Centers for Disease Control, 1986

[5] Parker B: Abuse during pregnancy: effects on maternal complications and birthweight in adult and teenage women. *Obstetrics and Gynecology* 84:323–328, 1994. This study showed that battered women sought prenatal care late, after the sixth month of pregnancy, and reported drinking alcohol, using drugs, or gaining too little weight, all of which predispose women to deliver low-birthweight babies. The implication, therefore, is that abuse may lead to behavior that causes low-birthweight babies.

[6] "Boy meets girl, boy beats girl." *Newsweek*, December 13, 1993, pp 66–68

[7] "Wife beating 'n the hood." *The Wall Street Journal*, July 6, 1993

[8] Randall T: Domestic violence intervention calls for more than treating injuries. *Journal of the American Medical Association* 264:939–940, 1990

[9] Stark E, Flitcraft A: Spouse abuse, in Koop E, op. cit.

[10] Straus MA, Gelles RJ, Steinmetz S: *Behind Closed Doors.* New York, Doubleday, 1980

[11] Stacy W, Shupe A: *The Family Secret.* Boston, MA, Beacon Press, 1983

[12]Lung CT, Dara D: Current trends in child abuse reporting and fatalities: the results of 1995 survey, National Committee to Prevent Child Abuse, April 1996

[13]Straus MA, Gelles RJ, Steinmetz S, op. cit.

[14]Currie E: A study by Dorothy Lewis cited in *Confronting Crime: An American Challenge.* New York, Pantheon Books, 1985, pp 205–206

[15]Peled I, Jaffe P, Edelson J (eds): *Ending the Cycle of Violence: Community Response to Children of Battered Women.* Thousand Oaks, CA, Sage, 1995; Wolfe DA, Jaffe P, Wilson SK, et al: Children of battered women: relationships of child behavior to family violence and maternal stress. *Journal of Consulting Clinical Psychology* 5:657–665, 1985

[16]Randall T: Domestic violence intervention calls for more than treating injuries. *Journal of the American Medical Association* 264:939–940, 1990

[17]Stark E, Flitcraft A, Zuckerman D, et al: *Wife Abuse in the Medical Setting.* Rockville, MD, National Clearinghouse on Domestic Violence, 1981

[18]CNN poll in *Time*, January 14, 1995

[19]Hu T, Bai J: *The Impact of Large Tax Increase on Cigarette Consumption: The Case of California* (Working Paper No 91-174). Berkeley, CA, University of California Berkeley, Department of Economics, July 1991

[20]Kizer K, Honig B: *Toward a Tobacco-Free California: A Status Report to the California Legislature on the First Fifteen Months of California's Tobacco Control Program.* Sacramento, CA, Department of Health Services, 1990

[21]The Advertising Research Foundation: *Inspiring Action and Saving Lives.* New York, Advertising Council Study, press release, April 8, 1991

[22]"Study says hospitals fail abuse victims." *San Francisco Chronicle*, August 18, 1993

[23]Sugg NK, Inui T: Primary care physicians' response to domestic violence: opening Pandora's box. *Journal of the American Medical Association* 267:3157–3160, 1992

[24]Kurz D: Emergency department responses to battered women: resistance to medicalization. *Social Problems* 34(1):69–81, 1987; Plichta S: The effects of women abuse on health care utilization and health status: a literature review. *Women's Health Issues* 2(3):154–163, 1992

[25]Sugg NK, Inui T, op. cit.

[26]Harris L, op. cit., 1993

[27]Goldberg WG, Tomlanovich MC: Domestic violence victims in the emergency department: new findings. *Journal of the American Medical Association* 251:3259–3264, 1984; Council on Ethical and Judicial Affairs, American Medical Association: Physicians and domestic violence: ethical considerations. *Journal of the American Medical Association* 267:3190–3193, 1992

[28]Correy S: "The menopause industry: how the medical establishment exploits women." *MS Magazine* 5(4):21, January/February 1995

[29]Bendtro M, Bowker LH: Battered women: how can nurses help? *Issues on Mental Health for Nurses* 10(2):169–180, 1989

[30]Council on Ethical and Judicial Affairs, American Medical Association, op. cit.

[31]Blair KA: Battered women: is she a silent victim? *Nursing Practitioner* 11(6): 38–47, 1986

[32]Parker B, McFarlane J: Physical and emotional abuse in pregnancy: a comparison of adult and teenage women. *Nursing Research* 42(3):173–178, 1993

[33]"Groups seek insurabilities for battered women." *New York Times*, May 12, 1994

[34]Schumer CE: *Schumer Charges Insurance Companies With Denying Coverage to Victims of Domestic Violence*. Washington, DC, Congressional press release, May 12, 1994

[35]Kellerman AL, Merce JA: Men, women and murder: gender specific difference in rates of fatal violence and victimization. *Journal of Trauma* 33: 1–4, 1992

[36]Kellerman AL, Rivera RP, Rushford NB, et al: Gun ownership as a risk factor in the home. *New England Journal of Medicine* 329:108–109, 1993

[37]"Exploding cost of gunfire." *Time Magazine*, October 11, 1993, p 59

[38]Harris LH: *Survey of Experiences, Perceptions and Apprehensions About Guns Among Young People in America*. New York, LH Research, June 1993; Recktenwald W, Harrington L: "Outrage over guns on rise: Harris Poll reports 52% favor ban on handguns." *Chicago Tribune*, June 4, 1993

[39]"Two cabinet voices, one echo: violence is a public health issue." *Washington Post*, April 6, 1993; "CDC's new chief worries as much about bullets as bacteria." *New York Times*, September 26, 1993; "Surgeons join outcry over guns and violence." *New York Times*, November 16, 1993

5

Diseases That Affect Only Women

Ruth Anne Queenan, M.D.
Lynne Beauregard

W omen have been included in research on diseases and conditions of the female reproductive tract by necessity, unlike many areas of health research. Despite this, there is still much we do not know about these exclusively female conditions. In this chapter, we discuss pelvic disorders; pregnancy-related illnesses, including the special problems of pregnancy caused by several sexually transmitted diseases (STDs); and diseases of the female reproductive tract. However, we begin with a discussion of contraception because, even though this does not fall into any of these categories, it is a paramount health issue almost always exclusive to women, who most often assume responsibility for birth control and bear the consequences not only of unwanted pregnancy but also of many of the STDs discussed below.

Contraception

The contraceptive options that have been developed in the past 40 years are probably the single most important advance in terms of improving the quality of women's health from a medical, social, and economic point of view. However, contraceptive research in the United States has slowed to a crawl because manufacturers fear liability lawsuits since the Dalkon Shield debacle, when litigation forced the recall of the product and ultimately caused the company to seek bankruptcy protection. Lawsuits over product liability to protect the consumer have led to financial gain for a small number of individuals and have limited contraceptive options for the rest of us as United States pharmaceutical companies have been slow to introduce new products. Other countries, particularly France and China, have far outstripped American research efforts.

There is no ideal contraceptive. This is clear from the fact that many women (and men) do not use any form of contraception despite the numerous methods available, leading to a large number of unwanted pregnancies in the United States. The birth control methods that do exist include permanent sterilization (tying off the fallopian tubes in women or the vas deferens in men); oral contraceptives that contain female hormones; injectable and implanted progestins (e.g., Norplant); barrier methods (male and female condoms, spermicides, diaphragms, cervical caps, and spermicidal sponges, foams, creams, and jellies); intrauterine devices (IUDs); withdrawal (removing the penis from the vagina before ejaculation); and periodic abstinence (avoiding intercourse during ovulation, commonly called the rhythm method). The effectiveness of each of these methods varies, running from almost 100% for permanent sterilization to about 97% for most oral contraceptives, 94% for IUDs, 88% for condoms, and only 79% for foams, creams, and jellies.

There are many reasons to continue contraceptive research. They include the need to

- Develop new methods that improve efficacy, patient acceptance, ease of use, and protection against STDs
- Lower the cost and increase the availability of existing contraceptives
- Develop educational programs to convince women to use birth control until they desire children and after they have completed their families

There is no doubt that developing more effective contraception would go a long way toward reducing the number of undesired children and abortions.

Infectious Diseases of the Reproductive Tract

Pelvic infections occur either in the lower genital tract (the vulva, vagina, and cervix) or the upper genital tract (the uterus, fallopian tubes, ovaries, and pelvic cavity). One of the dangers of infections of the pelvic cavity is that they can become systemic.

Some but not all pelvic infections are transmitted sexually. STDs, now epidemic in the United States, vary in their severity. Although some are only annoying, others can lead to systemic illness and may cause life-threatening infection. Several of the agents that cause STDs can predispose infected women to a number of gynecological malignancies and can therefore have long-term consequences. Certain STDs are never eradicated, even with optimal treatment. Therefore, the best defense against them is prevention. Condoms used with a spermicide during sexual intercourse reduce the risk of STDs. Women with multiple sexual partners are particularly vulnerable to STDs.

Lower Genital Tract Infections

Prevalent lower genital tract infections include candida or yeast vulvovaginitis (a fungal infection), bacterial vaginosis (a bacterial infection), trichomoniasis vaginitis (a parasitic infection), and herpes simplex vulvovaginitis (a viral infection). Candidal vulvovaginitis and bacterial vaginosis are not sexually transmitted, but trichomoniasis vaginitis and herpes vulvovaginitis are. Diagnosing lower genital tract infections is relatively straightforward. Treatment is quite successful and simple in most cases; however, certain infections persist even after multiple treatments.

Yeast infections.   A number of factors contribute to candidal vulvovaginitis, including antibiotics, excess moisture, synthetic undergarments, coexisting diabetes mellitus, pregnancy, and, sometimes, oral contraceptives. Recognizing these risk factors may facilitate early diagnosis and treatment and diminish the discomfort caused by this condition. Treatment includes various antifungal vaginal creams or suppositories. Recently, an oral antifungal agent has been approved for use. Research should be aimed at simplifying treatment, increasing the variety of effective medications, and decreasing the cost of treatment.

Bacterial vaginosis.   An overgrowth of certain bacteria typically present in the vagina causes bacterial vaginosis. In addition to localized symptoms that generate a great deal of discomfort, bacterial vaginosis has been implicated in several of the complications of pregnancy. These include premature rupture of the membranes, preterm labor, infection of the membranes (chorioamnionitis), and infection of the uterus after delivery (postpartum endomyometritis). Treatments for this condition include oral antibiotics and vaginal application of antibiotic creams.

Research that accurately identifies predisposing conditions is needed. The development of simpler and more accessible treatments could decrease discomfort. Clinically, the most important research would increase our understanding of the mechanisms that contribute to poor pregnancy outcomes and would reduce their incidence.

Trichomoniasis vaginitis.   Diagnosis of trichomoniasis vaginitis is rapid and simple, and treatment involves either oral antibiotics or antibiotic vaginal creams. Of all STDs, this condition is probably the least serious.

Human papillomavirus infection.   Human papillomavirus (HPV) infection is the most common sexually transmitted viral infection of the lower genital tract. There are many subtypes of this virus, and infections by different varieties lead to disparate clinical conditions. These include genital warts (condylomata acuminata), subclinical infection, abnormal growth of epithelial cells (intraepithelial neoplasia), and/or carcinoma of the vulva, vagina, and cervix. In fact, more than 60 subtypes of HPV have been identified, but only a few cause infections of the genital tract. Subtypes 6 and 11 are more often associated with genital warts (overt condylomata acuminata), but subtypes 16 and 18 are more likely to promote progression to premalignancies or malignancies.

HPV infection is widespread. As many as 60% of women tested for HPV DNA with sensitive molecular biology techniques (polymerase chain reaction, or PCR) are positive. Although the majority who test positive are asymptomatic, there is always the risk of reactivation, with subsequent serious consequences, because this virus remains in a woman's system for life once she is infected.

Health care providers diagnose warts by their typical appearance on physical examination. They can be flat or raised; pink, white, or other pigments; large or small; and they can appear singly or in clusters. Pap smears provide an important screening test to determine the presence of warts. One diagnostic method involves applying 5% acetic acid to the affected area and then examining it microscopically. A colposcopic examination offers a more definitive diagnosis. The surgical excision or biopsy of suspicious tissue and examination of it by a pathologist are often required.

Symptoms include occasional itching or bleeding but usually not much pain. In pregnancy, if the wart becomes large it can interfere with a vaginal delivery. Although rare, the vocal cords of vaginally delivered infants have become infected.

The most appropriate treatment depends on the location of the lesion, its extent, the severity of the disease, and whether the patient is pregnant. There are several chemical treatments (podophyllin, bichloroacetic acid, trichloroacetic acid, and 5-fluorouracil [5-FU]). Physical treatments include freezing the lesion (cryotherapy), laser therapy, electrotherapy, and surgical excision. Immunotherapy also is used in severe cases. Although each of these methods has a success rate that approaches 95% in properly selected patients, recurrences are common.

We need research to develop agents that would confer immunity, eradicate latent infection, improve the treatment of overt infection, and further clarify the association between this virus and malignancy.

Toxic shock syndrome.   Toxic shock syndrome (TSS) is a relatively rare women's disease. It is an infection caused by *Staphylococcus aureus*, a bacteria producing a toxin that enters the bloodstream. Symptoms of TSS run the gamut from a high fever, a diffuse red rash, scaly skin, vomiting, and diarrhea to much more serious manifestations, such as shock, multisystem organ failure, and, in up to 3% of patients, death.

High-absorbency tampons were the major cause of TSS. Some women tended to leave them in place for long periods, unwittingly providing an environment in which the bacteria could survive and multiply. After these tampons were removed from the market, the incidence of this disease dropped dramatically. Less absorbent tampons must be changed more frequently, preventing the bacteria from growing.

A different type of TSS, associated with adverse gynecological and obstetrical conditions, is caused by *Streptococcus pyogenes* and *Clostridium sordellii*. It is usually a consequence of infection following abortion, uterine inflammation following delivery (postpartum endomyometritis), and postoperative wound infections.

Treatment for menstrual-related TSS involves removing the tampon, culturing the infection site, and administering intravenous antibiotics.

Upper Genital Tract Infections

Upper genital tract infections occur in the uterus, fallopian tubes, ovaries, pelvis, and lower abdomen. Frequently referred to as pelvic inflammatory disease (PID), this clinical entity is a major health problem in the United States, with 1 million women affected annually. PID is usually transmitted sexually. It is associated with two bacteria—*Neisseria gonorrhoeae* and *Chlamydia trachomatis*—in more than 50% of cases. Vaginal microorganisms and respiratory pathogens also are infectious agents in PID.

Chlamydial PID.   Symptoms of chlamydial and gonococcal PID differ. Even though the symptoms of chlamydial PID may be subtler than those of gonococcal PID, chlamydia frequently causes much more permanent damage to the fallopian tubes. In fact, chlamydia is probably the most frequent cause of PID, with somewhere between 5% and 15% of sexually active women harboring the pathogen.

Chlamydial infections generally come on gradually but can cause inflammation of the fallopian tubes, the urethra, and the cervix, the latter associated with the production of mucus and pus. The most common symptom is a profuse yellow vaginal discharge that may cause irritation. The cervix may be tender during intercourse or during a pelvic examination. If the infection has spread to the fallopian tubes, mild or severe pelvic pain may be present. Some women with chlamydial infection notice no change in vaginal discharge and may only experience mild abdominal pain or backache. A burning sensation during urination may occur. Because the organism cannot be grown in the standard urine culture medium, a negative urine culture in a woman with symptoms of a urinary tract infection should suggest a chlamydial infection.

A subset of women with chlamydial infection may be entirely asymptomatic and receive no treatment. However, this asymptomatic clinical situation often leads, over time, to blocked fallopian tubes and infertility. It is important to diagnose and treat chlamydial infection during pregnancy, as the newborn can contract an infection if delivered vaginally through an infected genital tract.

A reddish inflamed cervix with a discharge of pus and mucus is often evidence of infection. The diagnosis is confirmed with a positive culture. But culturing the organism is expensive and time-consuming. Health providers also use tests indicating the presence of antibodies to the organism in cervical mucus or use enzyme-linked immunoassays. Research to develop a clinically useful PCR test to diagnose the infection is being conducted.

Gonorrheal PID. Gonorrheal PID has more striking symptoms, including severe pelvic and abdominal pain, chills and high fever, and a vaginal discharge. Sometimes there is vaginal bleeding as well, and women frequently experience nausea and vomiting. Physical examination most often reveals tenderness of the cervix, uterus, and abdomen. A bacterial culture of the cervical discharge frequently identifies the N. gonorrhoeae organism, but it takes time. Other signs of infection are an elevated white blood cell count and an abnormal sedimentation rate of red blood cells. Often, physicians perform an ultrasound examination to assess the pelvis for evidence of abscesses on the fallopian tubes and ovaries (tubo-ovarian abscess). Because the symptoms of gonorrheal PID mimic those of appendicitis and ectopic pregnancy, the physician should do a pregnancy test to eliminate this latter possibility. In fact, it is the similarities of the symptoms of ectopic pregnancy, appendicitis, and gonorrheal PID that make differentiating among them difficult. Yet, because their management is so radically different—appendicitis and ectopic pregnancy require surgery, whereas gonococcal PID needs a course of antibiotics—in unusual cases the physician may have to perform a laparoscopic examination to look at the pelvic organs.

Under certain circumstances, treatment of PID requires hospitalization. Indications for hospitalization include

- Ineffective outpatient treatment
- Presence of a pelvic abscess

- A young patient, or a patient who has not completed child-bearing, to decrease the possibility of tubal factor infertility
- Inability of the patient to tolerate oral medications
- Inability of the physician to obtain adequate follow-up 72 hours after initiating therapy
- Any uncertainty about the diagnosis
- Pregnancy

The mainstay of therapy for *N. gonorrhoeae* is a broad-spectrum antibiotic, as a multitude of pathogenic bacteria are present in this infection.

Approximately 25% of women with PID develop long-term consequences. Chronic pelvic pain is common in women with a history of PID. The incidence of ectopic pregnancy jumps 10-fold in women who have had previous episodes of PID. Infertility caused by blocked fallopian tubes is common among women with a history of PID; the incidence increases with the severity of the infection and the number of episodes of PID.

Research to develop tests that could supply a rapid diagnosis, as well as research on effective prevention, is the top priority for PID. Public health policy must address this problem because it has reached epidemic proportions.

Benign Diseases of the Female Reproductive Tract

Uterine Fibroids

Uterine fibroids (leiomyoma uteri) are encapsulated benign smooth muscle tumors that grow inside the uterus. These tumors occur in approximately 25% of women of reproductive age. Because of their frequency, they are responsible for most of the pelvic surgery performed in women. Typically, they remain asymptomatic, but, depending on their size and location, they can be associated with myriad symptoms.

Fibroids generally increase the blood supply to the uterus, causing the heavy menstrual bleeding that can lead to chronic anemia. Fibroids located just beneath the surface of the uterine lining (subendothelial) are the most likely ones to cause excess menstrual bleeding. They also are associated with decreased fertility because they distort the endometrial cavity, block off the opening to the fallopian tubes, or cause chronic inflammation of the uterine lining. Intramural fibroids are contained within the muscular wall of the uterus. Those located along the outer surface of the uterus are called subserosal fibroids and can cause adhesions to other pelvic structures, including the fallopian tubes, with resulting infertility. All types of fibroids can be responsible for pelvic pain or pressure—especially if they outgrow their blood supply and begin to degenerate—as well as painful menstrual periods (dysmenorrhea), urinary symptoms (especially urgency), or disturbances of bowel function. They occasionally degenerate during pregnancy, resulting in serious complications, including preterm labor or delivery, separation of the fetus from the placenta (placental separation), difficulty with vaginal delivery and consequent need for cesarean section, and bleeding after delivery (postpartum hemorrhage). Depending on their size, they can retard fetal growth, cause a contraction of fetal limbs because the fetus cannot move freely, and lead to fetal malpresentation.

Physicians can diagnose fibroids during pelvic examinations and confirm their diagnosis with a pelvic ultrasound examination. Often, the symptoms of pain or pelvic pressure, dysmenorrhea, and moderately heavy menstrual bleeding can be treated quite successfully with nonsteroidal anti-inflammatory agents. Acute bleeding can be controlled by hormonal preparations (progestins) or by scraping out the uterus (dilation and curettage [D&C]).

Sometimes surgery is the only effective therapy for symptomatic women. Women who choose surgical removal of the fibroids (myomectomy) usually do so because they wish to preserve their uterus for future childbearing. But myomectomy is often associated with heavy blood loss, and the risk of future uterine fibroids remains. Removal of the uterus (hysterectomy) provides permanent relief for women who have completed their childbearing and do not wish to preserve their uterus.

The gonadotropin-releasing hormone (GnRH) agonists, which include leuprolide, nafarelin, goserelin, and buserelin, produce a temporary medical menopause by blocking the action of the gonadotropins—the luteinizing hormone (LH) and the follicle-stimulating hormone (FSH)—thereby reducing estrogen production and interfering with ovulation. They are used in some women with uterine fibroids to decrease the size of the uterus preoperatively to lessen the anticipated blood loss at surgery or to allow enough shrinkage of the uterus to perform a vaginal rather than an abdominal hysterectomy. Profoundly anemic women also are treated with these medications and iron to achieve an improved blood count before surgery.

Physicians and scientists do not understand why fibroids grow. There is no medical therapy that can shrink fibroids without disturbing the uterus or the ovulatory cycle. Given the high incidence of these tumors, development of less invasive therapeutic options would have a tremendously beneficial impact on women's health.

Endometriosis

Endometriosis, which affects approximately 7% of women, occurs when the endometrial tissue lining the uterus migrates and grows at distant sites, usually on the filmy peritoneal covering of the pelvis or on the surface of structures within the pelvis—the ovary, fallopian tubes, bladder, uterine ligaments, and rectum. Endometrial tissue also can grow on the cervix, vagina, and vulva. When spread through the bloodstream, it may move to more distant sites and grow on the skin, lungs, central nervous system, and other structures, causing significant invasion and destruction.

Many women with endometriosis have no symptoms, and the reasons some women progress to symptomatic endometriosis are not clear. Some authorities postulate that immune mechanisms may play a role. The typical pain of endometriosis occurs just before the menstrual period and lessens after menstrual flow begins because the endometrial tissue growing outside the uterus responds to the hormonal fluctuations of the menstrual cycle just as it does within the uterus. The amount of endometriosis does not correlate with the severity of symptoms. Although involvement of the ovaries can result in persistent pain, endometriosis on the rectal wall may cause occasional pain limited to bowel movements or intercourse.

Severe endometriosis is a major contributor to infertility by causing dense pelvic adhesions or scar tissue. Other hypothetical explanations of the connection between endometriosis and infertility include the possibility that pelvic endometriosis produces severe inflammation, which produces substances that are toxic to eggs and sperm.

Physicians diagnose endometriosis in a variety of ways. The patient's medical history is important. Physical examination that reveals nodules behind the uterus or on the uterine ligaments or ovaries or decreased mobility of the uterus are indications that endometriosis is present. But a biopsy of the lesions or laparoscopic visualization of endometrial implants is needed to be sure of the diagnosis.

Any treatment plan must include consideration of the woman's age, the severity of her symptoms, and her reproductive desires and treatment goals. Women with relatively small amounts of endometrial tissue can choose laser or electronic laparoscopic surgery to remove the endometrial implants. For women with more extensive disease who wish to preserve their child-bearing capacity, surgery to remove as much endometriosis as possible while restoring the normal anatomy is the therapy of choice. Women who have completed their families or who do not wish to preserve their fertility can elect a total hysterectomy, with removal of the ovaries and fallopian tubes (bilateral salpingo-oophorectomy) and as much endometrial tissue as possible. Because this treatment produces a surgical menopause, the hormonal loss inactivates the remaining endometriosis. However, because menopause increases the risk of cardiovascular disease and osteoporosis, and because hormone replacement therapy may restart endometrial growth, this option requires a woman to consider the risks and benefits carefully.

Effective medications for the medical management of endometriosis include oral contraceptive pills, which reduce the stimulation of the endometrial implants and slow the progression of disease. Progestins also are used effectively in mild to moderate disease. Danazol, a synthetic steroid derived from testosterone, inhibits the action of LH and FSH, producing a low-estrogen state. It is most effective for short-term management of mild to moderate disease. It causes a pseudomenopause with serious side effects—hot flashes, cessation of periods, moodiness, depression, bone loss, and alterations in the levels of cholesterol and other lipoproteins that increase the risk of heart disease. Complaints about the masculinizing effects of testosterone, such as acne, hair loss, and weight gain, usually limit the duration this medication can be used.

The GnRH agonists previously described as a treatment for uterine fibroids also are used to treat endometriosis. They cause a temporary menopause with similar menopausal symptoms—hot flashes, decreased libido, vaginal dryness, mood changes, and insomnia. Although they avoid the acne, hair loss, and oily skin that are related to Danazol use, they are responsible for a decrease in bone density and cannot be used for longer than 6 months. A recently developed treatment called add-back therapy uses small doses of estrogen with these agents to help alleviate the profound symptoms of menopause without significantly reducing the benefits of the drugs. Add-back therapy can safely extend GnRH agonist use beyond 6 months.

Large, long-term studies are under way and are designed to clarify the factors that contribute to this disease, determine which agents provide the most appropriate medical management, find medical agents that women can tolerate better, and lessen the impact of this disease on infertility.

Chronic Pelvic Pain

Chronic pain in the pelvic area is another frustrating condition for women and their physicians. Pelvic pain is considered chronic if it has lasted for at least 6 months. The common gynecological causes include endometriosis, pelvic adhesive disease, and adenomyosis, a condition in which endometrial tissue burrows deep into uterine muscle. This type of pain also can be caused by gastrointestinal problems, such as inflammatory bowel disease, diverticulosis, and spastic colon, as well as urological, orthopedic, and neurological abnormalities.

Physicians treating women with this troublesome condition should search for whatever pathology may be causing the problem while also considering a psychological evaluation, which should include questions about previous physical or sexual abuse. Unfortunately, we do not yet understand the interplay of the patient's peripheral nervous system, psychological status, and physical symptoms. It is clear that depression is commonly found among patients who complain of chronic pelvic pain. As in other types of chronic pain, it is not easy to know whether pain causes depression or depression causes pain. Therefore, a multidisciplinary treatment approach carries the best chance of success. This can include pain killers (analgesics), behavioral and psychological therapies (biofeedback, self-hypnosis, and relaxation techniques), local anesthetics, and acupuncture or acupressure. Narcotic analgesics are not suitable remedies because they work for a limited time and can cause drug dependency. Surgical treatments include removing the adhesions, excising or vaporizing the endometriosis, and cutting the involved nerve. Some women seek help from multidisciplinary clinics, which coordinate the sometimes complex treatment plans. Research should concentrate on the physical and psychological causes of chronic pain and their interaction.

Premenstrual Syndrome

Premenstrual syndrome (PMS) is another condition that often requires a multidisciplinary approach to effective therapy. Although many women notice body changes and/or mood alteration before their menstrual periods, only a few will experience symptoms severe enough to consider the diagnosis of PMS.

There is a long list of characteristic symptoms associated with PMS. They occur in a cyclic pattern late in the menstrual cycle and disturb normal function. Physical symptoms include bloating, breast discomfort, headache, pelvic pain, gastrointestinal disturbance, skin eruptions, and fatigue. Psychological symptoms run the gamut from anxiety to irritability, depression, mood swings, clumsiness, and loss of concentration. Some women also experience behavioral changes, such as withdrawal and food cravings.

The causes of PMS are unclear. Many factors may be related to the condition, including an allergy to progesterone, low blood sugar (hypoglycemia), imbalances in certain neurotransmitters (such as serotonin and monoamine oxidase), vitamin B_6 deficiency, elevated prolactin levels, and increased prostaglandin activity. Because no clear causes have been identified, treatment is quite varied and most often includes a combination of nonmedical and medical therapies. Nonmedical therapies include changes in diet, exercise, vitamin supplementation, and stress reduction; medical therapies include nonsteroidal anti-inflammatory drugs, antidepressants, Danazol, oral contraceptive pills, and other hormonal manipulations to suppress ovulation. Until more is know about what brings on PMS, individualizing therapy offers the most success in reducing a woman's symptoms and improving her ability to function.

Prolapse

The ligaments that support the pelvic organs are subjected to an enormous amount of stress during a woman's life span. Damage to the pelvic support system can occur from trauma during childbirth, cigarette smoking, chronic coughing related to lung disease, occupations that require heavy lifting, lack of estrogen during menopause, and aging of tissue in the pelvic area. Prolapse, the descent of the pelvic organs—the bladder, uterus, rectum, or bowel—can be the result.

Because the trauma of childbirth tears and weakens these ligaments, prolapse usually occurs only in women who have had vaginal deliveries. Symptoms often begin after menopause, when decreasing estrogen levels further weaken supporting structures. Mild prolapse of the uterus causes the sensation of pelvic pressure. In cases of more severe prolapse, the cervix, uterus, and portions of the vaginal wall may descend through the vaginal opening, often interfering with walking, and bowel, bladder, or sexual function.

Bladder prolapse (cystocele) often causes malfunction of the urinary system, either the inability to empty the bladder adequately or incontinence. When the rectum falls (herniates), a condition known as rectocele occurs, compromising normal bowel function.

Treatment of these conditions depends on the severity of the prolapse and other symptoms, the woman's overall health or illness, and her own wishes. For mild cases of prolapse, altering the conditions that accelerate the weakening of the supporting structures will slow the progression of symptoms. This might include stopping smoking, switching to a less strenuous job, and taking cough suppressants and/or systemic estrogen replacement therapy. Estrogens also can be applied regionally to improve blood supply to estrogen-sensitive tissues of the pelvis. Treatment of constipation is often helpful in decreasing the need to strain with bowel movements.

Women who do not want surgery can use a pessary, a soft rubber or plastic device fitted around the cervix that adds support to the uterus.

The pessary remains in place except during intercourse and for a weekly cleaning to avoid infection. Occasionally, women who use a pessary will develop vaginal infections that require treatment.

Numerous surgical options are available and should be chosen based on the defect, the woman's age, her desire to preserve her fertility, and her overall health and ability to tolerate the procedure. The most common operation is a vaginal hysterectomy with repair of the structures that support the bladder, rectum, and uterus.

Preventive interventions include better obstetrical management so that the supporting pelvic structures are not damaged in the first place; pelvic exercises (Kegel exercises), particularly after childbirth, to improve the tone of muscles that support pelvic structure; and estrogen early in menopause to prevent deterioration or atrophy of vaginal tissues.

Cancers of the Reproductive Tract

Cancer is the leading cause of death in women between ages 35 and 75. However, survival rates for cancers detected at an early stage are improving. Although 80% to 90% of white women with stage I and II cervical cancer now survive the disease, African American and Hispanic women experience a much higher death rate, probably because of the barriers to medical care they experience, which prevent early diagnosis and treatment. The overall 5-year survival rate for cervical cancer is 68%, but for women diagnosed with localized disease, it jumps to 91%.[1] For endometrial cancer, the 5-year survival rate is 83%, but, if discovered early, it improves to 95%. When endometrial cancer is diagnosed at the regional stage, survival is 65%.[2] Ninety percent of women with vulvar cancer who undergo vulvectomy (removal of the vulva) are still alive 5 years after surgery. Overall, 75% of all women with vulvar cancer are cured. An estimated 10 million people in the United States have had cancer, and 7 million of them are alive 5 years after the disease was first discovered. Most of these can be considered cured—that is, with no evidence of disease.[3]

Cancer is not a monolithic condition but one that comes in many forms and has myriad causes. What all cancers have in common, however, is the uncontrolled growth of tissue that has become malignant, destroying normal tissue as it grows. Carcinoma refers to cancers that arise in the epithelial tissue that lines the surface of the body's structures. Sarcoma, however, is a cancer that occurs in muscle or bone. Malignant cells either enlarge locally and destroy essential organs, or they metastasize and travel through the bloodstream or the lymphatic system to distant parts of the body, usually the lymph nodes, liver, and lung, where they continue to grow and destroy tissue. The growth of malignant cells can be limited in part by the fibrous tissue surrounding them and by the immune system.

The conversion of cells from benign to malignant occurs because of a number of factors. Some patients carry a genetic trait causing malignancy of specific tissue, such as in the breast or colon. Exposure to carcinogens, including viruses, chemical toxins, or radiation can promote the disease. The malignant conversion of cells is a complex process. Genes that promote growth are typically held in balance by genes that are growth inhibitors. The immune system plays a major role in these control mechanisms. When this system breaks down, the body may lose its ability to stop uncontrolled growth. Recent advances in immunotherapy have been used to bolster the immune system to increase its protective function in preventing or eliminating malignancies.

Cancer of the Vulva

Vulvar cancer is a form of skin cancer and is, generally, a disease of women whose average age is 70. The incidence of vulvar cancer among young women is growing because infection with HPV, which causes genital warts, is increasing and has been clearly associated with this particular malignancy.

Physicians diagnose vulvar cancer by examining the vulvar skin or by a biopsy of suspicious lesions. Gynecologists treat early precancerous lesions, called vulvar intraepithelial neoplasias or dysplasias, with local surgery using laser or by applying chemotherapeutic creams. Invasive cancer of the vulva requires more extensive and individualized therapy. Minimally invasive cancer of the vulva can be successfully treated with local surgery. If the lesions have invaded deeper and display significant pathology, surgeons excise a wider area and remove selected lymph nodes for pathological examination. The treatment of choice for more extensive lesions is a simple or radical vulvectomy. A simple vulvectomy involves removal of the skin of the vulva. A radical vulvectomy dissects all tissue to the underlying muscle layer, usually removes the lymph nodes of the groin, and is followed by radiation therapy. Surgeons try to preserve urethral, vaginal, and anal openings so that their functions are not impaired.

Possible complications from this extensive surgery are blood loss, infection, and inadequate or slow healing. For patients who are poor surgical risks or who have extensive inoperable disease, the combination of chemotherapy and radiation therapy is used.

Typically, vulvar carcinomas are slowly growing tumors, which explains their high rate of cure if detected at an early stage of disease. Research should focus on better methods of early detection and less invasive surgical options.

Cancer of the Vagina

Vaginal cancer is an unusual tumor. Because of the vagina's proximity to other vital structures, such as the bladder and rectum, it is a difficult malignancy to treat. HPV infection is one of several conditions that predispose women to vaginal cancer. Another is exposure to diethylstilbestrol (DES) in utero, which causes clear cell carcinoma, a condition that is 20 times more common in DES-exposed daughters than in unexposed women. In this high-risk group, the incidence of vaginal cancer is 1 per 1,000 women.

Early preinvasive disease (vaginal intraepithelial neoplasia) is most often asymptomatic but can be detected by the Pap smear. As the disease advances, symptoms, such as vaginal bleeding and discharge, urinary or bowel problems, or pain, proliferate. Physicians diagnose vaginal cancer by physical examination, usually using the colposcope for microscopic enlargement, and by ordering a biopsy of suspicious lesions to obtain laboratory confirmation of the disease.

Treatment depends on the extent and invasiveness of the cancer. Local surgical removal of involved tissue using laser or the application of a chemotherapeutic cream such as 5-FU are most successful for superficial disease. Invasive disease is best treated either with radiation therapy or, in cases of small invasive lesions, radical surgery. Complications from these treatments include blood loss, infection, and chronic scarring and narrowing of the vagina, which may prevent sexual activity. The overall cure rate for vaginal cancer is approximately 50%.

Cancer of the Cervix

The cervix, the connection between the uterus and vagina, is accessible and easy to examine. For many years the Pap smear has been used to identify premalignant and malignant changes in the superficial layer of the cervix. The colposcope, a magnifying instrument, allows visualization and study of the cervical surface; biopsies of suspicious areas and pathological examination confirm the diagnosis. These two techniques are the basic tools in the detection and prevention of cervical cancer.

Pap smears usually detect abnormal precancerous changes in the cervix. A progression of these precancerous changes has become more apparent in recent years. As a result, a National Institutes of Health committee recommended abandoning the old "class" system for reporting Pap smear results in favor of the "Bethesda system," in which cytopathologists describe the abnormalities they see.

Over the past decade or so, scientists have become aware of the link between sexual intercourse, infection with HPV, and development of cervical neoplasias. For cervical cancer specifically, the HPV subtypes 16 and 18 are frequently involved. Cigarette smoking also contributes to the development of cervical cancer, probably through the secretion of teratogens.

An abnormal Pap smear requires colposcopy, curettage of the endocervical canal, and a biopsy of any suspicious tissue. The treatment for mildly abnormal tissue growth (dysplasia) is close observation with frequent Pap smears, approximately every 3 to 4 months. More persistent disease or worsening dysplasia requires repeat colposcopy. Approximately 80% of mildly dysplastic lesions will resolve spontaneously. For moderate or severe dysplasia (carcinoma in situ), more aggressive treatment is indicated as these lesions are at risk for developing into cervical cancer. The various treatment options include freezing the superficial abnormal cells (cryotherapy), removing the superficial abnormal cells with laser surgery, excising a cone of tissue (cervical cone biopsy) from the opening of the cervix if tissue is needed for better diagnosis, and hysterectomy.

Cervical cancer begins in the superficial layer of cells, spreads deeper into the cervix, and then spreads locally to the vagina, uterus, bladder, rectum, lymph nodes, and other pelvic structures. Distant spread occurs late in the disease.

Evaluation of the extent of the disease (staging) includes a thorough history and physical examination, a biopsy, routine laboratory tests, a chest X ray, X-ray studies of the kidneys and ureters, and use of an endoscope to view the bladder (cystoscopy) and the rectum and lower colon (sigmoidoscopy).

The earliest stage of cervical cancer is treated by hysterectomy. As disease stage advances, indicating a larger tumor and deeper penetration, the treatment choice is either a radical hysterectomy, which involves removal of the uterus, the surrounding supportive ligaments, and the upper vagina, with dissection of the lymph nodes, or radiation therapy. In early-stage disease, cure rates of 80% to 90% are roughly comparable for surgery and radiation therapy. Cure rates drop for later-stage disease, in which surgery is no longer as effective and the tumor has become too extensive to be treated optimally with radiation therapy. For late-stage inoperable cervical cancer in which the tumor has not become too large, radiation is the treatment of choice for palliation of symptoms. Chemotherapy has not been particularly successful in treating this disease.

Cancer of the Endometrium

Endometrial cancer, cancer of the glands lining the uterus, is the most common cancer of the female reproductive tract and is frequently characterized by unscheduled vaginal bleeding. It is most prevalent in women between age 50 and 60 years but may occur at any time after puberty. Endometrial cancer is diagnosed by a biopsy of the endometrial tissue. Usually, this is done in an office and is well tolerated by patients. Occasionally, because the diagnosis is uncertain or a satisfactory endometrial sample cannot be obtained in the office, the physician does a D&C as outpatient surgery. In this procedure, the physician uses a hysteroscope to view the endometrial cavity, opens (dilates) the cervix, and scrapes the lining of the uterus to obtain the necessary sample. Most cases are detected early, and, therefore, the overall survival rate is about 75%, making this one of the most curable of gynecological malignancies.

Like the cervix, the lining of the uterus passes through premalignant stages before becoming true cancer. During the menstrual cycle, high estrogen levels stimulate the lining of the uterus to divide rapidly in preparation for the implantation of a fertilized egg. Progesterone matures this process and then halts it, bringing on the menstrual period when no conception takes place. Throughout a woman's life, the endometrium will proliferate whenever it is exposed to estrogen, whatever the source, and this growth may escape normal control mechanisms. In its mild form, the uncontrolled growth of the endometrium, called hyperplasia, may revert to normal without treatment or with the administration of progesterone. Women with endometrial hyperplasia require careful follow-up with repeat biopsies for recurrent irregular bleeding. Those who have an intact uterus should not take estrogen without progesterone. For patients with persistent endometrial hyperplasia who do not wish to preserve their fertility, hysterectomy is one possible solution.

Menopausal women at increased risk are those who take estrogen without progesterone (unopposed estrogen) and obese women because fatty tissue is the major source of estrogen production after menopause. Women who experience heavy bleeding, longer episodes of bleeding, or irregular bleeding between identified menstrual periods are at greater risk for endometrial hyperplasia. By far the most ominous pattern is irregular bleeding or spotting after menopause.

Oral contraceptives containing both estrogen and progesterone are protective against endometrial cancer. In fact, oral contraceptives have been associated with a 50% reduction in the rate of endometrial cancer, probably because the combination pills contain enough synthetic progesterone to oppose the estrogen effect on the endometrium. A history of multiple full-term pregnancies also is protective. Conversely, infertility, late menopause, diabetes, hypertension, and obesity all increase the risk of this disease.

Staging of endometrial cancer includes careful physical examination and a chest X ray, followed by surgery. Total hysterectomy, which removes the uterus, the fallopian tubes, and the ovaries, cures about 85% of women. More extensive disease usually requires additional radiation therapy either before surgery, to reduce the size of the tumor, or afterward, to destroy any remaining disease. When finding suspicious tissue, the surgeon will examine and sample the lymph nodes in the abdomen and pelvis. Many advanced cancers of the endometrium that have spread beyond the pelvis respond to synthetic progesterone, which has few side effects. Chemotherapeutic agents given singly or in combination are effective for variable periods.

Sarcomas of the uterus are malignant tumors of muscle and connective tissue. Although considerably less common than carcinomas, they tend to behave much more aggressively and are therefore harder to treat. Uterine sarcoma occurs in only about 2 of 100,000 women. These rapidly growing tumors are difficult to distinguish from the common benign fibroid tumors of the uterus. In fact, physicians often recommend hysterectomy for a uterine fibroid that is enlarging for fear that a uterine sarcoma may actually be responsible for the growth. Total hysterectomy offers the only hope of cure. Although radiation therapy helps to reduce local recurrences, chemotherapy is of little documented use.

Cancer of the Ovary

This "silent" disease, so named because it has no early symptoms, is a major killer of women, accounting for 25% of all malignancies of the female reproductive tract, but 50% of all deaths. It has received much media attention over the past decade, largely after the entertainer Gilda Radner died from the disease, and her husband launched a campaign to increase awareness about ovarian cancer.

One woman in 70 will develop cancer of the ovary in her lifetime. The incidence is higher in infertile women, those with a family history of the disease in a first-degree relative (mother, child, sister), and white women. Oral contraceptives, used even for a short time, reduce the incidence by 50%, but women with other estrogen-sensitive tumors, such as breast or endometrial cancer, have a higher risk of developing ovarian cancer. Research suggests that these three cancers are related to a high-fat diet.

Careful pelvic examination, the most effective method of detecting cancer of the ovary, is not entirely satisfying as early malignancies can easily be missed. Pap smears occasionally contain malignant cells from the ovary but are not a reliable screening tool. Pelvic ultrasound yields information about tumors found during pelvic examination but does not always distinguish between benign and malignant tumors. Doppler studies added to ultrasound examination are helpful in visualizing blood vessel growth in tumors, which suggests malignancy. Currently, ultrasound has not demonstrated adequate specificity to be used for routine screening. Several tumor markers are elevated in the blood of patients with cancer of the ovary and other pelvic conditions such as endometriosis. The most familiar of these tumor antigens is CA-125. None of the tumor antigens is sensitive or specific enough for routine mass screening, but tumor antigens are valuable measures of response to chemotherapy and in surveillance for disease recurrence.

Symptoms of ovarian cancer, such as bleeding, abdominal fullness and discomfort, or the discovery of a mass through the abdominal wall, occur late in the disease, frequently when the tumor is large and extends over the surface of the pelvic structures. Other malignancies, especially from the breast and gastrointestinal tract, often spread to the surface of the ovary and need to be distinguished from primary ovarian cancer to guide therapy.

Several studies, most commonly chest X rays and blood studies for tumor markers, are useful in evaluating the effectiveness of treatment. These initial studies establish a baseline, with subsequent repeat studies indicating an increase or decrease in the size and spread of the tumor.

Surgery is the treatment of choice for cancer of the ovary. In most cases, physicians perform a total abdominal hysterectomy, removing the uterus, fallopian tubes, and ovaries, because this cancer commonly spreads to the opposite ovary and adjacent pelvic structures. Careful exploration of the pelvis and abdomen is necessary to identify sites to which the cancer has spread. In the rare case of early, limited disease in a young woman who wishes to preserve her fertility, the surgeon can take a more limited approach, sparing one ovary and the uterus or the uterus alone.

The surgeon removes as much of the tumor from all sites as possible to increase the effectiveness of subsequent chemotherapy or radiation therapy, which is almost always indicated. Studies have shown that chemotherapy significantly improves survival. Oncologists use many different chemotherapeutic schedules, all of which are aimed at using lower doses of multiple agents in an attempt to reduce toxic side effects. Platinum compounds and, more recently, Taxol (paclitaxel) are two effective agents for advanced ovarian cancer that have extended survival but cause substantial side effects. Some types of ovarian cancer respond to radioactive sodium phosphate (^{32}P) injected into the abdominal cavity.

Repeat surgery (second-look laparotomy) to assess the recurrence or persistence of the disease is somewhat controversial. It is frequently used to detect subclinical growth, which can then be removed, and to plan further chemotherapy or radiation therapy. Oncologists also use blood tumor antigen markers, which are useful in monitoring the woman's response to treatment.

Overall, ovarian cancer remains a frustrating disease, with only about one-third of cases being diagnosed in an early stage and almost half of the early tumors recurring. The newer techniques of chemotherapy are beginning to improve outcome. The widespread use of oral contraceptive pills should reduce the incidence of this malignancy. Women with a first-degree relative who has been diagnosed with ovarian cancer are at increased risk and should be monitored closely.

Cancer of the Fallopian Tubes

Cancer of the fallopian tubes is an exceedingly rare malignancy. A clear vaginal discharge is one distinguishing symptom of this cancer, but typically there are few if any symptoms and this condition is usually discovered late, often at the time of pelvic surgery for other reasons. The treatment and survival rates are similar to those for ovarian cancer.

Research Needs for Gynecological Malignancies

We need research to find much better methods of prevention and early detection. Studies of the genetic, infectious, hormonal, and immunological aspects of these cancers are important, as they should provide important clues for understanding, preventing, and combating these diseases. Such research should uncover genetic, hormonal, and immunological manipulations that would improve the course and cure rates of these conditions. Finally, research should focus on better surgical, chemotherapeutic, and radiation techniques to decrease deforming results and mitigate side effects.

Diseases and Conditions of Pregnancy

Gestational Trophoblastic Disease

Trophoblasts are cells of placental origin that normally burrow into the lining of the uterus in early pregnancy and form the placenta, which provides the fetus with oxygen and nutrients. This normal fetal tissue shares many characteristics of cancer because it invades other tissue and blood vessels. Yet, because it is under an exquisite and complicated control system, it rarely becomes malignant.

There are two forms of gestational trophoblastic disease. One is benign and takes the form of hydatidiform mole or molar pregnancy; the other is malignant and is called choriocarcinoma.

Hydatidiform mole.   In the benign form, which occurs in about 1 in 1,000 pregnancies in the United States and much more frequently in Asia, an improper exchange of genetic material occurs at conception, causing the placental tissue to form into abnormally small or large cysts. Most often fetal tissue cannot be identified.

A constellation of symptoms is related to hydatidiform mole, including vaginal bleeding, a rapidly enlarging uterus that is bigger than expected for the gestational age of the fetus, and a high level of a particular hormone of pregnancy called beta–human chorionic gonadotropin (HCG), which is detected by a blood test. There is often more of the nausea and vomiting common in pregnancy. Hyperthyroidism, ovarian cysts, and early preeclampsia—a serious condition characterized by high blood pressure, swollen extremities (edema), and protein in the urine—are all associated with this condition. Hydatidiform mole can be diagnosed with ultrasound or by a laboratory test evaluating the pathology of the tissue obtained at biopsy. After a thorough preoperative evaluation, including blood tests, thyroid tests, chest X ray, electrocardiogram, urinalysis, and blood type, the physician removes the molar placental tissue by suction curettage, which uses a plastic tube attached to a vacuum pump to empty the uterus. Approximately 20% of patients with a hydatidiform mole will develop the malignant changes of choriocarcinoma, which also can develop from a normal pregnancy. All women who have been treated for a molar pregnancy need to have a series of weekly pregnancy tests that evaluate the level of the pregnancy hormone beta-HCG until three sequential negative results are obtained; for the following year, the beta-HCG level should be evaluated every 3 months. It is important for these women to use contraception and avoid pregnancy during this period because if the beta-HCG level rises, it either indicates the persistence of the disease or another pregnancy, two conditions that are treated quite differently. Serial beta-HCG levels and transvaginal sonography should determine if a pregnancy is causing the elevated beta-HCG. If there is no pregnancy, the woman should have a D&C to determine the presence of malignant tissue.

Choriocarcinoma.   Once an invasive mole, choriocarcinoma, or collective gestational trophoblastic tumors at the placental site are diagnosed, physicians must evaluate the extent of the disease. This workup includes a thorough physical examination; a chest X ray; a computed tomography (CT) scan of the chest, abdomen, pelvis, and head; blood tests; and tests of antigen/antibody reactions (serology) and of beta-HCG level. These studies allow the physician to determine whether the disease is localized (nonmetastatic) or if it has spread (metastasized). Women with metastatic disease can then be subdivided into low- and high-risk subgroups and can choose from various treatment protocols.

When nonmetastatic disease occurs in a woman who has completed childbearing or does not want to become pregnant, hysterectomy is a therapeutic option. For women with nonmetastatic disease who want to preserve fertility, and in women who have low-risk metastatic disease, the treatment of choice is single-agent chemotherapy. The most common chemotherapeutic agent is methotrexate, but actinomycin D also is used.

For women whose beta-HCG levels remain persistently elevated despite single-agent chemotherapy, and for women with high-risk metastatic disease, the treatment is multiagent chemotherapy, using methotrexate, actinomycin D, and etoposide. Where there is central nervous system involvement, radiation therapy to the entire brain is added.

Serum beta-HCG levels should be monitored serially in all patients treated for gestational trophoblastic disease, more frequently at first, then less frequently as serial levels become negative. Contraception should be used for 1 year after completion of therapy.

Even with metastatic disease, the outlook for this tumor, which was fatal before the development of chemotherapy, is quite good. The cure rate for nonmetastatic disease and low-risk metastatic disease approaches 100%. The cure rate in high-risk cases of metastatic disease is 80% to 90%.

Molecular Biology and Pregnancy

The explosive progress in molecular biology in the past 10 to 20 years has had important implications for many medical specialties, but none more so than obstetrics. The development of advanced techniques has made possible the Human Genome Project, which is attempting to map all the genes in the human body by early in the next century, and has already provided an enormous growth in genetic information. This project has permitted scientists to identify sites in human DNA that account for inherited disorders. The ability to find carriers of significant heritable diseases and to diagnose fetuses who are afflicted with these conditions, sometimes even before the embryo implants on the uterine wall, may allow treatment and/or prevention of such illnesses.

Genetic Screening

Prenatal screening involves noninvasive procedures, such as ultrasonography and tests of maternal serum for certain markers—most commonly alpha-fetoprotein, beta-HCG, and the relatively weak human estrogen, estriol. There also are invasive procedures available for fetal screening. In chorionic villus sampling (CVS), for example, a biopsy of the villi, the short hairlike structures that the placenta grows, provides tissue with the same chromosomal content as the fetus, which can then be used for genetic evaluation. CVS sampling, obtained either through the vagina or abdomen, ideally occurs between 9 and 11 weeks of pregnancy, permitting an early abortion if the fetus is abnormal and the parents so desire. Amniocentesis, however, has to await the 15th or 16th week of pregnancy, until enough amniotic fluid collects in the uterus to permit the procedure. For this test, the physician inserts a thin needle through the abdomen to withdraw a small amount of amniotic fluid, using ultrasound as a guide to avoid injury to the fetus. The third invasive test obtains umbilical cord blood by taking a sample of fetal blood through the maternal abdomen. Such procedures, although generally quite safe, have some risk to the pregnancy. Ideally, it should be possible to evaluate fetal genetic information without invading the uterus. Researchers are seeking a reliable and consistent method of extracting fetal cells from the maternal circulation and using them to evaluate the fetus without any risk.

Prematurity

Despite major improvements in the survival of premature infants, the incidence of preterm labor and premature rupture of the membranes has not decreased. In most cases, the causes of these conditions are unknown. Many factors contribute, however, including subclinical infection, overdistention of the uterus from twins or triplets (multiple gestation) or from excess amniotic fluid, uterine abnormalities, previous cervical surgery, extremes of age, and low socioeconomic status.

A variety of agents have been used to try to arrest preterm labor, including magnesium sulfate, beta-adrenergic agents, calcium channel blockers, and prostaglandin synthetase inhibitors. The efficacy of these agents in prolonging pregnancy beyond 24 to 48 hours is questionable. Because oxytocin provides the major stimulus to the uterine contractions that bring on labor, research is under way to develop oxytocin inhibitors or agents that block its effects.

Probably the most significant contribution in the past decade has been administering corticosteroids to mothers who are at risk for early delivery. Maternal treatment with corticosteroids has been associated with a reduction in newborn mortality, respiratory distress syndrome, and infant cardiac (intraventricular) hemorrhage. The development of surfactant, a drug that is used effectively to treat premature infants with respiratory distress syndrome, has made a major contribution to improved neonatal survival.

Hypertension in Pregnancy

Although the hypertensive diseases of pregnancy, such as preeclampsia and eclampsia, still account for significant maternal and newborn illness and death, these conditions are generally well recognized and treated effectively in women receiving prenatal care. The causes of the eclampsias remain unknown, although some postulate that their development may be caused by immunological, genetic, nutritional, or biochemical mechanisms. We need research that will finally find the factors that contribute to these conditions and ways of altering their negative effects.

Diseases of the Breast

Benign Breast Disease

The breast is basically a milk-producing organ. At the cellular level, lobules that make milk connect to ducts that transport the milk out to the nipples. One-third of the breast is composed of fat, which surrounds the lobules and ducts, whereas the remaining two-thirds is composed of breast tissue. The amount of fat in the breast is what accounts for the wide range of differences in women's breast size, which is largely governed by genes.

The breast contains no muscular tissue, but rather is fixed to the pectoralis major muscle of the chest wall. Breast tissue extends beyond the visible area of the breasts, from the clavicle to the upper abdomen and from the sternum to the armpit (axilla). The axillary lymph nodes drain the lymphatic channels of the breast.

Benign breast conditions include cysts, solid masses, calcifications, fibrocystic breast changes, breast discharge, and mastitis.

Breast cysts.   Breast cysts are fluid-filled sacs that can be palpated. Ultrasound is used to diagnose them. Physicians can drain a cyst in an office. As long as the fluid obtained is clear and the cyst is no longer palpable after drainage, no further treatment or evaluation is necessary.

Fibroadenomas, lipomas, and nipple adenoma.   These conditions refer to solid masses that also can be palpated and confirmed as solid by ultrasound. To distinguish between benign and malignant masses, the physician either does a needle biopsy in the office or an excisional biopsy, usually performed in the ambulatory surgical unit of a hospital, which does not require an overnight stay. If the mass is benign, observation and excisional biopsy are options, depending on the size of the mass, the woman's symptoms, and her decisions regarding treatment.

Calcifications.   Mammography often reveals calcifications, which are microscopic deposits of calcium within the breast tissue and may not always be felt on breast examination. The vast majority of calcifications, about 85%, are benign and occur because of the normal aging of the breast. But some calcifications can be an early sign of breast cancer, and the presence of certain patterns requires further investigation. These include a cluster of calcifications (a group of five or more), a linear pattern of calcifications, or a cluster of calcifications that increase in size on sequential mammograms. Suspicious calcifications require biopsy.

Fibrocystic breast changes.   Fibrocystic breast changes are common and therefore should not be classified as a disease. This condition probably arises from an exaggerated response of normal breast tissue to the hormonal fluctuations of the menstrual cycle. Symptoms include breast tenderness, cystic masses felt in the breast, and, occasionally, a nipple discharge. Often there is a family history of similar symptoms. Physical examination reveals diffuse nodules, which are small cystic areas, in the breast tissue. Although many treatments have been tried, including vitamins, reduced caffeine intake, diuretics, and hormonal manipulations, no therapy has been proven uniformly effective.

Nipple discharge.   The nipples normally discharge fluid during pregnancy and lactation or whenever the breasts are stimulated. Occasionally, however, a discharge can signal a tumor of the pituitary gland, producing a hormone called prolactin, which stimulates lactation. Any evidence of a bloody component to the discharge, especially when the physician palpates a breast mass, raises the suspicion of either a benign intraductal tumor (papilloma) or a malignancy. Evaluation includes a physical examination, a blood test to exclude an elevated prolactin level as the cause of the discharge, and a mammogram to assess the breasts for masses or calcifications. If an elevated prolactin level is the problem, hormonal therapy and an assessment of the pituitary gland are indicated. Any suspicious masses require an excisional biopsy to determine whether they are benign or cancerous.

Mastitis.   Mastitis is an inflammation of the breast most often associated with breast-feeding. It occurs when a breast duct becomes blocked and subsequently infected. Antibiotic therapy usually takes care of the infection, and breast-feeding can continue. Should an abscess occur, surgical drainage is indicated.

Malignant Breast Disease

The commonly quoted risk of developing breast cancer over a woman's life span is one in eight. But this method of computing risk assumes that every woman has an equal chance of developing breast cancer and that every woman will live to be 110 years old. It is therefore misleading. A more realistic assessment is that the chance of developing breast cancer for the average 40-year-old woman is 1 in 1,000 per year, or 0.1%, and for the average 50-year-old woman, the figure doubles to 0.2%.[4] The American Cancer Society estimate of new cases of breast cancer in women for 1996 is 185,700.[5]

The factors that increase a woman's risk of developing breast cancer include a family history of breast cancer in a first-degree relative (mother or sister), a first pregnancy after age 35, the onset of menstruation before age 10, and late menopause. Early diagnosis is vital because oncologists can cure 75% to 80% of women with early-stage disease. The malignant cells that cause breast cancer arise in either the lobules or the ducts. Ninety percent of breast cancer is ductal in origin, whereas approximately 10% arises in the lobules.

Carcinoma in situ.   Carcinoma in situ, frequently diagnosed during the biopsy of a dominant mass, is not breast cancer. There are two forms of carcinoma in situ—lobular and ductal. These two conditions have different implications. Lobular carcinoma in situ is an increase in the number of cells lining the milk-producing lobules of the breast. Because it produces no abnormalities in the breast, this condition is usually discovered as an incidental finding during a biopsy done for another reason. But it does represent an increased risk for breast cancer. Approximately 25% of women with this condition will develop invasive breast cancer in either breast over the next 25 to 30 years. If the biopsy reveals clean margins—that is, that the edges of the incision are free of pathology—a woman can be followed up closely, with twice-yearly examinations and annual mammograms. The alternative treatment—the surgical removal of both breasts (bilateral mastectomy) to prevent cancer from developing in the future—is extremely radical for a precancerous condition.

Ductal carcinoma in situ progresses in stages. Normally a single layer of cells lines the duct walls. Ductal hyperplasia occurs when the cells divide and grow to form more than one layer. In atypical ductal hyperplasia, a step closer to breast cancer, the cells multiply and have an abnormal appearance. Atypical ductal hyperplasia, diagnosed by biopsy, increases a woman's risk of developing breast cancer during her lifetime only slightly. It is when the cells become even more atypical, but remain inside the duct wall, that the lesion is diagnosed as ductal carcinoma in situ, also called intraductal carcinoma. Frequently detected by mammography, ductal carcinoma in situ will progress to an infiltrating carcinoma in as many as 50% of cases if left untreated. The standard therapy for in situ ductal carcinoma has always been a total mastectomy, which removes all breast tissue and has a cure rate of 99%. Because this surgery is quite an extensive treatment for a precancerous lesion, a less aggressive approach, using a wide local excision (partial mastectomy), can be performed. This procedure removes more breast tissue from around the original biopsy site to be certain that all of the ductal carcinoma in situ cells are gone. If the partial mastectomy reveals no additional ductal carcinoma in situ cells, or indicates only a small number of such cells, and the margins of the excision are free of pathology, the subsequent treatment is either close observation or radiation therapy. Radiation therapy involves nearly 2 months of five treatments per week. If the partial mastectomy reveals extensive ductal carcinoma in situ, or if the disease has extended to the margins of the area that has been excised (the resection), the best treatment is total mastectomy. Studies are in progress to determine whether total or partial mastectomy offers better long-term results.

Breast cancer.   When tumor cells have spread beyond the ductal system of the breast, the diagnosis is infiltrating or invasive ductal carcinoma. Invasive lobular carcinoma starts in the lobules but spreads to
adjacent breast tissue. The treatment for either of these malignant conditions, infiltrating ductal carcinoma and infiltrating lobular carcinoma,
is the same.

Invasive carcinoma of the breast has the potential to metastasize to
other sites, most commonly to the lungs, liver, and bones. Before therapy,
the oncologist performs a staging evaluation to be as certain as possible
that metastasis has not occurred. Routine tests include a chest X ray,
blood studies (including carcinoembryonic antigen marker [CEA], which
is sometimes elevated in patients with breast carcinoma), and liver function studies. Although it is uncommon for early-stage breast carcinoma
to involve the bones, physicians often order a bone scan because it can
serve as a baseline for future reference as therapy progresses. A bone
scan involves injecting a small amount of radioactive dye intravenously
and then imaging the skeletal system. There is considerable controversy among practitioners as to whether staging is necessary for early,
small breast carcinomas (less than 2 centimeters in diameter) because
the incidence of metastatic disease is low.

During breast surgery, the surgeon performs an axillary lymph node
dissection. Finding metastatic disease in lymph nodes indicates that there
may be microscopic bits of the tumor elsewhere that were too small to
be detected by the staging studies. However, the presence of lymph node
disease is not entirely accurate, because 30% of women with negative
lymph nodes have microscopic disease elsewhere and 35% of women
with positive nodes do not have distant disease. Another way to determine whether a tumor has spread is the pathological examination of
the tumor cells. Tumor characteristics that indicate a poor prognosis
include tumor cells that invade lymphatic vessels, poorly differentiated
tumor cells, a tumor larger than 5 centimeters in diameter, and tumor
cells that do not carry estrogen receptors.

There is no ideal treatment for breast cancer. Surgical therapy is
aggressive and disfiguring. Despite even the most aggressive therapy,
treatment is often ineffective. Lumpectomy, also called a partial mastectomy, involves removing the tumor and some additional breast tissue from around the original biopsy site to obtain a margin of normal

breast tissue (medically referred to as "negative" margins). Concurrently, through a separate incision at the lower end of the armpit (axilla), the surgeon performs an axillary lymph node dissection. This procedure removes 5 to 15 of the 30 to 40 lymph nodes of the axilla, including any lymph nodes that appear abnormal. Radiation therapy to the breast, for 6 to 7 weeks, five times per week, follows surgery. Each radiation treatment lasts approximately 15 minutes. For the first 5 weeks, the radiation oncologist irradiates the entire breast. During the final 1.5 weeks, a different instrument that can deliver a higher dose of radiation focuses the treatment directly on the tumor area. The main side effect of radiation therapy is profound fatigue. Frequently the skin over the breast becomes reddened, similar to a sunburn.

There are several types of mastectomies. A radical mastectomy removes all the breast tissue including the underlying chest wall muscle, the pectoralis muscle, and all the axillary lymph nodes. This is the most deforming procedure and is rarely used now. A modified radical mastectomy removes the entire breast plus some or all of the axillary lymph nodes, sparing the pectoralis muscle. A simple or total mastectomy removes the entire breast. The appropriate surgical procedure for the treatment of breast cancer is a highly individual decision. For early-stage disease, wide local excision (with negative margins) or a lumpectomy (partial mastectomy), with axillary lymph node dissection followed by radiation therapy, offers equivalent survival with better cosmetic results than the more aggressive surgical options of mastectomy. In some cases of early-stage disease, however, breast conserving surgery may not be the best option. Many factors need to be considered, including the patient's desires, the size of the tumor compared with the size of the breast, the ability to obtain a good cosmetic result from conservative surgery, the histological cell type, and the ability to obtain margins free of tumor. In more advanced stage disease, more aggressive surgical procedures are appropriate.

If microscopic cancer seems to be present elsewhere in the body, chemotherapy may be indicated. The goal of chemotherapy is to eradicate selectively those tumor cells that the surgeon was not able to remove. Most chemotherapeutic agents are associated with toxicity, and therefore, side effects, sometimes severe, are common. Many chemotherapeutic agents are available to treat breast cancer. They are often used together. One common combination, particularly for premenopausal women, includes Cytoxan (cyclophosphamide), methotrexate, and 5-FU, known as CMF. Methotrexate and 5-FU are administered intravenously, but Cytoxan can be taken either orally or intravenously. The treatment extends over a 6-month period in 3-week cycles. Side effects are common and include nausea, vomiting, fatigue, and temporary hair loss. Another combination of agents uses Cytoxan, Adriamycin (doxorubicin hydrochloride), and 5-FU. Again, Cytoxan is taken orally, whereas Adriamycin and 5-FU are administered intravenously. This group of agents is more potent and therefore often has more toxic side effects. Hair loss, which is usually temporary, always occurs. Nausea and vomiting are common. In addition, Adriamycin can sometimes damage the heart muscle. The efficacy of chemotherapy is measured in disease-free survival. Studies have indicated that premenopausal patients with positive lymph nodes have improved survival with the administration of chemotherapy.

The most appropriate therapy for patients with "node negative" breast cancer is somewhat controversial. The majority of these women are cured by mastectomy or lumpectomy and radiation and would not benefit from chemotherapy. However, the inspection of lymph nodes is not a perfect predictor of whether a cancer has spread. The potential benefit of chemotherapy must be weighed against the risks of chemotherapy. Several factors have been identified that allow division of patients with node negative breast cancer into a high-risk and a low-risk group. These factors include the size of the tumor, the pathological appearance of the cells, the chromosomal composition of the tumor cells, and the estrogen receptor status. Chemotherapy is most likely to benefit high-risk patients.

Recently, high-dose chemotherapy regimens have been developed. Because they are highly toxic, patients often require treatment to enhance their bone marrow function. This treatment is usually used in women with metastatic breast cancer. The long-term outcome in patients treated with such aggressive therapy is under investigation.

An alternative breast cancer therapy involves hormonal treatment with an estrogen antagonist, or blocker, called tamoxifen. This drug binds to estrogen receptor sites on the malignant cells and arrests the division of these cells. The pathologist determines the status of the patient's estrogen receptors during the original biopsy. Tamoxifen is most often used in postmenopausal women who have tumors with estrogen receptor positive cells and positive lymph nodes. Studies have shown that, in this subset of patients, tamoxifen improves survival. But how long a woman should take tamoxifen is another controversial issue. Most oncologists think it should be used for the rest of the patient's life. The side effects of tamoxifen include occasional hot flashes and intermittent uterine bleeding. The recently postulated links between the long-term use of tamoxifen and endometrial hyperplasia and carcinoma are worrisome. However, specialists generally believe that patients who will clearly benefit from tamoxifen therapy because of a history of breast cancer should take this medication, but such women need to be followed up closely with periodic biopsies to evaluate the endometrium for any evidence of endometrial bleeding. Some evidence indicates that tamoxifen may prevent the development of breast cancer in high-risk patients or prevent a second tumor in a woman whose previous tumor has been removed. Investigators are conducting trials to determine the effectiveness of tamoxifen for this purpose and to establish guidelines for its future use.

Breast Reconstruction

An important consideration in treating breast cancer, and one that should be planned during the initial stages of treatment, is reconstructive surgery. A plastic surgeon should evaluate the patient before extensive breast surgery. There are two major types of reconstructive surgery: implants and rotational flaps involving the patient's own nearby muscle, fat, and skin. Silicone implants consist of a plastic sac filled with liquid silicone and have been used for several decades either for reconstructive surgery or for cosmetic reasons to augment the size of the breast. They became highly controversial in 1991, when possible serious side effects were reported. These side effects included infection, pain, fibrosis of the surrounding breast tissue, false mammography results, silicone leakage, and autoimmune disorders. Initially many members of the medical community doubted the possibility of an immune reaction to silicone. But in August 1992, the *Lancet*, a prestigious British medical journal, reported on two children who had produced antibodies against silicone after experiencing severe reactions to implanted silicone-coated tubes, giving credence to the possibility of such reactions. As a result, the U.S. Food and Drug Administration (FDA) has halted the use of silicone implants for cosmetic reasons. The use of silicone implants is permitted in cases of reconstructive surgery in controlled clinical trials. The safety and effectiveness of saline-filled implants are also under investigation.

The psychological value of breast reconstruction must be weighed against the possible harm of silicone breast implants. The benefits of breast reconstruction include helping a woman's sense of self, restoring a sense of balance (particularly when only one breast has been removed), and avoiding the use of a prosthesis. Even under the best of circumstances, a reconstructed breast does not always look or feel like a normal breast.

Silicone implants are placed under the pectoralis major muscle that covers the chest wall, allowing the muscle and overlying skin to expand over the implant and form a breast mound. When the muscle and skin cannot accommodate the implant, the surgeon places a tissue expander (a plastic sac containing a small amount of saline solution) beneath the pectoralis major muscle. The surgeon then injects additional saline solution through a valve placed under the skin over a period of 2 to 3 months. This office procedure slowly expands the overlying skin and muscle. During a later operation, the surgeon replaces the valved saline-filled sac with a silicone implant. Another type of reconstruction involves the surgical creation of rotational muscle flaps. The two commonly used muscles are the rectus abdominis muscle of the abdominal wall and the latissimus dorsi muscle of the back. In this procedure, the surgeon dissects the muscle and overlying skin from the underlying tissue while keeping the blood vessels that supply the muscle intact. A tunnel is created under the skin into the area of the mastectomy. This allows the muscle and attached skin with their native blood supply to be rotated into position, creating a breast mound. Using skin from the inner thigh, the surgeon also can create a nipple-areola complex.

This procedure can be performed at the time of mastectomy, or later. The advantage of immediate reconstruction is that only one surgery, hospitalization, and administration of anesthesia are necessary. The disadvantage is that the operation takes longer and requires a more extended hospital stay. In addition, moving muscle from one part of the body to the mastectomy site creates a scar where the muscle was removed and causes a loss of function in the donor muscle. Because the rectus abdominis muscle helps to support the abdominal wall, its removal may increase the risk of hernia formation. Removal of the latissimus dorsi muscle may affect shoulder motion.

Although there is a great deal of breast cancer research, we still need research to find

- More effective educational programs that encourage women to use self-examination and routine screening
- Less aggressive surgical procedures
- The most appropriate adjuvant (assisting) treatment for each patient (e.g., chemotherapy, radiation therapy, immunotherapy)
- More information on hormonal therapy and the interaction of hormone replacement therapy and the development or recurrence of breast cancer
- Improved reconstructive methods that have fewer negative side effects and better cosmetic results

Systemic Sexually Transmitted Diseases

Three important STDs affecting both genders are hepatitis, syphilis, and human immunodeficiency virus (HIV). But they have a particular impact on women during pregnancy because each can be transmitted to the fetus during a vaginal delivery. Although these diseases do not remain localized in the female reproductive tract, they do gain access through moist mucous membranes and then spread to become significant and sometimes life-threatening systemic illnesses.

Viral Hepatitis

Viral hepatitis B is the most common sexually transmitted form of hepatitis. In about 90% of patients with hepatitis B, symptoms are ultimately resolved and patients develop a protective immunity against the virus. But those who do not acquire immunity become chronic carriers of hepatitis B; they are at risk for chronic liver disease, which can ultimately lead to liver failure. Hepatitis D frequent accompanies hepatitis B and, when present, increases the risk of chronic hepatitis and liver failure. Hepatitis C, also called non-A, non-B hepatitis, is the third form of sexually transmitted hepatitis and the one in which chronic liver disease occurs in up to 50% of patients.

These viral hepatitis infections are especially dangerous for women because of the risk of transmitting the disease to the fetus. The degree of risk depends on a number of factors—the timing of the infection, the immunological status of the pregnant woman, and the subtype of the virus. All women at risk for STDs and all women who have a diagnosed STD should be screened for hepatitis. Vaccination against hepatitis B is available and has become standard for all infants and toddlers. Hepatitis B immunoglobulin is routinely given to infants of infected mothers. As yet there is no vaccination against hepatitis C or D. Research should focus on developing ways to eradicate the chronic carrier state of these hepatitis infections and to develop a vaccine against hepatitis C and D.

Herpes Simplex Vulvovaginitis

Herpes is a serious venereal disease affecting an estimated 30 million people in the United States, with 500,000 new cases every year. An incurable, painful, and costly condition, the particular problem for women is pregnancy related. Women who experience an initial outbreak (primary infection) during labor run the risk of infecting vaginally delivered infants; in fact, a recurrent outbreak (secondary infection) in a woman who knows she has herpes at the time of labor is an indication for a cesarean delivery. Although the risk to the infant is not clearly established, reports of central nervous system infection and blindness are common. Research directed at finding an agent that would confer lifetime immunity to this virus is ongoing.

The typical small blisters of herpes appear 3 to 14 days after intercourse with someone who has the disease and rapidly lose their tops, becoming painful, especially when irritated by urine. Voiding may be so excruciating that a woman cannot pass urine except in a tub of warm water. Ulcers, areas where the top layer of skin has been lost, most often follow the tiny blisters. Severity varies among women, with some only having one or a few sores, some having many, and some remaining asymptomatic. The virus is most prevalent and infectious during an outbreak of the open ulcers. Therefore, men and women should avoid intercourse and oral sex during this time.

Although an experienced health care provider can make an accurate diagnosis by examining the genital lesions, definitive diagnosis requires a viral culture of the suspicious lesion. Antibodies in the blood indicate contact with the virus but do not reveal when this may have occurred. Because the virus has been cultured in vaginal secretions when no lesions are present, health care providers recommend that all individuals who have ever had herpes and their partners use condoms for life, unless a couple is trying to conceive a child. If there are infected areas in the vagina or on the cervix, there may be a profuse vaginal discharge. The vulva may swell, and there may be fever as well as tender and enlarged lymph nodes in the abdomen.

The initial infection lasts about 10 to 12 days. The lesions gradually clear and the virus particles travel up the nerve fibers to hibernate in nerve cells near the spinal cord. Whenever the person's immunity to infection is low, the virus migrates back down the nerve fiber to the site of the previous infection, precipitating a similar but shorter outbreak. Herpes type II virus is most often the culprit in genital herpes. Herpes types I and II are closely related, but it is the type I virus that causes the common fever blisters. Both viruses can grow either in the mouth or in the genital area, but the type II virus usually causes more general symptoms, such as fever, aching, and swollen lymph nodes. Infection with type I virus seems to make subsequent infection with type II less severe. Although the herpes virus predisposes to cancer in animals, and women with herpes have a higher than average risk of precancerous conditions and cervical cancer, it is still less likely to cause such problems than is the wart virus.

Oral acyclovir, a relatively nontoxic antiviral agent, is the treatment of choice to mitigate symptoms and shorten attacks. Early treatment is the most effective. Acyclovir cream is not as effective as the pills. But, despite this symptomatic therapy, this virus persists throughout an infected patient's lifetime, as does the risk of recurrent infection. If recurrences are a major problem, acyclovir capsules taken three times a day will usually reduce the frequency and severity of infections. The drug has now been used in this way for up to 3 years without severe side effects. But acyclovir is expensive, costing $50 to $100 per month for preventive care. Recurrences are likely to appear at times of physical stress, such as after riding a bicycle, or with emotional stress or when a woman has another illness. Some women have recurrences each month just before their periods. Each woman must depend on her own immune system to keep the infection in check.

Needed Research on Herpes

We urgently need research on prevention, not only on better methods of prevention, but also on how to educate women and men about the necessity of using barrier methods of contraception to avoid spreading the disease. Obviously we need research to find a cure. Meanwhile, a less expensive drug to treat this condition would be helpful in reducing the cost to individuals and the entire medical system.

Syphilis

Unlike hepatitis, syphilis is a sexually transmitted disease with an effective treatment. The spirochete *Treponema pallidum* causes syphilis. The initial symptom is a painless ulcer involving the moist mucous membranes of the genital tract. Several weeks or months later, as the infection spreads through the bloodstream, secondary syphilis evolves, causing a rash on the palms of the hands and soles of the feet. The lymph nodes swell, and a genital wart (condylomata lata) appears. The infection then becomes latent, a phase that can last for many years, before it develops into tertiary syphilis, which causes lesions of the cardiovascular, central nervous, and musculoskeletal systems. The risk of transmitting syphilis to a fetus depends on the stage of disease, with the earlier infection phase with its higher spirochete load carrying a greater risk of transmission. Congenital syphilitic infection is associated with fetal malformations involving the long bones, nose, teeth, liver, and spleen. Other complications include preterm delivery and stillbirth. Over the past several years, an alarming rise in the incidence of syphilis among women and in the incidence of congenital syphilis has been documented.

Health care providers diagnose syphilis by examining the serous discharge of a primary lesion under a dark-field microscope or, more commonly, through serological tests. Under some circumstances, examining a sample of cerebrospinal fluid is necessary to assess the involvement of the central nervous system. The mainstay of therapy is injected penicillin, with the dose and duration based on the stage of disease. Treatment of syphilis is successful but requires aggressive screening programs to identify women who have contracted the disease and have few or no symptoms. All pregnant women are routinely screened for syphilis. Concomitant infection with other STDs, most notably HIV, is common. Syphilis complicated by HIV infection often progresses rapidly to the later stages of the disease. Research efforts should be aimed at finding the best means of prevention of this age-old condition.

Acquired Immunodeficiency Syndrome

Acquired immunodeficiency syndrome (AIDS), caused by HIV, is the bleakest of all STDs because there is no effective cure or vaccine, and treatment, until recently, has been largely palliative. Currently, AIDS researchers have devised a combined drug therapy that appears to be promising in terms of slowing disease progression. Over the past several years—as a result of a relative increase in the heterosexual transmission of HIV and the ability to transmit HIV from mother to newborn (vertical transmission)—there has been a gradual rise in the percentage of HIV-infected women and children. The good news is that, when an HIV/AIDS-infected woman receives zidovudine (AZT) during her pregnancy, the rate of infection of the fetus is reported to be as low as 12% if AZT is given during labor and the early months of the infant's life. In untreated patients, vertical transmission from mother to infant is thought to be somewhere between 20% and 50%.

AIDS is spread through intimate contact with bodily secretions, by exposure to blood products, or by an infected woman to her infant during labor and birth. Once infection has occurred, the retrovirus selectively invades a variety of cells that possess a certain receptor (CD4). Many cells of the immune system carry this receptor. When these cells become infected, their ability to function is greatly diminished or absent, leading to the clinical manifestations of disease. The length of time from the original infection to clinical symptoms varies markedly. As this disease becomes active, evidence of immune system dysfunction occurs. Ultimately, the AIDS patient is stricken with opportunistic infections, characteristic malignancies, weight loss and diarrhea, and central nervous system dysfunction.

A blood test that identifies the antibody against HIV confirms the diagnosis even before any symptoms occur. A number of pharmaceutical agents can help to prevent or treat the various opportunistic infections and malignancies. Several drugs (zidovudine and dideoxyinosine) are somewhat effective in delaying the progression from latent to active infection. As mentioned earlier, zidovudine has been used in pregnancy and during the early months of life to lessen perinatal transmission.

AIDS has reached epidemic proportions worldwide, with millions already infected with HIV. The current research effort is aimed at developing a vaccine to confer immunity to this virus, finding new medications to alter the course of the infection, and creating effective preventive education programs.

Infertility

A couple is considered infertile if they have failed to conceive after 1 year of unprotected intercourse. Because fertility declines with age, the definition now includes women who do not conceive within 6 months of unprotected intercourse if they are older than 35. In the past several years, the number of patients who have sought infertility treatments has increased for several reasons. One is the large number of women (the so-called baby boomers) who have waited until their mid-to-late reproductive years to start their families. Another is the increased incidence of STDs, which have contributed to infertility from blocked fallopian tubes. Forty percent of the causes of infertility can be attributed to problems in the female, another 40% to the male, and 20% to a combination of the two. All infertility workups should start with the couple and proceed from the least invasive approach to more invasive components of the evaluation.

Causes of male factor infertility include hormonal abnormalities, testicular abnormalities, and obstruction to the flow of sperm. Female infertility can be caused by ovulatory disturbances, impediments in the tubes or in the lining of the abdominopelvic walls (peritoneum), or uterine and cervical factors.

An infertility workup can be quite extensive, expensive, and stressful. It starts with an initial assessment that includes a comprehensive history and physical examination of both partners. Typical studies on the woman include blood tests for circulating levels of estradiol, FSH, and LH; basal body temperature charts; tests that indicate blood hormone levels; a biopsy of the endometrium to ascertain evidence of ovulation in the female; examination of the uterus to discover any uterine cavity abnormalities; and examination of the fallopian tubes to discover whether they are open, using an X-ray dye study called a hysterosalpingogram. Male capability is ascertained through semen analysis and evaluation of the quality of sperm motion in the presence of cervical mucus during ovulation.

Treatment for infertility depends on the cause of the problem and may therefore be different for each couple. Therapy may include manipulating hormones in either partner or procedures aimed at bypassing or alleviating the contributing causes. These procedures include

- Reversing a vasectomy (tying off the vas deferens) or tubal ligation (tying off the fallopian tubes)
- Sperm washing and separation
- Ovulation induction using oral or injectable medications
- Inseminating the woman with sperm injected into the uterus
- In vitro fertilization (IVF), fertilization that occurs outside the body in a test tube or Petri dish, followed by the transfer of the embryo back to the uterus (transcervical embryo transfer)
- Gamete intrafallopian transfer (GIFT) using laparoscopy, a high-tech procedure that transfers the gametes (egg and sperm) directly to the fallopian tubes
- Zygote intrafallopian transfer (ZIFT), another high-tech method of transferring the fertilized ovum to the fallopian tubes before it divides
- Intracytoplasmic sperm injection (ICSI), the newest technique, which involves injecting a single sperm directly into the protoplasm of the cell that surrounds the nucleus of the egg; this approach has revolutionized the treatment of male factor infertility and has a high success rate.

The success of infertility treatments depends on many factors, including the ages of the couple and the cause(s) of the problem.

One major advance of genetic screening is that specialists are now able to diagnose genetic abnormalities in embryos before implantation.

This is particularly important for men and women who are known carriers of a genetic disease because it allows the parents to choose an unaffected embryo for embryo transfer and avoid having a baby with abnormal chromosomes that cause serious illnesses.

There are vast unknown areas regarding infertility. Research should concentrate on factors that contribute to subfertility and infertility, as well as changes in current treatment methods to improve success rates. Better medical management, less invasive surgical therapy, and more successful fertilization techniques are needed to spare couples the currently invasive surgical therapies, the lengthy and costly treatment regimens, and the anxiety and emotional upheaval inherent in this problem.

Endnotes

[1] American Cancer Society: *Cancer Facts & Figures—1996.* Atlanta, GA, American Cancer Society, 1996
[2] Ibid.
[3] Ibid.
[4] Love S: *Dr. Susan Love's Breast Book.* Reading, MA, Addison Wesley, 1990
[5] American Cancer Society, op. cit.

6

Diseases That Are More Prevalent in Women

Ruth Anne Queenan, M.D.
Lynne Beauregard

Separate from the gynecological and obstetrical conditions that affect women exclusively, there are the many medical conditions and diseases that are more prevalent among women. Oddly, although a number of these conditions have an autoimmune component, there is as yet no unifying theory that explains this phenomenon. In addition, there are the diseases that are influenced by female hormones and therefore affect women disproportionately. The following discussion is not meant to be exhaustive, but rather attempts to identify some of the common diseases more prevalent in women and to highlight areas of needed research that would improve the health of large numbers of women.

Bone, Joint, and Rheumatic Diseases

Osteoporosis

Osteoporosis is a condition that weakens the body's skeleton because of a loss of bone density, causing fractures from even the slightest injuries.

The most common fracture sites are the hip, wrist, and spine. Crush fractures of the spine can produce loss of height and deformation of the upper back. Authorities estimate that 15 to 20 million people in the United States have this condition, the majority of them older women. Osteoporosis is responsible for more than 1.3 million fractures annually, causing pain, deformity, and loss of independence and adding $7 to $10 billion to annual medical costs in the United States. Because the population in the United States is aging, this expense will double over the next 30 years—unless there is a program of prevention and treatment.

Some of the causes of bone loss are clear from a consideration of the structure of bone at the cellular level. Trabecular bone is concentrated in the spinal column and within the ends of long bones. This is the main site of osteoporotic fractures. Cortical bone is the compact bone of the bone shaft that surrounds the bone marrow cavity. Women lose approximately 50% of their trabecular bone and 30% of their cortical bone over their life span, whereas men lose only 30% and 20%, respectively. The majority of bone loss occurs around the time of menopause, when there is a dramatic fall in the level of estrogen, a hormone that supports bone structure. Osteoporosis is therefore eight times more prevalent in women than in men; in fact, 25% of all women develop osteoporosis during their later years.

Bone is living tissue that constantly rebuilds or remodels itself. Remodeling takes place in bone-remodeling units where, at the start of each remodeling cycle, osteoclasts replace the cells that line bone. Each osteoclast is a miniature excavating machine that creates a hollow on the surface of trabecular bone or a cavity inside cortical bone. Osteoblasts gradually refill these spaces, replacing the osteoclasts. The rate of bone turnover depends on 1) the number of remodeling units active in the skeleton (normally about 1 million) and 2) the remodeling balance, that is, the relative amounts of bone lost and formed at each unit.

Bone loss occurs when osteoclasts excavate an excessively deep cavity, when osteoblasts fail to refill a normal cavity, or when both processes occur concurrently. People with osteoporosis experience both these abnormalities. Increased osteoclastic activity, occurring during the immediate postmenopausal period, is more damaging structurally than is decreased osteoblastic activity. This is because excessive osteoclastic activity may destroy the entire trabecular system that normally supports the bone structure of the vertebrae, thereby impairing the bone's ability to rebuild itself. Decreased osteoblastic activity, however, merely thins the trabeculae without destroying it.

Women who are fair, slender, small, and of northern European or Asian background are at greater risk for osteoporosis. A family history of a first-degree relative (mother or sister) with the disease also increases risk. A high-protein diet may be a factor because it raises the amount of calcium excreted in the urine. Two additional risk factors are insufficient calcium consumption, particularly before age 25 when the body is most efficient at absorbing this mineral, and lack of exposure to the sunlight the body needs to get enough vitamin D, which it uses for calcium metabolism. Medications that increase the chance of developing osteoporosis include antacids containing aluminum, thyroid pills, corticosteroids, phenytoin, and heparin. Other abnormal conditions elevate risk; they include the absence of menstrual periods (amenorrhea), premature menopause, anorexia nervosa (a disease that causes extreme weight loss), genetically abnormal sex chromosomes, diabetes mellitus, some types of kidney disease, increased activity of the parathyroid glands (hyperparathyroidism), and excessive thyroid gland action (hyperthyroidism). Too much alcohol consumption, smoking, and the lack of physical activity also increase the risk of developing osteoporosis.

Treatment

The treatment of osteopenia, a thinning of the bones that precedes osteoporosis, centers on two methods: augmenting bone formation with increased calcium intake and weight-bearing exercise during and after menopause, and decreasing bone loss (resorption) with hormone replacement therapy (HRT) at and after menopause. The best prevention of osteopenia and osteoporosis, however, is a sufficient calcium intake and plenty of weight-bearing exercise throughout life, particularly during adolescence.

Physicians use the same methods to treat osteoporosis but may also add certain drugs that improve bone mass. Currently, there are two types of these drugs—those that decrease bone loss, called antiresorptive agents, or those that increase bone formation. The former include estrogen, calcitonin, and calcium. The drugs that increase bone mass—

the biphosphonates—do so by boosting both the activation rate of new bone remodeling units and the action of individual osteoblasts. Most agents that increase bone formation are still experimental, but in 1995 the U.S. Food and Drug Administration approved the use of alendronate sodium after studies involving 2,000 women showed that the drug, to be marketed under the name Fosamax, not only stops bone loss but also restores some of the bone mass lost to the disease.[1]

Estrogen.   At menopause, more bone loss than bone formation exists. In fact, one-third to one-half of all bone loss in women is probably caused by menopause. Most of this loss occurs in the first 3 to 6 years after menopause, but bone loss related to decreased levels of estrogen may continue for 20 years. Prolonged absence of menstruation, as is usually seen in athletes and those with eating disorders, causes bone loss in younger women and requires medical attention.

Estrogen replacement therapy (ERT) prevents the early phase of bone loss if started soon after menopause and decreases the incidence of osteoporotic fracture by 50%. ERT also is effective in women who already have osteoporosis because it increases the mean vertebral bone mass by more than 5% and cuts the rate of vertebral fracture in half. The negative side effects of estrogen therapy include an increase in the rate of endometrial cancer, which can be eliminated by adding progestin to the ERT regimen. It is not clear if ERT increases the risk of breast cancer. Most studies show that the risk may escalate after 15 years of therapy. However, the most recently reported study found a substantially increased risk of breast cancer among women who used HRT for 5 years compared with women who never used HRT. Researchers at Harvard Medical School studied 122,000 nurses from 1978 to 1992 and found a 30% higher risk among women who used estrogen alone and a 40% increased risk among women who used a combination of estrogen and progestin. Among women between ages 60 and 64 years, who normally have a higher rate of breast cancer, the elevated chance of getting breast cancer was 70%.[2] A definitive answer to the relationship between HRT and breast cancer incidence may emerge from a large, long-term study of 140,000 women that is part of the Women's Health Initiative (WHI), but results will not be available for 10 years. WHI also is evaluating one positive side effect of HRT—a possible 50% reduction in the risk of heart disease with long-term therapy.

Calcium. The typical American diet is low in calcium and has been implicated in the increasing incidence of osteoporosis in the United States because, if the amount of absorbed calcium is not enough to make up for calcium lost in urine and feces, bone loss occurs. The ideal amount of calcium required to maintain bone mass and whether diets should be supplemented with calcium are controversial topics. The peak amount of an individual's bone mass is largely controlled by genetic factors, but there is some evidence that increased consumption of calcium can enhance it. One study of identical twins done at the Indiana University School of Medicine showed as much as a 5% increase in bone density in the twin given twice the recommended dietary allowance (RDA) of calcium, but only before puberty; no effect was seen in older children.[3] Another study of adolescent girls found that increasing daily calcium intake from 80% of the RDA to 110% through supplementation with calcium citrate malate resulted in significant increases in total body and spinal bone density, amounting to a gain of 1.3% of skeletal mass per year during the adolescent growth spurt.[4] Even among normal postmenopausal women, calcium supplementation of 1,000 milligrams daily significantly slowed bone loss throughout the skeleton.[5] Dr. Robert Heaney, commenting on a review of 43 studies published since 1988, said 26 of them reported that calcium intake was associated in some way with bone loss or fracture, yet 16 did not. However, in 19 of the 43 studies, the investigators controlled the amount of calcium intake, and 16 of those 19 showed that calcium slowed or stopped bone loss. In an accompanying editorial in the *New England Journal of Medicine*, Dr. Heaney concluded that there is now enough evidence to recommend supplementing the diets of postmenopausal women with 1,000 to 1,500 milligrams of calcium and 400 to 800 international units of vitamin D daily.[6]

Calcitonin. Calcitonin, a peptide hormone, has few side effects but must be administered by injection and is prohibitively expensive for preventive purposes. It is currently being tested in clinical trials in the United States.

Calcitriol. Calcitriol, a metabolite of vitamin D, acts to increase calcium absorption, which lessens after age 35. It also may stimulate osteoblast function. Calcitriol therapy improves calcium balance and decreases the rate of vertebral fracture, and some studies show that it increases bone mass temporarily. However, the spread among the low doses that are effective and those that produce too much calcium in the blood (hypercalcemia) and in the urine (hypercalciuria) is small, making it easy to overdose. Agents that function like calcitriol (calcitriol analogues) with greater margins of safety have been developed and are scheduled to be tested soon in clinical trials.

Biphosphonates.   Biphosphonates inhibit bone loss but may cause gastrointestinal irritation. One that has been studied, etidronate, prevents bone loss but also impairs the mineralization of newly manufactured bone and thus cannot be taken continuously. Studies of an intermittent regimen of 2 weeks of etidronate followed by 11 to 13 weeks of calcium supplementation led to an increase of about 2.5% per year in spinal bone mass and may have decreased the number of fractures during the first 2 years of treatment. Other biphosphonates are currently being tested. This class of drugs is potentially a low-cost, orally administered alternative to estrogen and calcitonin for treating osteoporosis.

Questions surrounding this disease remain unanswered; thus, there are many options for future research. Studies should focus on the development of a genetic test that predicts who is at risk, as well as drugs that rebuild bone mass with fewer side effects. More studies of increased calcium intake in children (particularly girls) are needed to determine whether that improves bone density and whether the improvement is sustained through adulthood and to answer the question of whether the calcium RDA should be raised. Additional research also should investigate whether routine screening of perimenopausal women with noninvasive bone density studies is effective in identifying women at risk and is affordable financially for large numbers of women because these tests cost more than $100 per study. Further studies should examine the role of weight-bearing exercise in preventing and treating osteoporosis, whereas others should explore why African American women do not commonly develop osteoporosis.

Arthritis

Arthritis is a condition that results from chronic joint inflammation. There are many forms of arthritis that, according to estimates of the

Arthritis Foundation, affect 20 million persons in the United States, the majority of whom are women. Symptoms include pain, stiffness, tenderness, swelling, and soreness of the joints; tingling in the toes and fingers; and unexplained fatigue and weakness. In some forms of arthritis, many organ systems are involved with the disease process.

Osteoarthritis

Osteoarthritis, also called degenerative joint disease, is the most common form of arthritis, affecting an estimated 16 million people. It worsens with age but rarely causes serious disability. Characterized by mild aches and stiffness in overused joints that have experienced the most stress—especially the stress of bearing the body's weight—it particularly occurs in the spine, hips, knees, toes, and fingers. Several conditions accelerate the development of osteoarthritis: obesity, joint injuries from trauma, and athletic or occupational activity that stresses the affected joints. Typically patients complain of stiffness in the involved joints after use, but these symptoms often improve with rest. Physicians diagnose this condition from the symptoms reported by patients, a physical examination, and the results of X-ray studies.

Collagen is the main building unit of cartilage, which covers and shields the bony articulating surfaces in joints. In 1990, researchers identified a genetic defect that produces an abnormal collagen called type II collagen in members of a family in which many individuals were afflicted with osteoarthritis. Thus, the production of abnormal collagen may play a major role in the development of osteoarthritis. In the family studied, afflicted members had one normal and one abnormal gene for type II collagen, causing the disease. Researchers speculate that many other genetic mutations or defects are probably involved, because thousands of DNA building blocks compose the gene that is responsible for the production of collagen II.

Treatment of osteoarthritis is based on the severity of the symptoms. Local measures such as heat, ice, and physical therapy often improve symptoms. For more significant symptoms, medications such as acetaminophen and nonsteroidal anti-inflammatory agents are used. In patients with relentless symptoms, whose mobility is decreased because a large joint is involved, orthopedic surgeons can replace either the hip or knee joint, whichever is causing the problem.

Rheumatoid Arthritis

Rheumatoid arthritis is an autoimmune disease affecting three times as many women as men, which usually starts between ages 25 and 50. The hallmark of this condition is chronic inflammatory destruction and the subsequent deformity of the affected joints. Patients most often complain of morning stiffness, with symptoms improving as they use the joints during the day. Most commonly impaired are the small joints of the hands, feet, wrists, elbows, and knees. Other organ systems can be involved in this disease, including the lung, heart, eyes, skin, peripheral nervous system, and blood (hematological) system. The progression of this condition is highly individual, with some patients becoming gradually worse and others experiencing symptoms for a limited time followed by remission.

Physicians diagnose rheumatoid arthritis from a patient's history and physical examination. Eighty percent of these patients have an elevated rheumatoid factor, that is, a particular immunoglobulin in their blood. X rays of affected joints reveal characteristic findings that support the diagnosis.

There are many treatments for rheumatoid arthritis, including physical therapy to maintain an adequate range of motion, occupational therapy to preserve the function of the joint involved, and surgery to replace joints that are severely deformed. Many medications are used in treating this disease, but the principle of therapy is to decrease the destructive inflammatory process. Medications that help to do this include aspirin (salicylates), nonsteroidal anti-inflammatory agents, gold, hydroxychloroquine, methotrexate, and corticosteroids. Therapy is usually highly individualized, depending on what works best for each patient.

Systemic Lupus Erythematosus

Systemic lupus erythematosus (SLE) is a chronic disease of unknown cause that is highly variable and affects many organ systems. Five hundred thousand people in the United States have SLE; nine times as many females as males and three times as many African American women as white women have SLE. Most people afflicted with this condition are women of childbearing age.

SLE can cause general systemic symptoms, such as weight loss, fatigue, and general malaise, as well as inflammation of specific organ systems, including the central nervous system, heart, lungs, kidneys, joints, and gastrointestinal system. Often, the skin breaks out in a typical rash. Patients have a low white blood cell count, anemia, and a low platelet count. Their immunological systems show altered complement levels and swollen lymph nodes. High blood pressure (hypertension) frequently develops, and many SLE patients have antibodies to their own organ systems (self-antibodies), the most common being the antinuclear antibody (ANA).

Women with SLE also experience a host of reproductive consequences. They have more spontaneous abortions and a greater incidence of preeclampsia and hypertension in pregnancy. Their fetuses have growth restriction while in utero, and they have more preterm deliveries and stillbirths. Often, it is difficult to distinguish an exacerbation of SLE from worsening preeclampsia, because both processes cause hypertension, kidney disease characterized by protein in the urine, abnormal kidney function, low platelet count, and seizures.

Physicians diagnose SLE if several of the organ systems previously listed are involved and if the patient's clinical course is consistent with the disease. Detecting the ANA alone is not sufficient to make the diagnosis. As in other rheumatic diseases, treatment is highly individualized, based on the severity of the patient's symptoms and the degree of organ system dysfunction. Pharmaceutical agents in use include aspirin and other salicylates, nonsteroidal anti-inflammatory agents, hydroxychloroquine, and immunosuppressive agents (corticosteroids, azathioprine, cyclophosphamide, and chlorambucil).

The outlook for patients with SLE has improved dramatically in recent years because of more sophisticated diagnostic methods that lead to earlier diagnosis of milder disease and more effective and aggressive therapeutic options. In the past, 50% of patients died within 5 years; now more than 90% of SLE patients are alive 10 years after their illness is diagnosed. Despite these improvements, this disease still poses many questions. We still do not know why some women and African Americans are more susceptible. Medical treatment has slowed the disease process but has found neither the cause(s) nor a cure. More research is obviously needed.

Endocrinological Diseases

Diabetes Mellitus

An estimated 10 to 12 million Americans have diabetes, more of them women than men. If the condition is well controlled, individuals can live normal and productive lives for many years. The disease can, however, lead to significant vascular problems resulting in hypertension, poor vision, accelerated heart disease, kidney disease, neurological impairment, and even death. Forty thousand Americans die annually from diabetes itself, and many more succumb to its complications.

Diabetes, one of history's oldest diseases, is a family of disorders caused by a malfunction of the endocrine system, which impairs the metabolism of blood sugar (glucose). Glucose is the body's major fuel, essential to all tissues to survive and function properly. In fact, because the absence of glucose rapidly damages brain cells, it is as necessary to the brain as oxygen. Of the three major nutrients in food, carbohydrates, proteins, and fats, it is carbohydrates—sugars and starches—that are most readily transformed into glucose, providing quick energy for work, for exercise, and to deal with emergencies. The body also turns proteins and fats into glucose for energy that it uses over time, to promote growth and healing and to provide sustenance during times of food shortage or famine. When we consume more calories (fuel) than we need, the body stores the excess, either as glycogen in the liver and muscle cells or as body fat.

The pancreas, a crucial gland located behind the stomach, manufactures hormones that regulate how the body uses its fuel. It contains beta cells, which produce insulin, and alpha cells, which manufacture glucagon. It is the interaction of these two hormones that permits the body to maintain the correct level of sugar in the blood. Insulin—the major hormone that controls the use of glucose at the cellular level—is really the gatekeeper, allowing glucose to enter most of the body's cells to be burned for energy. Glucagon converts the glycogen stored in the liver to glucose and releases it into the bloodstream as needed.

There are many types of diabetes but they all have one thing in common—a defect in the way the body handles insulin, either failing to produce all of it, not producing enough of it, or being unable to use what insulin it does manufacture, a condition known as insulin resistance.

Type I Diabetes Mellitus

Type I diabetes mellitus, or insulin-dependent diabetes mellitus (IDDM), affects an estimated 300,000 to 500,000 people in the United States. In this disease, the beta cells of the pancreas are destroyed and do not produce insulin. Although the exact causes of IDDM are unclear, there is a predisposition to inherit a susceptibility to this disease. IDDM also is, in part, an autoimmune disease, because the body's immune system contributes to the destruction of the beta cells. Scientists have suspected for some time that a virus or toxin may activate the immune system to destroy its own beta cells because IDDM is often diagnosed after a viral infection. However, except for the virus that causes German measles, other environmental or infectious agents have not been identified. Recent research suggests that there may be several triggers that provoke the immune system, and, in fact, one team of scientists has identified a specific beta cell enzyme, glutamic acid decarboxylase (GAD), as a possible stimulus.

IDDM occurs early in life; the mean age at onset is 20 years. These diabetic patients, who are typically slender, require daily injections of insulin and careful attention to diet to maintain an effective balance between insulin and glucose. Physicians diagnose the illness by measuring the glucose level in the blood, which is normally 50 to 115 milligrams per deciliter (mg/dL). Two tests showing a value greater than 140 mg/dL in the fasting state confirm the diagnosis. For patients with borderline readings between 115 and 140 mg/dL, who also exhibit the familiar symptoms of uncontrolled diabetes—excess thirst and urination—physicians usually order provocative diagnostic glucose challenge tests.

Type II Diabetes Mellitus

Type II diabetes mellitus, or non–insulin-dependent diabetes mellitus (NIDDM), typically occurs in middle age. NIDDM is 10 times more common than IDDM, affecting 95% of all diabetic patients, although as many as half of them do not know they have the disease. NIDDM is more prevalent among minority populations: it afflicts twice as many African American women as white women and is two to five times more common among Native American women than women of other ethnic groups. In fact, 68% of Pima Indian women between ages 55 and 64 have NIDDM. Mexican Americans are two to four times more likely to develop NIDDM than are white Americans; in fact, Hispanic Americans generally have three times the risk of developing NIDDM than do non-Hispanic white people.

In NIDDM, the body does not use insulin effectively at the cellular level, hence, the name insulin resistance. Obesity is a primary contributing factor to developing the disease, and most patients are overweight. However, many NIDDM patients can control their blood glucose levels and thus mitigate the negative impact of the illness with weight loss, proper diet, and exercise, although frequently they also need medications that increase the release of insulin from the pancreatic beta cells. When these interventions are not successful, they require insulin therapy.

Subtypes.   There are numerous NIDDM subgroups that include both lean and obese patients. In addition, secondary diabetes is associated with pancreatic disease or exposure to certain drugs or chemicals. The World Health Organization (WHO) identified a version of diabetes common in tropical countries as malnutrition-related diabetes mellitus (MRDM). Finally, there is gestational diabetes, which occurs during pregnancy because of the antagonism of certain placental hormones with insulin but usually resolves after delivery. However, women with gestational diabetes have an increased risk of developing diabetes, usually NIDDM, later in life.

Symptoms.   There are several classic symptoms of NIDDM, including

- Excessive thirst (polydipsia) because the extra circulating blood glucose causes water to shift from the body's cells into the blood
- Frequent urination (polyuria) to get rid of the additional water consumed
- Sugar in the urine (glycosuria) because high blood glucose levels make the kidneys spill glucose into the urine
- Excessive hunger because without insulin the body cannot absorb glucose so that, at the cellular level, the body is actually starving

Patients with IDDM commonly lose weight even if they overeat because, unable to use glucose in the absence of insulin, their bodies turn instead to stored protein and fat for energy. Ketoacidosis, which disturbs the body's normal chemical balance and can cause a life-threatening diabetic coma, occurs when the liver metabolizes substantial quantities of fat and manufactures ketones as a by-product. Whereas the muscles and other body tissues can use some of the ketones for energy, the excess enters the blood and is excreted in the urine. A particular ketone, acetone, produces a typical fruity smell on the breath that is one of the well-recognized signs of diabetic ketoacidosis, or impending diabetic coma, in patients with poorly controlled IDDM. Because of this odor, diabetic ketoacidosis is often confused with drunkenness, which can delay diagnosis.

In patients with NIDDM, overeating has the opposite effect. Because insulin is available, the body eventually uses the consumed calories and can store varying amounts of excess glucose as body fat. This is one reason for the obesity that plagues most patients with NIDDM.

Complications.   Complications of diabetes include hypertension, high blood cholesterol, heart attacks because of clogged coronary arteries, stroke, and circulatory disorders characterized by an inadequate blood supply to the extremities, particularly the legs. This causes chronic ulcers on the arms and legs. In many cases, inadequate circulation can lead to gangrene and require amputation of the afflicted limb. In addition, diabetes affects the nervous system, causing a deterioration in nerve function characterized by numbness or tingling in the fingers and toes, slowed reflexes, and coordination problems. Male diabetic patients often experience sexual impotence. This disease also is the major cause of blindness among American adults because it damages the blood vessels of the retina. Patients with diabetes develop cataracts at a younger age, which progress more rapidly than in the general population. In addition, diabetes is a primary cause of kidney failure and, among African Americans, is the most common cause of the need for dialysis. Finally, this disease makes patients more vulnerable to infection in the urinary tract, respiratory tract, vagina, skin, mouth, and other structures, and the poor circulation that is a hallmark of the condition slows the healing process.

Genetic causes.   NIDDM is much more heritable than IDDM. Among identical twins, NIDDM afflicts both twins 91% of the time, yet IDDM affects both twins only 36% of the time. Although the formal genetics of IDDM are unknown, studies have confirmed an association between IDDM and certain human leukocyte antigens (HLAs). Researchers have identified a specific family of antigens, substances capable of producing antibodies to fight infection, which are much more common among type I diabetic patients than in the normal population. Ninety-six percent of patients with IDDM have one or both of these HLAs, compared with only 50% in the general population. HLA genes are almost always inherited in groups and are unique in each individual. Recently, researchers have found other genetic markers for NIDDM that are similar to the HLAs associated with IDDM.[7]

Genetic researchers at the University of Alberta have been studying a Mennonite extended family that has lived separately from the dominant population, intermarrying among themselves and permitting marriages between first and second cousins, which concentrates the gene pool. They are an ideal population for investigators because they have large families and keep excellent genealogical records. In the six generations of the family, researchers have found 10 individuals with IDDM, 3 with NIDDM, and several family members with other autoimmune diseases, including thyroiditis, arthritis, multiple sclerosis, and blood disorders. In this Mennonite clan, IDDM is accompanied by additional abnormalities of carbohydrate metabolism, including low blood sugar (hypoglycemia), gestational diabetes, and a form of NIDDM that requires insulin administration when individuals reach middle and old age. One exciting aspect of this research is the possibility of preventing IDDM. Researchers are conducting clinical trials to study the effectiveness of certain drugs in interrupting the usual course of IDDM and delaying the onset of the disease in newly diagnosed patients. If such therapy proves practical, crucial to its success will be the ability to identify patients at high risk for developing the disease.[8]

Prevention.   Because obesity can trigger NIDDM in genetically susceptible people, prevention involves avoiding weight gain, weight loss for those who are overweight, and regular exercise. One study of 6,000 men from the University of California at Berkeley found that regular exercise can actually prevent NIDDM. In fact, the risk of developing NIDDM dropped by 6% for every additional 500 calories that were burned each week during exercise. The more rigorous the exercise, the more protection it provided so that jogging, tennis, and swimming were more beneficial than golf. The bottom line was that those who burned 3,500 calories per week exercising cut their chance of developing NIDDM in half. The problem, of course, is that no women were in the study. Therefore, we need similar research on women to quantify the effects of rigorous exercise in females.[9]

One protective factor exclusive to women is breast-feeding, which seems to shield offspring from IDDM. Swedish investigators found that an increase in breast-feeding reduced the annual incidence of IDDM, and these results have been corroborated by studies in Australia and Colorado. Researchers do not know exactly how breast-feeding might protect people from IDDM. Some evidence indicates that cow's milk consumed by infants during the first year of life may play a role in establishing an immune reaction to the infant's pancreatic cells, eventually destroying them and causing diabetes. Human milk, however, has certain antimicrobial properties, which may protect some individuals. In addition, breast milk contains antibodies against the very viruses that can destroy the pancreatic cells that make insulin, and this may be the protective element.[10] If future research confirms the association between breast-feeding and a lower incidence of IDDM, then the next step would be to study patients who were breast-fed but developed diabetes anyway to determine whether a genetic profile exists that makes them highly vulnerable. Meanwhile, because breast-feeding has numerous other advantages and few drawbacks, it would be wise for all mothers, and particularly those from families in which diabetes is prevalent, to nurse their infants.

Investigators are studying the efficacy and practicality of transplanting pancreatic islet cells into patients with IDDM, which cures as many as two-thirds of the patients on whom it has been tried. Research also has developed improved systems for delivery of insulin and better methods to monitor the blood glucose levels of patients with diabetes.

Thyroid Disease

The thyroid gland regulates the body's metabolism—the rate at which the body uses oxygen and nutrients. It does so by producing the hormone thyroxine. An underactive thyroid gland causes cretinism in infants and a deficiency in thyroid activity (hypothyroidism) in adults. Conversely, an overactive thyroid gland produces increased thyroid gland action (hyperthyroidism) in adults. Thyroid disease affects approximately 5% to 10% of women throughout life, and autoimmune thyroid disease is 15 times more common in women than in men.

Hypothyroidism

Hypothyroidism, a condition caused by the underproduction of thyroxine, causes a variety of symptoms, including fatigue, increased sleep requirement, weight gain, intolerance of cold, constipation, dryness and scaling of the skin, hair loss, muscle aches, facial puffiness, swelling of the lower extremities, and depression. Patients with long-standing untreated hypothyroidism are often pale and have a slow resting heart rate and delayed reflexes. Long-standing severe hypothyroidism can lead to psychiatric disease and even "myxedema coma." Hypothyroidism interferes with ovulatory function in women because of a complicated interaction among the thyroid-stimulating hormone (TSH), prolactin, and the ovulation-stimulating hormone in the hypothalamus and pituitary glands. Impaired ovulation causes infertility in some patients, and those who do become pregnant have an increased rate of spontaneous abortion. Because of this ovulatory disturbance, patients, when they menstruate, have either irregular excessive bleeding (menometrorrhagia) or markedly reduced bleeding (oligomenorrhea). Some do not menstruate, a condition known as amenorrhea.

Physicians diagnose hypothyroidism from the signs and symptoms previously discussed. In early hypothyroidism, evidence of disease may be subtle but can be confirmed with a blood test that evaluates thyroid function. It is particularly important that medical caregivers note any symptoms that indicate hypothyroidism because it is so common in women, the early signs and symptoms can easily be missed, and it is successfully remedied with orally administered thyroid replacement hormone. Once treatment starts, physicians use periodic tests of thyroid function to ensure that the patient's metabolic balance is maintained.

Hyperthyroidism

Hyperthyroidism, however, means there is too much thyroid hormone. It has several different causes. In Graves' disease, for example, autoantibodies against receptors for the TSH within the thyroid gland stimulate that gland to release excess thyroid hormone. A toxic nodular goiter causes a release of excess thyroid hormone. Less commonly, a small, benign thyroid hormone–producing tumor may be present within the thyroid gland. In the latter two conditions, thyroid hormone production escapes the normal regulatory mechanisms. There are other extremely rare causes of hyperthyroidism.

Hyperthyroidism increases the body's metabolism. Symptoms include weight loss, sweating, heat intolerance, nervousness, fatigue, weakness, increased frequency of bowel movements, and palpitations. Patients often have an enlarged thyroid gland, an elevated resting heart rate, and a number of eye symptoms—a bulging of the eyes from the sockets (exophthalmos), retracted eyelids, and weakness of the eye muscles. Profound hyperthyroidism can be life threatening and may be associated with irregular heart rates (arrhythmias), congestive heart failure, and difficulty breathing. Symptoms vary, and the ones that predominate depend on the patient's age, how long the disease has been present, and the degree of thyroid hormone excess. Hyperthyroidism also has negative reproductive consequences, including ovulatory disturbances, irregular menstrual periods, infertility, and an increased risk of spontaneous abortion, premature delivery, and fetal growth restriction. Occasionally, transient hyperthyroidism occurs in women after they have delivered a baby. The fetuses of pregnant patients with this condition have a small risk of developing fetal and neonatal hyperthyroidism from antibodies crossing the placenta and stimulating the fetal thyroid. There also is a slight risk they may develop hypothyroidism from the antithyroid drugs the mother takes that cross the placenta and suppress the fetal thyroid. Both of these risks can be minimized by the careful monitoring of pregnant patients with hyperthyroidism.

Physicians diagnose this illness from the patient's symptoms and physical findings. They confirm it by blood tests that evaluate thyroid function and determine the presence of antithyroid antibodies. The medical treatment of hyperthyroidism includes different classes of drugs. Beta-blockers are used to treat the symptoms of high metabolism. Salicylates or nonsteroidal anti-inflammatory drugs are used if an inflammation exists. Antithyroid drugs help to decrease production of the thyroid hormone and to impair the conversion of certain thyroid hormones into more active forms. These specifically targeted drugs restore a normal thyroid state within several months, but the therapy is usually continued for only 1 to 2 years. Once therapy is discontinued, physicians monitor patients closely. Approximately 50% of those receiving antithyroid drugs go into remission. Hyperthyroidism can be cured with radioactive iodine, but the majority of patients so treated will develop hypothyroidism after treatment. It cannot be used during pregnancy. Occasionally, surgery is recommended in cases of large goiters, solitary functioning thyroid nodules, or patients who cannot tolerate medical therapy.

Neurological Diseases

Migraine Headaches

Migraine headaches, another condition occurring more frequently in women than men, are caused by changes in blood vessels that produce symptoms. Initially a narrowing of the arteries (vasoconstriction) occurs, which leads to the typical premonitions or aura of a migraine headache. This is followed by an opening (vasodilation) of the same arteries, which brings on the throbbing pain. These severe headaches generally last less than 24 hours, often produce nausea and vomiting, and get worse for most patients when they are exposed to light or noise. The pain can be located on one or both sides of the head. The premonitory symptoms include fatigue, visual disturbances, neurological symptoms such as weakness or numbness, or problems with speech. For many women, migraine headaches are connected to the menstrual cycle, occurring just before or during the menstrual period. Oral contraceptive pills play a role, typically causing headaches on the days when a woman takes the placebo pills, just before the onset of bleeding. In fact, oral contraceptives are contraindicated for women with recurrent migraine headaches. At menopause, women often have more frequent attacks. In all of these circumstances, authorities think that the migraine headache is associated with falling estrogen levels. In certain patients, hormonal manipulations lessen symptoms. For most women, migraine headaches tend to disappear after menopause.

Patients should avoid medications and foods that have been associated with migraines. The former include nitrates, oral contraceptive pills, and certain blood pressure medications; the latter are chocolate, certain cheeses, and alcohol. Aspirin (salicylates) and acetaminophen are effective treatments for mild headaches, but more severe migraines require alternative medications, including ergotamines, which cause continued vasoconstriction once an attack has started, and narcotic analgesics. Many agents are used to prevent migraines, including beta-blockers, calcium channel blockers, antianxiety agents, antidepressants, anticonvulsants, and serotonin antagonists.

Multiple Sclerosis

Multiple sclerosis (MS) is an autoimmune disease that affects twice as many women as men. MS typically attacks young adults between ages 20 and 40. For unknown reasons, it is more prevalent in less temperate climates, afflicting 1 in 5,000 people in the northern United States but only 1 in 20,000 in the South. MS is a degenerative disorder of the central nervous system characterized by episodes of neurological deficits at a specific focus. The cause is unknown, but there is evidence that something prompts the body's lymphocytes to attack myelin, the fatty substance that surrounds and coats nerves. Theories have proposed various initiators of this autoimmune reaction, among them a virus, an allergy, or a toxin. By destroying the myelin, the transmission of impulses and therefore the function of the affected nerves is significantly impaired. MS attacks different nerves at different times; between episodes there is frequently enough repair of the myelin to allow a complete resolution of symptoms in some patients. Over time, however, after many attacks, most patients do develop permanent deficits. The most common ones involve the optic nerve, causing visual disturbances; the spinal cord, causing weakness; sensory changes; bowel and/or bladder dysfunction; and alterations in the brain, causing emotional and intellectual difficulties.

Despite substantial research efforts, there is no cure for MS. Physicians attempt to relieve symptoms during the acute phase of an attack with corticosteroids and other anti-inflammatory agents. Although these drugs do lessen the severity of symptoms and speed recovery time, they do not change the basic course of the disease. There also are medications designed to counteract the neurological deficits, including antispasmodics, muscle relaxants, and anticonvulsants. Physical therapy sometimes helps to overcome weakness and loss of physical function. Physicians counsel patients to avoid fatigue by getting plenty of rest and to consume a balanced diet. Recently an immune modulator, beta-interferon, has been genetically engineered and, in preliminary studies, has been shown to suppress the immune system, thereby slowing the progress of the disease. Studies of the use of the steroid hormone dehydroepiandrosterone (DHEA) in MS patients found that 64% of the study group experienced alleviation of the fatigue syndrome that accompanies this disease.[11]

Alzheimer's Disease

An estimated 4 million people in the United States have Alzheimer's disease; slightly more women than men have the disease. This condition starts with a loss of intellectual ability (dementia) that interferes with the patient's ability to function and continues over time. Initially patients show signs of impaired memory and emotional disturbance. As the disease progresses, other neurological deficits occur, including language problems, intellectual deficits, personality changes, disturbances in purposeful movement, and gait abnormalities. The brain shrinks as the cerebral ventricles enlarge. The cause of Alzheimer's disease is unknown, but a clear genetic predisposition is involved. Recently, genetic defects that make brain cells disintegrate and die have been reported. These defects occur at a crucial position in the formation of a protein precursor of amyloid, a normal brain protein that is found in the destructive plaques characteristic of Alzheimer's disease. There is no known cure or effective treatment for this illness. Patients almost always require institutionalization and continuous care. Estrogen replacement has recently been shown to have a protective effect, but the mechanism by which it works remains poorly understood.

Psychiatric Diseases

Depression

Because women are twice as likely as men to develop depression, it is a common condition among the patients of gynecologists. Depression may be caused by a number of factors, including a history of physical or sexual abuse, the stress related to single parenting, or the difficulties of combining parenting with a career. There is a strong and well-recognized relationship among infertility, poor pregnancy outcome (pregnancy or neonatal loss), menstrual problems, menopause, and depression. Symptoms of depression are numerous. Patients complain of sleep disturbances, weight variations, changes in appetite, decreased ability to concentrate, irritability, decreased sexual drive, anxiety, tearfulness, and lack of interest in their normal activities. Depression can lead to alcohol or drug abuse, and some depressed patients become suicidal. Patients often stress their physical complaints when talking to a health care provider as they tend to become more prominent in the presence of depression. Major life changes, such as the death of a loved one, divorce, job loss, and the inability to conceive, are frequently associated with depression.

Treatment includes both medication and psychotherapy. When patients have mild symptoms without ideas of suicide, they can be effectively treated and monitored by their primary care provider. More serious episodes of depression with suicidal thoughts, or a failure to respond to initial therapy, should by treated immediately by a mental health care provider. Recently, a small study of the efficacy of acupuncture in treating depression in women found that partial or complete remission of symptoms occurred in 65% to 70% of patients (personal correspondence to B. Jacobson from John J. B. Allen, Ph.D., coprincipal investigator, Department of Psychology, University of Arizona at Tucson, September 27, 1995). (See Chapter 7 for more on depression.)

Eating Disorders

Anorexia nervosa and bulimia are common conditions among middle-class adolescent girls and young women. Anorexia nervosa is characterized by weight loss, behavioral changes, excessive exercise, food aversion, distorted body image, and a profound fear of weight gain. These young women frequently stop having menstrual periods. Approximately 50% of anorectic patients also have bulimia. In bulimia, binge eating is often followed by the use of laxatives and/or diuretics to induce purging. Anorexia nervosa can lead to a number of metabolic derangements, some of which are life threatening. These include disturbances in blood counts and electrolyte levels; alterations in function of the thyroid gland, the hypothalamus, and the adrenal gland; and disturbances in heart rhythm. Bulimic patients who use self-induced vomiting may experience electrolyte imbalance, esophagitis, and poor teeth. Those with hypothalamic dysfunction, which causes low estrogen levels, are at risk for developing osteoporosis. Treatment includes medications, hospitalization, psychotherapy, behavior modification, and nutritional support. Therapy is more effective if the condition is recognized early, before profound metabolic and psychiatric disturbances have been established.

Gastrointestinal Diseases

Gallbladder Disease

The major diseases of the gallbladder include the formation of gallstones (cholelithiasis) or inflammation of the gallbladder caused by infection and associated with gallstones (cholecystitis). These two conditions affect two to three times more women than men.

The liver makes bile, composed of cholesterol, bile acids, and phospholipids, which the body either stores in the gallbladder or excretes into the first part of the small intestine. When the balance of these three components is disturbed, stones can form in the gallbladder. The majority of gallstones are cholesterol stones, which usually remain in the gallbladder without causing symptoms. Approximately 20% of people with gallstones do not know they have them. Cholesterol stones are more likely to form in obese patients, diabetic patients, pregnant women, highly fertile women, and women taking estrogen preparations, such as oral contraceptives or ERT. Estrogens may contribute to gallstone formation by diminishing the flow of blood or other body fluids to the gallbladder. Symptoms of gallstones include heartburn; indigestion; abdominal pain, especially after consuming a fatty meal; nausea; and vomiting. Paroxysms of pain (biliary colic) are caused by the passage of gallstones from the gallbladder along the bile duct. The intermittent obstruction caused by the stones worsens the abdominal pain and causes nausea, vomiting, and, sometimes, fever. If the bile duct remains obstructed, acute inflammation and infection of the gallbladder can develop, with more severe and persistent abdominal pain, fever, nausea, and vomiting. Recurrent bouts of acute cholecystitis may lead to chronic inflammation of the gallbladder. Gallstone disease has several less frequent consequences, among them inflammation of the pancreas when a stone is passed, infection of the entire biliary tree, liver abscess, gangrene of the gallbladder, and an increased risk of developing a malignancy of the gallbladder.

Physicians diagnose gallbladder disease from a patient's history and physical examination in combination with certain laboratory tests. Ultrasonography is useful in visualizing the gallbladder and evaluating it for the presence of stones. A radioisotope study, which can distinguish between a normally functioning gallbladder and an inflamed organ, is useful in establishing the diagnosis of acute cholecystitis. Treatment of gallbladder disease depends on the age of the patient, the size and number of stones, the severity of symptoms, and the presence of infection or inflammation. When symptoms are mild, there is no evidence of infection, and the stones are relatively small, physicians prescribe medications that slowly dissolve the stones. Therapeutic sonography (lithotripsy), which pulverizes gallstones, is a new treatment. Surgery is recommended for patients with large symptomatic gallstones, cholecystitis that is unresponsive to medical therapy, and chronic cholecystitis. It is always preferable to remove the gallbladder when it is not inflamed. Laparoscopy, which is less invasive than open surgery, has become the most common procedure for gallbladder removal.

Irritable Bowel Syndrome

Irritable bowel syndrome (IBS) is the most common functional gastrointestinal disorder seen by health care providers. Two-thirds of all patients with IBS are women. Symptoms include abdominal pain; altered bowel habits, such as diarrhea, constipation, or an alternating combination of both; and no identifiable pathology. Patients often complain of excess gas, heartburn, and abdominal distention. Most patients with IBS also have a psychological disturbance, most commonly depression, anxiety, and cancer phobia. IBS can cause chronic pelvic pain and may be confused with lactose intolerance. A careful history combined with the absence of pathology on physical examination indicate a diagnosis of IBS.

Treatment of IBS needs to be multidimensional. Patients should be reassured that no harmful pathological condition exists. Dietary advice to avoid foods that exacerbate the symptoms is important. Medications that decrease spontaneous movement (motility) and gas production while increasing bulk in the diet or that avoid spasms help certain patients. To be most effective, psychological counseling is an important addition to these treatments.

These gastrointestinal diseases display striking similarities. Many have autoimmunity as their primary cause or as a component in their development. Others occur because of alterations in the hormonal milieu. It is thus not surprising that women are affected more often than men, given the remarkable fluctuations in their hormonal status throughout their reproductive years and the dramatic changes that occur at menopause.

Research is needed to understand the interactions among immunological factors, the use of estrogen and progesterone, and a woman's gynecological and nongynecological organs. As women make the transition from reproductive life to their postmenopausal years, we need to know how estrogen and progesterone deprivation or replacement affects these medical conditions.

Urological Problems

Urinary Tract Infections

Urinary tract infections (UTIs) are much more common in women of all ages than in men and either affect the bladder (cystitis) or the kidney (pyelonephritis). Women get more UTIs because they have a short urethra, the tube running from the bladder to the urinary opening, which is close to the vagina and rectum, allowing easy access of bacteria and other infectious agents from those sites into the female urinary tract. Pregnancy makes matters worse because the high level of progesterone tends to open (dilate) the ureters, the tubes that connect the kidney and bladder, increasing the risk of UTIs. These infections may increase the risk of a preterm delivery.

Symptoms of cystitis include burning on urination, urinary urgency and frequency, and blood in the urine. When the kidney is infected (pyelonephritis), a woman may experience fever, chills, back pain, nausea, and vomiting in addition to the symptoms of cystitis. Urine analysis confirms the diagnosis. Treatment includes

- Increasing liquid intake (hydration) about 8 ounces every hour— particularly cranberry juice, which, according to a recent study published in the *Journal of the American Medical Association*, may reduce the amount of bacteria in the urine[12]
- Avoiding caffeine, acidic foods, spices, citrus fruits, tomatoes, alcohol, and chocolate
- Consuming one teaspoon of baking soda dissolved in one-half cup of water once or twice a day
- Taking antibiotics that kill the bacteria causing the infection

In recent years, antibiotic options have improved, and physicians have used shorter treatment courses involving higher doses of antibiotics, which are effective because patients comply better with short-term therapy.

Incontinence

Another common problem with a tremendous impact on women's health is urinary incontinence, defined as a clinically significant, involuntary loss of urine. Incontinence is caused by the same stresses on the pelvic structures that lead to prolapse, but here the stress mainly affects the bladder. Patients complain of leakage of urine, frequency of urination, and/or inability to empty the bladder entirely.

Physicians diagnose incontinence from the patient's history and symptoms. This is an important point because many women with urinary difficulties are embarrassed by them and do not tell their health care providers about the problem. The diagnosis can be confirmed during an office visit by asking the woman to perform the physical actions (that is, coughing or laughing) that bring on incontinence. More detailed tests, called urodynamic studies, can identify which of the many types of incontinence each particular patient has. Causes of urinary incontinence include pelvic relaxation (an anatomical disturbance), instability of the muscle of the bladder leading to involuntary contraction, and neurological impairment. Noninvasive urodynamic studies evaluate pressures at different sites within the urethra, bladder, and abdomen; measure the capacity of the bladder; observe urinary flow; and assess the distribution of nerves (innervation) to the lower urinary system.

Physicians choose treatments based on the severity and cause of the problem. Women with mild stress urinary incontinence can benefit from nonsurgical approaches. Methods include medications, pelvic floor strengthening exercises (Kegel exercises), and mechanical devices to restore normal pelvic floor anatomy. Surgical intervention is reserved for patients who have significant stress urinary incontinence. Surgeons use either vaginal or abdominal procedures to restore the normal anatomy and improve pressure in the urethra. When incontinence is caused by bladder instability, or irregular unpredictable contractions of the bladder, therapy choices include bladder retraining, which involves voiding on a regular schedule, biofeedback, medications, and, rarely, surgery.

Research is needed on methods to improve obstetrical procedures so that they cause less damage to the pelvic structures. Solid educational programs, particularly during pregnancy, about the value of pelvic floor support (Kegel) exercises after delivery and throughout a woman's life would go a long way to reducing the incidence of UTIs and the other consequences of pelvic stress. Education about the pros and cons of HRT early in menopause would help, as would research to develop better medical and surgical interventions.

Endnotes

[1] Leary WE: "New osteoporosis drug wins FDA approval." *New York Times*, October 3, 1995

[2] Colditz GA, Hankinson SE, Hunter DJ, et al: The use of estrogens and progestins and the risk of breast cancer in postmenopausal women. *New England Journal of Medicine* 332:1590–1593, 1995

[3] Johnston CC, Miller JZ, Slemeda CW, et al: Calcium supplementation and increases in bone mineral density in children. *New England Journal of Medicine* 327:82–87, 1992

[4] Lloyd T, et al: Calcium supplementation and bone mineral density in adolescent girls. *Journal of the American Medical Association* 270:841–844, 1993

[5] Reid IR, Ames RW, Evans MC, et al: Effect of calcium supplementation on bone loss in postmenopausal women. *New England Journal of Medicine* 328:460–464, 1993

[6]Heaney R: Thinking straight about calcium. *New England Journal of Medicine* 328:503–505, 1993

[7]Simopoulos AP, Herbert V, Jacobson B: *Genetic Nutrition: Designing a Diet Based on Your Family Medical History.* New York, Macmillan, 1993

[8]Ibid.

[9]Ibid.

[10]Ibid.

[11]Calabrese VP, Isaacs ER, Regelson W: Dehydroepiandrosterone in multiple sclerosis: positive effects on the fatigue syndrome in a non-randomozed study, in *Dehydroepiandrosterone (DHEA)*. Edited by Regelson W, Kalmi M. Berlin, Germany, Walter de Gruyter, 1990, pp 95–99

[12]Avorn J, Monane M, Gurwitz JH, et al: Reduction of bacteriuria and pyuria after ingestion of cranberry juice. *Journal of the American Medical Association* 271:751–754, 1994

7

Diseases That Manifest Differently in Women and Men

Nancy Fugate Woods, Ph.D., R.N.
Beverly Greenberg Jacobson

A number of diseases exist that affect women and men differently. Most notably, women get cardiovascular disease 10 to 20 years after men, with more serious consequences. Mental disorders, particularly depression and anxiety, are twice as prevalent in women as men. Finally, obesity has both physical and psychological consequences that are different for women than they are for men.

Cardiovascular Disease in Women

Heart disease has long had a reputation as a man's illness. It is now clear, however, that although women are unlikely to have heart disease or experience a heart attack before menopause, afterward they quickly catch up. By the sixth decade of life, women have the same degree of risk as men. Cardiovascular disease is the most serious female affliction later in life, hospitalizing 2.5 million women annually and killing 500,000 of them.[1] African American women are especially vulnerable because they die of cardiovascular disease at a much higher rate than white women do.[2] Thus, heart disease takes a considerably greater toll on women than any other illness, including breast cancer, which, with its annual death toll of approximately 44,000 women,[3] frightens them far more but kills them far less frequently.

Coronary Heart Disease

Half of the total mortality from cardiovascular disease is caused by coronary heart disease (CHD).[4] The heart is a four-chambered muscle that pumps blood to the body, bringing tissues vital oxygen and taking away carbon dioxide. All of the body's blood, about five to six quarts, passes through the heart every few minutes. But, while the body receives the oxygen and nutrients it needs to survive from the blood the heart pumps through its chambers and into the general circulation through the major blood vessels, the blood nourishing the heart itself enters through the small coronary arteries that encircle it like a crown. The female heart is smaller than the male heart, and its coronary arteries are smaller and narrower as well.

If any of the coronary arteries become blocked or narrowed, the heart muscle in the area fed by the damaged coronaries does not get enough oxygen. This condition is known as *myocardial* (meaning heart muscle) *ischemia* (lack of oxygen). It can cause angina pectoris, a Latin phrase for chest pain. The pain of angina usually appears suddenly after exertion and is often severe. But a lack of oxygen also can exist without symptoms, in which case it is called silent ischemia.

If a coronary artery becomes completely blocked, a heart attack may occur. The medical term for this is *myocardial infarction* (MI), which simply means severe damage to the heart muscle. If enough of the heart muscle is destroyed, then the pump itself may stop functioning, causing sudden death. If some heart muscle dies during a heart attack, the heart can keep working but with less efficiency, the way a car engine built with six cylinders but only operating on three performs. Sometimes the destruction of heart muscle makes the heart lose its regular rhythmic beat and quiver uncontrollably, failing to pump out its blood, a condition called *ventricular fibrillation*. Unless rapidly reversed by electrical shocks from a defibrillator, death occurs.

Blood vessels can become narrowed or blocked because of debris— plaque composed of deposits of white cells, fibrous tissue, and choles- terol—that stick to the blood vessel walls. In addition, the muscle may thicken, aggravating the obstruction. This process, called *atherosclero- sis*, occurs slowly over many years, just the way water pipes in an old house can corrode with rust over time. Atherosclerosis causes CHD.

Women with CHD have a worse prognosis than men for medical and surgical therapies. The rate of early death after MI is higher for women even when they receive clot-destroying drugs. When inva- sive techniques are used, women experience substantially greater in- hospital mortality than men. These techniques include

- *Coronary angioplasty:* passing a catheter with a deflated balloon on its tip into the narrowed coronary artery, then inflating the balloon to flatten the obstruction against the arterial wall
- *Coronary artery bypass graft surgery (CABG):* a detour around the blocked section of the coronary artery is surgically created with one of the internal mammary arteries or a blood vessel taken from another part of the body
- *Coronary atherectomy:* the surgical excision of the clot

Researchers do not know if this excess mortality is caused by women's smaller coronary arteries, their older age, the frequency of coexisting illnesses, or inadequate or delayed medical care.[5]

In fact, treating cardiovascular disease in women has been ham- pered by a lack of information about prevention, efficacy of diagnostic testing, and women's response to medical and surgical therapies. The reasons include

- The historic perception that women do not get heart disease
- The historic existence of an underlying bias in which males are considered the "normative group"[6]
- The exclusion of pre- and postmenopausal women from clini- cal treatment trials because of fear of unplanned pregnancy and fetal damage among the former and because of frequent coex- isting medical conditions among the latter; this means that most of the information about heart disease has come from studies of men

It is encouraging to note the recently revised policies of the National Institutes of Health (NIH) and the U.S. Food and Drug Administration (FDA) calling for the inclusion of women in clinical studies; the establishment of the Office for Research on Women's Health (ORWH) at NIH in 1991 and its Women's Health Initiative (WHI), which will investigate cardiovascular disease and its prevention in perimenopausal and older women; and the 1992 National Heart, Lung and Blood Institute (NHLBI) conference on "Cardiovascular Disease and Health in Women," designed to highlight new information from epidemiological and clinical research appropriate for clinical use and to identify gaps in knowledge for which research is needed.

Recommendations for Clinical Practice

Angina. The NIH conference recommended educating health professionals and women about the dangers of angina pectoris, which in the past has been regarded by some as benign. The clinician's complete evaluation should include a thorough clinical history and electrocardiographic exercise testing. For women with normal resting electrocardiograms who complain of chest pain, electrocardiographic testing involves taking an electrocardiogram during exercise. When the resting electrocardiogram is abnormal and the history suggests atypical angina, the conference participants advised using thallium or other perfusion imaging, which improves the quality of exercise testing in women. (Thallium is a radioactive substance that allows practitioners to trace the flow of blood through the heart to find blockage.) When not enough oxygen is reaching the heart, the conference recommended exercise and dipyridamole echocardiography. (Echocardiography uses sound waves to visualize the structure of the heart; dipyridamole opens the coronary arteries.) This test is apparently accurate in single-vessel coronary disease, which is common in women. It shows the development of new wall-motion abnormalities that occur when the heart fails to receive enough oxygen and is thus an accurate measure of ischemia. If the exercise test results are abnormal, referring the woman for coronary arteriography— visualizing the coronary arteries after injecting a radioactive dye—should be considered. For women unable to exercise, the conference recommended pharmacological stress testing. Two classes of drugs are used: the first forces the heart to beat harder, requiring more oxygen and exposing the injured areas, and the second opens (dilates) the coronary arteries so much that blood courses rapidly through them but fails to reach impaired areas, allowing those areas to be identified easily. None of these tests was thought useful for large-scale screening for CHD in asymptomatic patients.[7]

The conference participants acknowledged that not much is known about silent myocardial ischemia. Several conditions were identified as being more common in women, among them unrecognized heart attacks, variant (Prinzmetal) angina when angiography reveals normal coronary arteries, and insufficient blood reaching the heart even when the coronary arteries appear normal on angiography. The latter condition may represent small vessel disease, but this is not yet a proven concept. Although variant angina has a favorable prognosis, prognosis data conflict about insufficient oxygen even with normal coronary arteries. Survival is excellent, but left ventricular dysfunction occurs in some patients.[8] Left ventricular dysfunction requires treatment with drugs or procedures that bring more blood (revascularize) to the heart.

Treatment Differentials

Studies have shown that women undergo fewer invasive procedures, which raises the question of whether the rate of use is inappropriately low among women or too high in men. Although women experience more functional limitation caused by chest pain than men, fewer women are referred for diagnostic coronary arteriography, coronary angioplasty, or CABG. Although the number of coronary arteriograms performed in women has almost doubled in the past decade and the frequency of coronary artery bypass surgery in women nearly tripled,[9] women are still referred less often than men for diagnostic and therapeutic procedures, particularly coronary arteriography,[10] and the question of referral bias among medical practitioners remains. One study found that, on average, sex accounted for approximately 25% of the variance in rates of diagnosis and treatment, suggesting that sex may be a factor in physician decision making.[11] But another study of the referral practices of academic cardiologists found that the different referral rates of their female and male patients with possible coronary artery disease (18% to 27%) was appropriate because of lower pretest probability and a reduced rate of positive exercise test results among their female patients.[12] We need more research to determine how much of the sex referral differential represents physician bias and how much is a result of an appropriate conservatism because of negative exercise test results or because women are older and sicker by the time they seek treatment. If inappropriate, how can referral patterns be changed so that physicians provide suitable patient care?

Although men and women survive at similar rates after clot dissolving therapy for acute MIs, women have more bleeding problems, possibly because of differences from men in clotting. Women are less likely than men to be eligible for this therapy because they delay seeking treatment for their symptoms, are older, and are sicker. We need to find effective ways of educating female cardiac patients and those at risk to seek medical care promptly for chest pain.[13]

Not much data about sex differences exist in other drug therapies because women have been excluded from clinical trials. Some studies indicate similar effectiveness in men and women of aspirin and beta-blockers in preventing second heart attacks.[14] The Nurses' Health Study found that low-dose aspirin reduces the risk of a first heart attack in women by about 30%. The Physicians Health Study of 22,000 male physicians showed a 44% lower risk for the first MI among men who took aspirin.[15] Because the nurses study was not a randomized trial and the nurses only took aspirin sporadically, a prospective, randomized, placebo-controlled trial of aspirin in women is now in progress.

If the older age and sicker condition of female cardiac patients are reasons for less aggressive treatment, physicians' lack of confidence in data from exercise-based diagnostic tests is another. In addition, the reported excessive mortality and generally poorer outcomes for women after CABG—including twice the complication rate during and just after bypass surgery in women as compared with men—is a third reason.[16] However, when adjustments are made for clinical variables of CABG patients, including age and body surface area, these sex-based differentials fade, and survival up to 18 years after CABG has been equal in men and women.[17] Similarly, although women experience a higher mortality during and immediately after coronary angioplasty, their long-term survival appears to equal that of men.[18] Again, women's more severe disease and smaller coronary arteries may contribute to these statistics.

Women also get fewer referrals for exercise rehabilitation even though they benefit from this therapy as much as men. Some studies show that, when women are referred for exercise rehabilitation, they have poorer attendance than men, possibly because of coexisting illness, family responsibilities, or unidentified psychosocial factors.[19] We need research on what those psychosocial factors are and how to overcome them. For example, many of these programs are not geared to women's needs, from the times they are scheduled to transportation problems, child care, and the exercises themselves, which are often based on a male exercise model.

One study from Boston University found similar compliance rates for women. Although women had less exercise capacity than men initially, both groups achieved a comparable training effect; women increased their exercise time by 31% and their exercise tolerance by 30%, whereas the figures for men were 21% and 16%, respectively.[20]

The conference recommended increased prevention for women. Health care providers should assess risk factors in women, such as blood pressure, body weight, waist-to-hip ratio, dietary fat intake, physical activity, cholesterol levels, diabetic status, and smoking status, and should design preventive interventions as part of regular health care. Regarding smoking, more adolescent girls than boys now smoke, particularly among economically disadvantaged populations, and women tend to use smoking as a means of weight control. This is a powerful incentive, particularly for white adolescents. A study of 659 high school students found that weight control was a significant factor among those who became regular smokers, with 58% of white females and 38% of white males stating they use smoking to curb weight gain. The comparable figures for African American females and males were 4% and 2%, respectively, indicating that they are smoking for different reasons.[21] To be successful, smoking prevention and cessation programs must be geared not only to a targeted group (that is, teens, older women, white and African American women) but also to the perceptions that cause smoking in the first place. Women also smoke more so-called low-yield brands in the mistaken idea that they are safer, despite research that shows similar MI risk for smokers of low- and high-yield brands.

Stopping smoking has major survival benefits for MI patients. Educational materials designed to explain the advantages of proper diet, lower cholesterol, weight control, exercise, and smoking cessation should be designed for women. Although women are less successful in stopping smoking than are men, programs designed specifically for women, such as those that are part of selected prenatal programs, have had better success rates than generalized programs. One controlled study at the University of Alabama found a 14% quit rate among pregnant women in the program specifically designed for them compared with a quit rate of 6% in the group using the American Lung Association's *Freedom From Smoking Manual* and a 2% quit rate among control subjects.[22]

Hormone Replacement, Oral Contraception, and CHD

Epidemiological data indicate that estrogen replacement therapy (ERT) appears to cause a 40% to 60% reduction in the risk for CHD. In addition, coronary angiography indicates a reduced severity of atherosclerosis among postmenopausal women in the Lipid Research Clinics Program who are taking ERT.[23] Because estrogen alone increases a woman's risk of endometrial cancer, women who have not had a hysterectomy should use combined estrogen and progestin regimens, called hormone replacement therapy (HRT), to prevent developing this disease. For many years, the issue of whether the addition of progestin reduces or eliminates estrogen's protective effect has been unanswered. But a recent report from the Postmenopausal Estrogen/ Progestin Interventions (PEPI) Trials published in the *Journal of the American Medical Association* goes a long way toward establishing that adding progestin does not erase the benefits of estrogen to the heart. This 3-year NIH-sponsored study of 875 healthy women between ages 45 and 64 found that, although estrogen alone provided the greatest protection, estrogen combined with micronized progesterone contributed somewhat less advantage, and estrogen plus synthetic progesterone (the most widely used form of combined therapy) supplied only a slightly less striking benefit than micronized progesterone. Estrogen, either alone or with progestin, improved the levels of the so-called good high-density lipoprotein cholesterol (HDL-C) and lowered fibrogen levels without negative effects on either blood pressure or insulin. Because unopposed estrogen produced high rates of endometrial growth (hyperplasia), it should only be used by women without a uterus.[24] Physicians should follow closely their women patients with high triglyceride levels who are taking estrogen to ensure it does not raise these levels even higher.

Another unknown area requiring research is the effect of hormone therapy on cardiovascular health when it is instituted or reinstituted in old age. WHI is currently studying the long-term effect of estrogen and estrogen plus progestin on heart disease, breast and uterine cancer, and fracture incidence, but results are years away.

No evidence exists that the use of low-dose oral contraceptives increases the risk of CHD among women younger than 30 and among nonsmoking women without other coronary risk factors who are between ages 30 and 50.[25] The evidence regarding the possible adverse effects of smoking for women taking oral contraceptives is, however, worrisome.

The Role of Iron

A Finnish study published in *Circulation* in 1992[26] reported that the level of stored iron in men may be a stronger risk factor for heart attack than cholesterol, blood pressure, or diabetes. This research found that every 1% increase in serum ferritin, the form in which the body stores iron, was associated with a more than 4% increase in heart attack risk. A high ferritin level, 200 micrograms or more per liter of blood, more than doubled the relative risk of heart attack.

Although the study was done in men, American researcher Dr. Jerome L. Sullivan, who has studied iron, says that the regular iron loss women experience during their reproductive years through menstruation may play a role in the premenopausal woman's cardiac health, particularly because blood iron levels and the incidence of cardiovascular disease rise after menopause.[27]

But a study conducted by the National Center for Health Statistics of 4,516 men and women who participated in the first National Health and Nutrition Examination Survey Epidemiological Follow-Up Study did not find an increased risk of CHD or MI among participants with higher transferrin saturation levels.[28] The accompanying editorial by Drs. Ascherio and Willett of the Harvard School of Public Health points out, however, that transferrin saturation levels indicate the amount of circulating iron available to tissues but are poorly correlated with body iron stores except at the extreme ends of the iron scale, when body stores are either depleted or overloaded. The authors conclude that these new data leave "the relations between iron stores and the risk of coronary disease far from settled."[29] Clearly more research is needed on this subject.

Behavior and Cardiovascular Disease in Women

Women experience higher rates of depression, anxiety, and other psychiatric conditions, and, in the past, many physicians have tended to dismiss physical symptoms, such as chest pain and tachycardia, as psychogenic in origin. The NIH conference warned against this bias and urged practitioners to complete a thorough diagnostic evaluation of women presenting with these symptoms. Physicians also should be aware of the cardiac side effects of psychotropic drugs and the psychiatric effects of cardiac medications.[30]

Smoking is used as a way of coping with stress. Studies in the United States and Sweden of white collar workers found that the relationship between work-related stress and smoking was greater for women than men, and, among female nurses, those who smoked reported higher levels of job stress than did their nonsmoking colleagues. Although the cause-and-effect relationship of stress to cardiovascular disease has been a matter of controversy, one recent well-designed study suggests an association between a stressful heavy work load and increased levels of cardiovascular risk factors. Another study showed a relationship between hostility and the severity of atherosclerosis, which was stronger for women than men. We need research to find the mechanisms that cause these interactions, particularly whether smoking to relieve such stress is a factor.[31]

Because at least two studies have shown a relationship between employment and women's health, it seems important to examine further the relationship of a woman's job to her health. One study found that women who were employed and married had the best health, with or without children. Good health was associated with more complex challenging jobs and autonomy. Support from husbands was important for good health, task sharing for employed women, and emotional support for homemakers.[32]

Another study reported that clerical workers, especially if their supervisors were demanding and their job situations did not let them express anger, were at greatest risk for developing heart disease. This was especially true for women with children and husbands with blue-collar jobs. Time pressure was associated with poor health.[33]

Although women in lower socioeconomic levels are at increased risk for CHD, the reasons are not clear. They may have a poor risk profile, experience more stress, lack medical services, or exhibit poor use of existing services. For such women, it may be inappropriate to define their socioeconomic status by occupation, the determinant used for men, because they do not work outside the home. Rather, educational level may provide a better measure, but more research is needed.[34]

Cardiovascular Disease and Pregnancy

Encouraging results came from investigations of the use of low-dose aspirin to decrease the risk of pregnancy-induced high blood pressure (preeclampsia), but recommendations must await the results of ongoing clinical trials. Research is needed on the role of calcium supplementation to prevent preeclampsia. For women with suspected blood clots in the veins (venous thromboembolism), the conference recommended a number of noninvasive diagnostic tests because the diagnosis must be certain before anticoagulant therapy begins. These tests include

- Impedance plethysmography, which uses an instrument to evaluate the amount of blood passing through a vein
- Duplex sonography, which uses ultrasound of blood vessels to detect narrowing and impediments to blood flow
- Magnetic resonance imaging, which is used to visualize the veins
- Ventilation-perfusion scanning, which uses two different isotopes that respectively measure ventilation and perfusion

When the results of these tests are inconclusive, physicians should use contrast venography and pulmonary angiography, procedures that inject a dye into blood vessels to visualize a clot.[35]

For the 300,000 women in the United States with congenital cardiovascular malformations, maternal and fetal outcomes are good except for the following conditions:

- Eisenmenger's syndrome, which has a 30% maternal mortality
- Primary pulmonary hypertension or moderately severe to severe secondary pulmonary hypertension
- Aortic stenosis, in which an abnormal aortic valve blocks the flow of blood out of the left ventricle, and other obstructing lesions
- Lesions associated with left ventricular dysfunction or congestive heart failure before pregnancy
- Weakness or ballooning of the aorta or pulmonary arteries (i.e., Marfan's syndrome)
- Prior pulmonary blood clot (embolism)[36]

When the mother has an isolated cardiovascular malformation without diabetes or other risk factors, the risk of a similar defect in the fetus is low. But when the defect is part of a syndrome or associated with defects in many systems, the fetus is at a higher risk, and prepregnancy evaluations are needed. Women with prosthetic heart valves taking anticoagulation therapy, those with implanted tissue valves, and those whose ventricles function poorly need individualized care. The increase of rheumatic fever among immigrant populations and the consequent rise in rheumatic heart disease among women of childbearing age may require surgical intervention for mitral stenosis. In this condition, the mitral valve that guards the exit from the left atrium to the left ventricle is scarred and thickened from the streptococcal infection that causes rheumatic fever. Physicians should evaluate whether valve repair is better than valve replacement and whether a tissue or a mechanical value is best in view of the risk of anticoagulation therapy during pregnancy.[37]

Noncoronary Cardiovascular Disease in Women

Stroke.   Nearly 90,000 women die from strokes annually.[38] Risk factors include

- Elevated systolic blood pressure. (The systolic reading is the higher of the two numbers that define blood pressure, that is, the 120 of the 120/80, and reflects the maximum force of the blood as the heart contracts. The lower number identifies the diastolic pressure, the minimum force that occurs as the heart relaxes.) High systolic pressure can be reduced with diuretic therapy, which increases urination and removes excess fluid from the body.

- Glucose intolerance and diabetes (higher for women than men).
- Smoking.
- Atrial fibrillation (the disruption of normal atrial heart beats).

Although HRT does not increase the risk of stroke, aspirin therapy lowers the risk. When atrial fibrillation is present, anticoagulation reduces the risk.[39]

Aortic stenosis (abnormal aortic valve). Women are evaluated later in life than men for this condition and incur more emergency surgery. The conference recommended echocardiography to select patients for diagnostic cardiac catheterization and elective surgery.[40]

Congestive heart failure. Women are older than men when congestive heart failure is diagnosed, and CHD is less frequently the cause of their ventricular dysfunction. Women experience higher mortality than men that is not attributable to age or cause of heart failure.[41]

Sudden death. Not much is known about sudden death in women,[42] and more research is obviously needed.

Needed Research on Cardiovascular Disease in Women

The following items suggest areas that are needed for research on cardiovascular disease in women:

- Research long-term survival statistics of female patients with CHD (currently lacking as a result of exclusion from clinical trials).
- Study the role of myocardial ischemia in women and why unrecognized heart attacks, variant angina, and myocardial ischemia with normal coronary arteries are more common in women.
- Research the causes of sudden death in women.

- Research the cause, effect, and treatment of blood vessel spasms (vasospasm) in women.
- Evaluate information from clinical trials to compare features of CHD in men and women regarding baseline characteristics, clinical manifestations, responses to treatment, and clinical outcomes.
- Study clot-dissolving therapy with respect to women's smaller size, the relative dose, and the incidence of hemorrhage.
- Study whether women with single-vessel disease and good ventricular function get more complete relief from angina and better exercise test performance after coronary angioplasty than from medical therapy, as is the case for men.
- Study why women get cardiovascular disease, CHD, and stroke later than do men; confirm the protective role of estrogen; and study menstruation and iron loss.
- Study why women have high mortality after MI and revascularizing procedures.
- Research drug therapy for pregnancy-induced hypertension, predictors of same, and maternal and fetal outcomes.
- Research the management of chronic hypertension and the evaluation of various drugs, exercise, and smoking.
- Study nonpharmacological therapies, such as relaxation training, biofeedback, and self-management, to reduce CHD risk factors and manage hypertension.
- Research how to promote healthy lifestyle changes in women, such as diet, exercise, and nonsmoking.
- Study the patterns of obesity and fat deposition in women and their relation to cardiovascular disease.
- Research the relation of personality, behavior, and cardiovascular disease in women. Studies on panic disorders and anxiety, both more common in women, and the behavioral and psychosocial characteristics predisposing women to CHD are needed.
- Study why female hormones protect against heart disease and what the effects of estrogen therapy are on stroke and peripheral vascular disease. Study the effect of ERT and HRT on older women.
- Study the barriers to invasive diagnostic care for women and how to remove them (for example, patient preference, physician bias,

other illnesses, insurance coverage, and access to health care services).

- Establish a national registry of current observational and clinical studies that include women to encourage easier analysis of sex differences.[43]
- Because most studies on the relationship between employment and women's cardiovascular health have been done on middle-class women, determine how low-income women have balanced work and child care and their consequences for heart disease.[44]
- Establish funding priorities; for example, how much should be spent on cardiovascular disease in women? If breast cancer research is now getting $300 million a year, and advocates are calling for $500 million a year for a disease that kills 44,000 women annually, how much is needed to lower illness and death from cardiovascular disease, which hospitalizes 2.5 million women and kills 500,000 of them every year? Study how to reduce competition for research funds among advocates for research on different women's diseases.
- Study the reasons that cardiovascular disease incidence differs for women in disparate racial and ethnic groups. Those studies that have been done have focused on biology, but we need to know more about the role of oppressive social and economic circumstances in the development of cardiovascular disease.

Emotional Disorders

Affective disorders in general and anxiety disorders in particular are twice as common in women as men older than 18.[45] Women also have more depression, fear of open spaces (agoraphobia), simple phobia, obsessive-compulsive disorder, schizophrenia, and panic disorder than do men. Women are more likely to convert mental experiences into bodily symptoms (somatization disorder) than are men. In addition, more women than men use outpatient facilities to treat mental illness. Women receive more prescriptions for psychoactive drugs (tranquilizers, sedatives, and stimulants) than men do and account for 43% of drug-related deaths in the United States.[46]

Depression

Depression is a major problem for women in the United States. The symptoms of depression include changes in eating patterns, usually loss of appetite or overeating; sleep disturbances, either inability to sleep or sleeping too much; restlessness and hyperactivity or severe lack of physical activity; loss of interest or pleasure in one's usual pursuits; decreased sex drive; loss of energy and fatigue; feelings of worthlessness, self-reproach, or excessive guilt; diminished ability to think or concentrate; recurrent thoughts of death or suicide; and attempted suicide. The life events that can precipitate depression include the death of a spouse, lover, or a close family member; marriage problems, including sexual difficulties, pregnancy, separation, reconciliation, and divorce; personal illness or injury or sickness of a family member; and job loss, retirement, business readjustment, a jail sentence, or a change in financial status.[47]

The American Psychological Association's (APA) National Task Force on Women and Depression reported in 1990 that about 7 million women have diagnosable depression—double the rate for men.[48] However, the National Mental Health Association reports that 17.6 million adult Americans have a depressive illness each year, twice as many of them women as men, which would make the figure much higher.[49] Among elderly people, depression is almost four times more common in women than men.[50] This condition leads to 30,000 suicides annually and costs society an estimated $16 billion a year.[51] Depression also is the most frequent mental health–related cause of hospital admission for women.[52]

The APA task force identified certain groups of women at higher risk for depression: ethnic minorities, adolescents, older women, professional women, lesbians, abused women, women with few financial resources, and women who have eating disorders or substance abuse disorder. Six factors that contribute to women's elevated risk were noted, including reproductive events (menstruation, pregnancy, childbirth, abortion, and menopause), personality and other psychological attributes (self-esteem, coping and explanatory styles, and a sense of control), family roles and intimate relationships, work roles, victimization, and poverty.[53]

The question, then, as far as these debilitating psychiatric disorders are concerned, is not whether women suffer more, but why. Are the causes to be found in women's biology, in the way society is organized, or both? Many authorities believe women's difficulties in this area are connected to the hormonal alterations in women's reproductive biology. But a 1989 review of four psychiatric syndromes specifically linked to women's reproductive functions found this was not a valid assumption, at least for the conditions studied. These included depression after childbirth (postpartum depression), premenstrual syndrome (PMS), posthysterectomy depression, and menopausal depression (involutional melancholia). The authors found that two of them—posthysterectomy depression and menopausal depression—are simply fading "into psychiatric history."[54] It would be interesting to study why this has happened and to ascertain the effects of the women's movement. For example, is the fact that older women are now able to make significant contributions to society by going back to school and/or work responsible for many of them reporting being relieved after hysterectomy, particularly when it removes painful symptoms? Did women become melancholic at menopause in the past because there was no role beyond motherhood for them or because society devalued the old? Is this still happening to women who have neither the economic resources nor the educational level to train or retrain for a new work experience?

Studies reported that the women most likely to experience postpartum depression were those who had had prepregnancy depressions. In fact, given the huge drop in hormone levels right after birth, the authors expressed surprise that so many women are able to adapt to such changes without incident rather than surprise at the occasional experiences of postpartum depression. They found that postpartum blues and moderate depression, the milder forms of postbirth depression, were more often connected to the stress of caring for a newborn and lack of an adequate support system. For postpartum psychosis, beyond psychiatric history, risk factors included having a first baby, being unmarried, having a cesarean section delivery, and fetal or infant death.[55]

Many difficulties exist in studying PMS, including poor definition of symptoms, many retrospective studies, few controlled treatment trials, and conflicting results of the few studies that were sound methodologically. A review of research that investigated theories of a hormonal basis for PMS—postulating everything from excessive estrogen to insufficient progesterone to a higher estrogen-to-progesterone ratio or to the effects of prolactin levels, prostaglandins, and aldosterone—did not prove the validity of any of them. The studies that examined the relationship between emotional illness and PMS—although they did not all agree—did find a higher rate of moderate and severe PMS among women with previous psychiatric illness.[56] The APA study identified several cultural causes of depression, citing unhappy marriage, reproductive stress (particularly infertility), and sexual and physical abuse as strong factors in accounting for the gender difference. Although women are more depressed because of the way they experience being female in our contemporary culture, women's depression must be viewed from a "biopsychosocial" perspective.[57] A review article in the *American Journal of Psychiatry* reporting on European studies of depression in women also stressed cultural events, finding that a diagnosis of cancer and having a mastectomy caused depression. Women who had mastectomies for breast cancer were much more prone to psychiatric problems than were those who had the less disfiguring lumpectomy and radiation; many women who had had mastectomies said they wished they had opted for lumpectomy. Among mastectomy patients, however, those who had breast reconstruction experienced less distress, and the sooner they had the procedure, the better they felt.[58]

Feminist writers blame society for the high rate of depression among women. Gretchen Grinnell, a Canadian psychotherapist, reviewing the literature on the social roots of female depression, points out that society asks women to believe that male supremacy and the male belief in competition are "natural" tendencies, disallowing the female style of experience, which is subjective and intuitive. She calls this the "global folie." She says that the contemporary organization of society accepts what she calls the "testosterone imperative," excusing men from responsibility for their "hostile aggression and sexual imperialism." She maintains that this process starts in childhood, when boys are trained to suppress their tenderness, natural altruism, and empathy toward other boys, whereas girls are taught to suppress their erotic and aggressive urges and "depress themselves." This lays the groundwork for gender competition, with boys fighting one another and girls learning to mistrust their own assets. It establishes a societal hierarchy, a "vertical, upwardly striving, goal-oriented modality," with men on top and women on the bottom and thus "inferior." In such a construct, women acquire "a chronic subconscious sense that there is something wrong with them." Grinnell denies the idea that depression is a disease as expounded in the *Diagnostic and Statistical Manual of Mental Disorders* and the psychiatric literature and maintains that women are subject to depression because they are in a double-bind conflict. They want to change both themselves and society and get away from the forces that are entrapping them, but another message—that change is dangerous because it threatens the status quo and the relationships with the men in their lives—hampers their ability to act.[59]

Grinnell outlines five steps she uses with depressed women that have been effective. First, she explains the "folie" and tells the woman she is not at fault, which, she says, most women immediately recognize as true. Next, she asks the woman to abandon the vertical construct for a horizonal mode, allowing her to stop thinking in terms of success or failure, and substituting a continuum in which she imagines "what she wants and where she is going in her life." She recommends that the woman read Gilligan's 1982 book, *In a Different Voice*, which illustrates women's ways of decision making that reveal gender differences in how women view relationships. She validates the woman's altruism toward herself as being as important as altruism toward others, encouraging her to take back her own power even if her actions bring on verbal reprisals from the others she has been serving, a process she calls ego-validation. She then works with the woman to outline the gradual steps that will help her get where her needs call her. The fourth step involves showing the woman how she has become addicted to the influence of those who have dictated to her in the past and asks her to find substitutes for that person(s) with whom she feels comfortable. Finally, Grinnell encourages the woman to read and honor her body signals, recognizing what makes her comfortable and moving away from those who try to sabotage her feelings of self-worth. She tells the woman that quitting a destructive relationship can be an intelligent step if her moral, intellectual, or psychological life is on the line. This process takes time and continual support from the therapist, who must regard the woman as someone who can heal herself rather than as a person who is "crippled" by "illness." Grinnell warns other therapists not to become impatient with slow progress, which she calls "the male model." She believes that "we"—meaning women, therapists, and all who are concerned with these problems—can move away from vertical constructs by stressing the natural order of things in action and language. She points out that nature is not hierarchical, that all activity involves opening and closing, that breathing in and out is the true flow of life, and that sexuality involves swelling and shrinking, excitement and calm. She maintains we can ignore vertical thinking.[60]

Psychotherapy and antidepressants have been the main treatments for depression. Currently, the Office of Alternative Medicine at NIH is funding a small controlled acupuncture treatment study for depression in women at the University of Arizona. Initial results are that 70% of the women who have completed the study have experienced significant relief from the symptoms of depression, with approximately 65% achieving full remission. This treatment success rate compares favorably with antidepressant medication and psychotherapy, each of which has success rates that range from 50% to 70% for those who complete treatment (personal correspondence, letter to B. Jacobson from John J. B. Allen, Ph.D., coprincipal investigator, summarizing initial results of this study, September 27, 1995). A larger study is needed to determine whether these results can be replicated.

Research Needed on Emotional Disorders

Because women are much more vulnerable to affective and anxiety disorders, depression, agoraphobia, simple phobia, obsessive-compulsive disorder, schizophrenia, panic disorder, and somatization disorder, we need research to sort out the relative importance of biology (that is, genes, hormones, reproduction) and the environment (that is, family and work conflicts, self-esteem, interpersonal relations, explanatory styles, coping mechanisms) in causing emotional disorders in women. Looking only at biology excuses us from examining oppression, a problem whose origin is found in the way society is organized. For depression, we have the results of the work of APA's National Task Force on Women and Depression, which identified a number of risk factors, many of them—such as minority status, adolescence, age, poverty, substance abuse, battering, or eating disorders—characterized by a lack of control. Other risk factors included societal nonacceptance, such as lesbianism, or stress from overly high expectations, such as that experienced by many professional women.

We need research to determine how lack of control, high expectations, and society's disapproval cause depression and how women can overcome these deficits. We also need to study the negative effects of illness and aging on mental health and how to combat them.

Obesity

Overweight and obesity are major problems in the United States. According to government health surveys conducted between 1988 and 1991, one-third (33.4%) of all adults in the United States older than 20 were estimated to be overweight.[61] For women, the news from this survey is not good. Although just under one-third (32.9%) of non-Hispanic white women were overweight, nearly half of all Mexican American women and non-Hispanic African American women carried far too many pounds (46.7% and 48.6%, respectively). This represents a dramatic increase of 8% over the previous health survey done between 1976 and 1980 for all race and sex groups. During the 1988 to 1991 period, for adult men and women aged 20 to 77, mean body weight increased by 8 pounds. Other studies confirm these results. One, the Minnesota Heart Health Program, found that from 1980 to 1987 the prevalence of obesity for adults between ages 25 and 74 increased 4.6% for men and a startling 6.1% for women.[62] The effects of obesity are different in men and women. The effects are more dangerous physically to men because men carry their extra weight on the abdomen, which puts them at greater risk for heart attack. But women have more psychological damage as they struggle to conform to the American ideal that thinness equals beauty. The increasing prevalence of bulimia and anorexia—with current estimates indicating that 10% to 15% of girls and young women have these syndromes—is a symptom of this struggle for litheness.[63]

Menstruation and Pregnancy

Menstruation and pregnancy both affect a woman's weight. During the menstrual cycle, estrogen levels are high and progesterone is low at ovulation, but the reverse is true during the last part of the cycle before bleeding begins, which is called the luteal phase. When estrogen levels are high during ovulation, food intake is low. But the amount of food a woman consumes and her body weight increase during the luteal phase, when estrogen levels are low relative to progesterone. One study showed that women consumed 283 more calories a day during the luteal phase than they did when ovulating. Investigators measuring the basal metabolic rate (BMR), the rate at which the body burns calories at rest, found that the BMR increased just before menstruation and decreased to its lowest point during ovulation. Although researchers do not know whether the increased BMR during the luteal phase stimulates the need for extra food or whether the increased food intake speeds up the BMR, the effect of these physiological changes on dieting is significant. During the luteal phase, dieting women will not lose weight, will lose less, or will gain. Women struggling with weight control for valid health reasons—that is, to reduce their risk of disease—should be aware of these differences so that they do not become discouraged and give up their attempts to lose weight.[64]

During pregnancy, the average woman gains about 27 pounds, which is within the 25- to 30-pound range recommended by the National Academy of Science. It is important for women to gain enough weight to produce a normal-weight baby (7 to 8.5 pounds) and to avoid a low-weight baby (under 5.5 pounds) because low-weight infants have a greater incidence of illness, abnormalities, and death. It is vital to get enough protein (60 grams daily during pregnancy and 65 grams daily during the first 6 months of lactation), enough folic acid (800 micrograms a day during pregnancy and 500 micrograms while nursing), sufficient calcium (1,200 milligrams daily during pregnancy and lactation), and iron (30 to 60 milligrams daily). However, women who are already overweight may be wise to gain fewer pounds, in the range of 20 to 25 pounds or 300 extra calories daily for the last 6 months of pregnancy, while maintaining the correct intake of vital nutrients. This is because many women date their initial weight gain to their first pregnancy, with additional increases with each succeeding pregnancy. It is important for women to try to return to the prepregnancy weight after delivery to avoid this spiral of weight gain with each pregnancy. Nursing helps this process because, even if a woman consumes the recommended 500 extra calories a day when breast-feeding her infant, she burns 600 calories daily producing enough milk to feed that infant. Studies have shown that women can produce enough milk on intakes of 2,000 to 2,200 calories daily.[65]

Health Risks of Obesity

Obesity is a health hazard for women. A study of more than 115,000 nurses who were 30 to 55 years old in 1976 and free of CHD, stroke, and cancer found after 8 years that those who weighed the most had the highest rates of heart attack, angina, and death from CHD. Even mildly to moderately overweight middle-aged women had an increased risk of developing CHD. Weight gain also causes increases in blood pressure, a risk factor for heart disease. Obesity is an established risk factor for non–insulin-dependent diabetes. The relationship between cancer and obesity is still unclear, but one study of 750,000 men and women showed that those people 40% or more above average weight had high death rates from cancer, with women developing cancer of the gallbladder and biliary passages, breast, cervix, endometrium, uterus, and ovaries.[66]

Genetics of Obesity

The genetics of obesity are only just emerging. A major breakthrough occurred in 1994 when researchers found the *ob* gene, a genetic mutation that disrupts the body's appetite control center so that it fails to tell the brain when enough food has been consumed to meet the body's energy needs. Without this vital signal for fullness, people can continue to overeat even if they are already full and overweight. Researchers warn that translating this discovery into an effective therapy for weight control may take 5 to 10 years. But, in theory at least, they may create a drug eventually that will mimic the action of the missing protein that this faulty gene fails to produce. Scientists do not yet know how much of the widespread problem of overweight people this mutant gene causes. It is important to remember that obesity is probably caused by a complex mix of numerous genes and environmental influences. For example, the obese mouse, which was the animal model that led scientists to the human *ob* gene, has at least six genes that contribute to obesity. Therefore, it will not be surprising to find that humans have more than one obesity gene.[67] Subsequently, researchers have found a protein—glucagon-like factor-1 (GLP-1)—that tells the brain when it is time for the body to stop eating. Both this discovery and a previous one that identified another protein, leptin, which keeps the body's weight at a set level, may be bringing researchers even closer to more effective obesity treatments for humans.[68]

Earlier research found that inherited differences in the enzymes of the liver or other tissues influence how efficient we are at burning fats. Some people have a "fat burner" as part of their genetic code. Animal work has shown that a novel receptor in the fat cells of rats appears to control how efficiently these animals burn fat. The levels of this atypical receptor were 71% below normal in the fat tissue of genetically obese rats. Researchers are searching for the human equivalent of this receptor. Other animal research has established that the weight of obese mice seems to be standardized at a higher level than in lean animals. When obese rats fail to get enough food, their metabolism slows down to maintain as much of their body weight as possible.[69] Human research studies have discovered that some genetically obese people convert food rapidly to body fat and find it much harder to turn the body fat they store back into energy. Other obese individuals produce excess amounts of the enzyme lipoprotein lipase, which cells use to absorb lipids (fats) from the blood and deposit it as body fat. Research also has shown that obese children have more fat cells than lean children do. Investigators have quantified some aspects of energy expenditure, the amount of calories we burn, which are under genetic control. A recent report indicates that about 25% to 30% of the variation in our spontaneous level of activity—whether we are fidgety or indolent—is controlled by genes. Also, the amount of energy burned during moderate exercise is even more subject to genetic control. A recent study of twins found that 45% of the variation in their levels of output was caused by their genes. Interestingly, the genetic influence vanished when these subjects exercised at six times their resting level, indicating that one can overcome one's genetic limitations.[70]

In two recent studies of twins, scientists established that genes influence body composition and fat distribution. Although the first study investigated the effect of long-term overfeeding on 12 pairs of male identical twins, the results may have some validity for women. These 19- to

27-year-old men ate an extra 1,000 calories a day for 84 days, living under controlled conditions with members of the research staff supervising their activities. They did not drink or smoke and limited their physical activity to reading, playing video games and cards, watching television, and taking one 30-minute walk daily. The amount of weight gained ranged from just under 10 pounds to almost 30 pounds. The difference in weight gain occurred between the pairs of twins, not between the twins in each pair. The similarity between twins was particularly evident for regional fat distribution and the amount of abdominal visceral (deep) fat; there was six times more variance between the pairs of twins than within each pair for these two factors. Because identical twins share the same genes, genetic factors had to be largely responsible for these variations. The researchers do not know what caused this difference in weight accumulation and fat distribution. It might be the way the twin pairs stored their extra calories, with some pairs turning them into lean tissue and others converting them into fat. Or it might involve the variations in energy expenditure during rest between twin pairs. Either way, this study underlines the importance of inheritance in how people respond to overeating. It also shows that some people are more prone than others to store fat on the trunk, in the abdominal cavity, or in both places because of their genetic makeup. This is particularly important to clinicians and their overweight and obese patients because of the relationship between the abdominal spare tire and the greater risk of diabetes, elevated levels of fat in the blood, hypertension, and heart disease that this type of fat accumulation signifies.[71]

The second study looked at the genetic versus environmental influences on the weight of fraternal and identical twins of both sexes, some of whom had grown up together and others who had been reared apart. These investigators found that genes accounted for 70% of the differences in how much the twins weighed later in life and that childhood environment had little or no influence.[72]

Needed Research on Obesity

We need more information on the genetics of obesity. Is there more to the control of the appetite center than the important discoveries made since 1994? If so, what else may be involved, and will the genetics of obesity, when fully unraveled, pave the way for treatments to control this condition? How does the genetic-environmental interaction affect overweight humans and their difficulty in losing weight?

We need studies on how humans burn or accumulate fat and the role of the enzyme lipoprotein lipase in causing obesity. Genetic screening tests are needed to identify persons at risk because preventing weight gain is vital as losing weight is so difficult. Research on the most effective behavioral changes needed to achieve and maintain weight loss is essential. We need to investigate the effects of society's standards of beauty and body image on women, who sets and disseminates these standards, the influence of advertising, ways to determine healthy standards for women, and ways to distribute that information to women. We need to find effective ways of educating the public about the dangers of obesity, the particular ill effects of yo-yo dieting, and the nature of a healthy diet and how to achieve it on a limited income.

Endnotes

[1]Wenger NK, Speroff L, Packard B: Cardiovascular health and disease in women. *New England Journal of Medicine* 329:247–256, 1993

[2]Blumenthal S, Barry P, Hamilton J, et al: *Forging a Women's Health Research Agenda.* Washington, DC, National Women's Health Resource Center, 1991

[3]American Cancer Society: *Cancer Facts & Figures—1996,* Atlanta, GA, American Cancer Society, 1996

[4]Wenger NK: Coronary heart disease in women: an overview (myths, misperceptions, and missed opportunities). *CVR&R,* December 1995, pp 24–41

[5]Wenger NK, Speroff L, Packard B, op. cit.

[6]*Cardiovascular Panel Report: Section 1: Epidemiology and Scope of the Problem:2.* January 1992

[7]Wenger NK, Speroff L, Packard B, op. cit.

[8]Ibid.

[9]Wenger NK, op. cit.

[10]Chesney MA: Behavioral barriers to cardiovascular health in women. *CVR&R* March:19–33, 1994

[11]Travis CB, Gressley DL, Phillippi RH: Medical decision making, gender, and coronary heart disease. *Journal of Women's Health* 2(3):269–279, 1993

[12]Mark DB, Shaw LK, DeLong ER, et al: Absence of sex bias in the referral of patients for cardiac catheterization. *New England Journal of Medicine* 330:1101–1106, 1994

[13]Wenger NK, Speroff L, Packard B, op. cit.

[14]Ibid.

[15]American Heart Association, "Aspirin appears to reduce risk of first heart attack in women." *Heartstyle* 1(4), 1991

[16]Wenger NK, Speroff L, Packard B, op. cit.

[17]Fetters JK: Gender issues in coronary artery disease. *Cardiac Trends*, Winter 1995

[18]Ibid.

[19]Wenger NK, Speroff L, Packard B, op. cit.

[20]Cannistra LB, Balady GJ, O'Malley CJ, et al: Comparison of the clinical profile and outcome of women and men in cardiac rehabilitation. *American Journal of Cardiology* 69:1274–1279, 1992

[21]Chesney MA, op. cit.

[22]Windsor RA: The effectiveness of smoking cessation methods for smokers in public health maternity clinics: a randomized trial. *American Journal of Public Health* 75:1389–1392, 1985

[23]Wenger NK, op. cit.

[24]The Writing Group for the PEPI Trial: Effects of estrogen or estrogen/progestin regimens on heart disease risk factors in postmenopausal women. *Journal of the American Medical Association* 273:199–208, 1995

[25]Wenger NK, Speroff L, Packard B, op. cit.

[26]Salonen JT, Nyyssöhen K, Korpela H, et al: High stored iron levels are associated with excess risk of myocardial infarction in Eastern Finnish men. *Circulation* 86:803–811, 1992

[27]*Scientist Says New Study Supports His Theory That Stored Iron May Be Potent Heart Hazard.* Chicago, IL, American Medical Association, news release, September 8, 1992

[28]Sempos CT, Looker AC, Gillum RF, et al: Body iron stores and the risk of coronary heart disease. *New England Journal of Medicine* 330:1119–1124, 1994

[29]Ascherio A, Willett WC: Are body iron stores related to the risk of coronary heart disease? *New England Journal of Medicine* 330:1152–1154, 1994

[30]Wenger NK, Speroff L, Packard B, op. cit.

[31]Chesney MA, op. cit.

[32]Fogel CI, Woods NF (eds): Women and their health, in *Women's Health Care*. Thousand Oaks, CA, Sage, 1995

[33]Ibid.

[34]Ibid.

[35]Wenger NK, Speroff L, Packard B, op. cit.

[36]Ibid.

[37]Ibid.

[38]National Institutes of Health: *Opportunities for Research on Women's Health*, Part 1. Hunt Valley, MD, September 4–6, 1991 (hereafter called Hunt Valley, Part 1 or Part 2)

[39]Wenger NK, Speroff L, Packard B, op. cit.

[40]Ibid.

[41]Ibid.

[42]Ibid.

[43]Ibid.

[44]Fogel CI, Woods NF, op. cit.

[45]Hunt Valley, Part 2, p 57

[46]Ward D: Women and health care, in *Women's Health Care*. Edited by Fogel CI, Woods NF. Thousand Oaks, CA, Sage, 1995

[47]Gray MJ, Haseltine F, Love S, et al: *The Woman's Guide to Good Health*. Yonkers, NY, Consumer Reports Books, 1991

[48]McGrath E, Keita G, Strickland B, et al: *Women and Depression: Risk Factors and Treatment Issues*. Washington, DC, American Psychological Association, 1990 (hereafter called APA report)

[49]*Clinical Depression Fact Sheet*. National Mental Health Association's National Public Education Campaign on Clinical Depression, 1996

[50]Hunt Valley, Part 1

[51]Gladwell M: "Study finds women twice as likely as men to suffer depression." *Washington Post*, reprinted in *The Burlington Free Press*, December 6, 1990

[52]Fogel CI, Woods NF, op. cit.

[53]APA report. *Psychiatric Times*, January 1991

[54]Gitlin MJ, Pasnau RO: Psychiatric syndromes linked to reproductive function in women: a review of current knowledge. *American Journal of Psychiatry* 146:1413–1422, 1989

[55]Ibid.

[56]Ibid.

[57]APA report, op. cit.

[58]Goleman D: "Wide beliefs on depression in women contradicted." *New York Times*, January 9, 1990

[59]Grinnell G: Women, depression and the global folie: a new framework for therapists, in *Women and Therapy: A Feminist Quarterly*. Edited by Braude M. New York, Haworth Press, 1987, pp 41–58

[60]Ibid.

[61]Overweight in this survey was defined as a body mass index (BMI) over 27.8 for men and 27.3 for women. These values, used by the NIH Consensus Development Conference on the Health Implications of Obesity, represent approximately 124% of desirable weight for men and 120% of desirable weight for women, defined as the midpoint of the range of weights for a medium frame from the 1983 Metropolitan Height and Weight tables.

[62]Kuczmarski R, Flegal K, Campbell S, et al: Increasing prevalence of overweight among US adults. *Journal of the American Medical Association* 272:205–211, 1994

[63]Gray MJ, et al., op. cit.

[64]Ibid.

[65]Ibid.

[66]Ibid.

[67]Angier N: "Researchers link obesity in humans to flaw in a gene." *New York Times*, December 1, 1994

[68]Blakeslee S: "Signal to stop eating is found." *New York Times*, January 4, 1996

[69]Simopoulos AP, Herbert V, Jacobson B: *Genetic Nutrition: Designing a Diet Based on Your Family Medical History*. New York, Macmillan, 1993

[70]Ibid.

[71]Bouchard C, Tremblay A, Despres JP, et al: The response to long-term overfeeding in identical twins. *New England Journal of Medicine* 322:1477–1482, 1990

[72]Stunkard A, Harris J, Pedersen HL: The body mass index of twins who have been reared apart. *New England Journal of Medicine* 322:1483–1487, 1990; Simopoulos AP, Herbert V, Jacobson B, op. cit.

8

Women's Health and the Environment

Lynne Beauregard

According to dozens of studies, women believe environmental risks are more pronounced than men do.[1] This belief is hardly the product of hysterical thinking, and women have good reason to be concerned. Some of the unmistakable environmental hazards affecting men and women alike are cigarette smoke, alcohol, lead, suntanning, and substance abuse. There also is a legitimate basis for women's suspicions about lesser-known environmental agents, but authorities cannot tie them irrefutably to health problems. Exposure to certain pesticides, prescription drugs, air pollutants, and other environmental agents, often occurring over the course of years, may trigger a cascade of physical changes, yet inadequate human surveillance and insufficient animal testing typically frustrate efforts to establish firm linkages.

Fueling the gender difference in risk perception is this simple fact: women have greater physical vulnerability to many environmental insults. Because of their smaller size, the same exposure (for example, to alcohol or drugs) usually has more rapid and/or stronger physiological

The author acknowledges the important contribution of Miriam Davis, Ph.D., to the development of this chapter as a source of information and perspective. Any comments and conclusions, however, are solely those of the author.

effects. A fundamental principle of toxicology is that the higher the dose, the greater the impact. Furthermore, many environmental toxins are stored in body fat. Because women possess a greater percentage of body fat than do men, they may be more heavily burdened. Pregnancy, breast-feeding, dieting, menopause, and aging can serve to release stored toxins into the blood, posing health risks to women and their offspring.

Estrogen

Another problem is the female hormone estrogen. Long-term estrogen exposure, although beneficial to reproductive health and protective against bone loss and heart disease, also may place women at risk for endometrial and breast cancer. Scientists believe that estrogen-like substances in the environment, such as diethylstilbestrol (DES), Kepone, and other pesticides, may add to the body's own estrogen levels, mimicking its effects or altering its production or metabolism. This cumulative exposure may increase the risk of these cancers. Finally, women have higher rates of many painful and debilitating conditions such as osteoporosis, multiple sclerosis, osteoarthritis, and most autoimmune diseases (see Chapter 1). Environmental factors can contribute to the onset and course of these conditions.

Traditionally, concern about environmental toxins focuses on chemical and physical pollutants. Yet the environment also can involve lifestyle and social milieu, such as the ravages caused by poor nutrition, substance abuse, and domestic violence, conditions arising from poverty and powerlessness that disproportionately afflict women and their children (see Chapter 4 on domestic violence). Lifestyle and social factors can aggravate the effects of conventional environmental exposures. For example, the consequences of lead exposure, typically found in poorly maintained, older housing with deteriorating lead-based paint, are heightened by poor nutrition. Thus, this chapter looks at the environment through a wide-angle lens, examining a variety of environmental threats and their impact on women's health, including estrogen-like pesticides, dioxin, prescription drugs, lead, smoking, sunlight, electromagnetic fields, occupational hazards, and lifestyle and social issues, such as nutrition and substance abuse; highlighting new research findings; and recommending needed research.

Estrogen-like Pesticides in the Environment

Can exposures to substances in the environment that mimic estrogen add to the body's estrogen level and thereby heighten the risk for breast cancer and reproductive disorders? This is the intriguing hypothesis underlying a relatively new line of research on how estrogen-like pesticides and other substances contribute to risk.[2] Some authorities think that these substances, sometimes structurally similar to estrogen, act like estrogen or alter estrogen's production or metabolism.

Cumulative, long-term exposure to the body's *own* estrogen (estradiol-17β) may increase the risk of breast cancer.[3] Women whose ovaries have been removed—the major source of the internally produced (endogenous) estrogen—have a far lesser risk of breast cancer than do women who have a late onset of menstruation or an early menopause. Conversely, women who menstruate early and/or have delayed menopause are at far higher risk for breast cancer.[4] Meanwhile, the studies on the link between postmenopausal estrogen replacement therapy (ERT) and breast cancer are equivocal; some show a negative effect and some do not. One of the largest and most recent studies shows an increased risk of breast cancer with short-term use of ERT of 5 years or more,[5] but a month after it was published, yet another study failed to find a similar result.[6] We should have a definitive answer to this vexing question when the Women's Health Initiative, the largest study of cardiovascular disease, breast cancer, and osteoporosis among postmenopausal women ever conducted, is finished, probably within the next decade.

Momentum is building for research on estrogen imitators in the environment. Scientists are struggling to explain the worrisome yet poorly understood demographics: young girls are reaching puberty earlier, endometriosis appears to be on the rise, and breast cancer rates are soaring. Breast cancer incidence has risen by 24% since 1973 in a manner that cannot be explained solely by better detection (Figure 8–1). Thirty percent to 50% of women with breast cancer, the second most common cancer in women, have no recognized risk factor.[7]

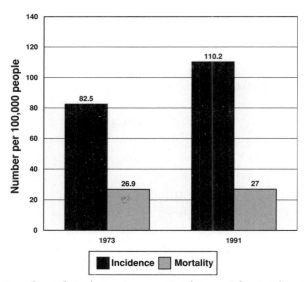

Figure 8–1.   Growth in breast cancer incidence and mortality, 1973–1991. *Source.* National Cancer Institute Surveillance, Epidemiology, and End Results Program.

Estrogen-like compounds are plentiful in the environment, in part because they can be extremely persistent. For example, the pesticide DDT, and its metabolite DDE, are among a class of pesticides called organochlorines that lodge in fat tissues and move up the food chain.[8] Even though DDT was banned in the United States in 1972 after studies showed it to be an animal carcinogen and reproductive toxin, residues are still found in our food supply, wildlife, human fat, and breast milk. DDT is still produced and used in India and other developing countries, representing a threat to women's health worldwide. At least one organochlorine pesticide marketed in the United States has estrogen-like effects, the pesticide endosulfan.[9]

PCBs—or polychlorinated biphenyls—are a class of more than 200 different compounds that have been produced commercially since 1929 for use as fluid electrical insulators. Their manufacture was banned in the United States in 1979 when they were found to be carcinogenic in experimental animals. It is not surprising that there are still trace quantities in the environment because PCBs are stable and resistant to thermal degradation. PCB-containing products may still be in use. Many, but not all, PCB compounds have estrogen-like effects.[10]

Research Advances

When a compound mimics estrogen, it binds to the body's estrogen receptors, an action that can trigger a cascade of hormonal effects, including enhanced cell division in reproductive tissues. As cells divide more rapidly, there may be an increased chance of genetic mutations that can lead to cancer.[11]

Examples of environmental agents that bind to estrogen receptors and mimic estrogen's effect on cell division are the plant estrogens coumestrol and genistein, the fungal product zearalenone, and the prescription drug diethylstilbestrol (DES).[12] However, before jumping to conclusions about the first three agents, which are found in our diet, it is important to point out their multifaceted effects. Even though they can induce breast cell proliferation in cultured cells, epidemiological studies suggest that diets rich in these compounds lower the risk of breast cancer. Unusual properties also apply to the drug tamoxifen, which is used to treat breast cancer. It has antiestrogenic effects on breast tissue but estrogenic effects on uterine tissue.[13]

When estrogens and antiestrogens enter the body through diet and drinking water, scientists suspect they may act additively, synergistically, or even antagonistically to alter estrogen levels.[14] The conceptual leap underlying the hypothesis that alterations in estrogen levels may cause more alarming reproductive and carcinogenic effects stems from early research on wildlife. Rachel Carson's landmark 1962 book *Silent Spring* brought to national prominence DDT's devastating consequences for bird reproduction. An overwhelming reduction in the alligator population of Florida's Lake Apopka has been traced by researchers to an extensive spill of DDT and other pesticides in the early 1980s. Young female alligators had abnormal ovaries and twice the estrogen levels of their normal counterparts, young males had unusually low testosterone levels, and more mature males had abnormally small penises. All these developments were consequences of marked endocrine disruption.[15] These and other accidental spills attest to some of the potentially irreversible effects of environmental toxins on wildlife and their offspring.

The human consequences of environmental spills also have been poignantly documented. Episodes of PCB contamination in Taiwan have led to adverse health effects in children born to women who consumed the PCB-contaminated rice oil. The consequences have ranged from IQ and behavioral deficits to alterations in genitalia. Women exposed to a similar type of PCB contamination in Japan have elevated breast cancer rates.[16] Although tragic, environmental spills can serve to generate, but not typically to confirm, scientific hypotheses. More rigorous research depends on experimental studies in animals and on epidemiological studies in humans.

A recent, widely cited epidemiological study in New York linked DDT, but not PCBs, to breast cancer.[17] It demonstrated that 58 women with the disease had significantly higher levels of DDE in their blood. Their blood had been sampled and stored up to 6 months before they developed breast cancer. The women were matched to control subjects to exclude the possibility that known risk factors, such as age and family history, could have explained the findings.

An even larger epidemiological study, conducted in San Francisco and reported a year later, did not find elevated breast cancer risk in relation to either DDE or PCBs.[18] There were hints of an elevation in breast cancer rates with higher levels of DDE in two of three subgroups (white and African American but not Asian women), but the findings lacked statistical significance. This study of 150 women had the advantage of using blood samples from up to 20 years before diagnosis, a time when DDT was still in use and when cancer induction could have begun. (Scientists think cancer involves a series of molecular changes to DNA that take place over the course of many years before a tumor eventually develops.) The DDE levels averaged across all San Francisco blood samples taken in the late 1960s were four to five times higher than those in the New York study, in which blood was drawn just months before diagnosis in the late 1980s and early 1990s. Despite higher levels of DDE in women in the San Francisco study—which should have induced more cases of breast cancer—there was no relationship between breast cancer and DDE levels. Thus, the San Francisco findings suggesting that DDE did not play an important role conflicted with the New York study.

Those who doubt the role of environmental estrogens point out that the dose and the estrogen-like potency can be so weak—sometimes thousands of times less than the action of estrogen itself—that the impact is negligible.[19] Estrogen-like effects can be measured relatively easily in new cell culture assays. Environmental agents can be tested for their ability to stimulate cell division of human breast cancer cells: in a recent study, three pesticides were found to enhance cell division but at a rate six orders of magnitude lower than estrogen.[20]

Many scientists view as provocative, yet unresolved, the possible association between estrogen-like agents and breast cancer. Conflicting findings almost always occur as new scientific leads emerge. Important answers may come from a large prospective study of the environmental causes of breast cancer now under way at the Long Island Breast Cancer Study Project. Results of this study, sponsored by the National Cancer Institute, are expected by the late 1990s. In addition, new research identifying the mutated gene in the inherited form of breast cancer may lead to genetic insights.

Dioxin

Dioxin is one of the most controversial environmental pollutants. A contaminant of the now-banned herbicide Agent Orange, it became notorious because of its use during the Vietnam War. Veterans exposed to Agent Orange complained of a variety of illnesses ranging from skin conditions to leukemia and lymphoma. For years, their complaints were dismissed until research findings began to provide legitimacy to some of their concerns.[21]

Dioxin is found in the environment now as a contaminant of organochlorine pesticides, in waste water from paper and pulp companies, and in air and soil from incineration, auto exhaust, and industrial uses.[22] Although research done in the past 20 years has shown dioxin to be a carcinogen, neurotoxin, immunotoxin, and reproductive toxin in animals, its effects in humans have been elusive. Recent investigation has shown that high levels of dioxin exposure contribute to a variety of human cancers, including respiratory cancer, soft tissue sarcoma, and liver cancer.[23] The occupations and environments that provide high exposure affect few women, and, therefore, few have been studied. A small study of German workers did show females who were exposed to dioxin at work had higher rates of breast cancer, but interpretation of the study was limited by the problem of other chemical exposures.

Research Advances

Dioxin refers to a class of more than 200 compounds, the most potent of which is TCDD, or 2,3,7,8-tetrachlorodibenzo-p-dioxin. Also included in this class are the furans, which are contaminants formed in the manufacture of PCBs. Dioxins and furans are undesirable by-products of manufacturing or combustion.

It is now well established that dioxin's actions in the body can occur only after dioxin interacts with a special receptor inside the cell, called the Ah (or aryl hydrocarbon) receptor. Following dioxin's binding to this receptor, critical changes occur, such as altered gene expression.[24]

Dioxin is somewhat unusual in having both estrogenic and antiestrogenic effects, depending on the species, target tissue, dose, or timing of exposure during development. One of its estrogenic effects is to feminize adult male animals.[25] Yet one of dioxin's most significant antiestrogenic effects is to block the growth of breast cancer cells in a test tube, in the presence or absence of estrogen.[26] This is an important finding because of the treatment implications; researchers are eager to find out how this antiestrogenic effect occurs and whether similar, but less toxic, compounds might be useful therapeutic agents for humans. After binding to the Ah receptor and activating certain gene sequences, dioxin can exert antiestrogenic effects in a variety of ways. One way is to enhance the action of enzymes responsible for metabolizing estrogen. Another way is to decrease the number of estrogen receptors, which in turn lowers the effective amount of estrogen in the body. Reductions in estrogen levels might possibly explain the findings of an animal study in which long-term dioxin exposure led to *fewer* uterine and mammary gland tumors.[27]

Dioxin has been recently linked to endometriosis, a poorly understood condition that causes pain and infertility in 5 million women in the United States. Tissue from the uterine lining migrates outside the uterus—to the fallopian tubes, ovaries, the abdomen, and beyond. The migration may take place as a result of a heightened immune system reaction—possibly an autoimmune disorder, but scientists do not understand the mechanism. Few risk factors had been identified until recently, when research on rhesus monkeys demonstrated that prolonged dietary exposure to dioxin led to endometriosis.[28] Up to 10 years after discontinuing the dioxin exposure, endometriosis was detected in the animals in a dose-response fashion—that is, the higher the dose, the greater the response or effect. Dose-response is one of the hallmarks used to establish the cause of a condition. Seventy-one percent of the animals exposed to the greatest dose of dioxin (25 parts per trillion) developed endometriosis, in comparison with 43% exposed to the lowest dose and an even smaller percentage of unexposed control animals.

The *extent* of human exposure to dioxin is the topic of intense research, and the *significance* of the exposure generates incendiary debate. The average estimated adult intake, mostly from beef and dairy products, is exceedingly small—in the picogram range—yet studies suggest that it exceeds the safe level that the Environmental Protection Agency (EPA) has established. Breast-feeding may expose infants to dioxin in amounts dependent on the mother's level. In a recent comprehensive eight-volume draft report that reassesses the risks of dioxin, EPA estimates that infants who are breast-fed for 1 year receive 4% to 12% of their total lifetime dioxin exposure through contaminated breast milk.[29] It is an unfortunate irony that lactating women can lower dioxin levels in their breasts by up to 50% through transfer to their infants. EPA's draft report concludes that dioxin should still be considered a "probable" human carcinogen, the second highest carcinogen rating.

Continued research on dioxin is needed to determine its relationship to endometriosis, its interaction with estrogen, and its effects on infants exposed through mothers' breast milk.

Prescription Drugs

Women are heavy consumers of prescription drugs, many of which can prolong life and improve its quality. Even though drugs undergo rigorous evaluation before they are allowed on the market, it is often difficult and expensive to test for long-term effects on women, particularly pregnant women, and on the unborn. Even if serious, long-term effects are identified after a drug has been approved for sale, the overall benefits may still supersede the risks.

Diethylstilbestrol

DES, a potent, estrogen-like, synthetic drug, was prescribed for more than three decades to an estimated 4 million women to prevent miscarriage.[30] It was withdrawn from the market for use during pregnancy in 1971 after a study was published showing that the daughters who were exposed to DES in utero developed a rare form of vaginal and cervical cancer. Later, researchers determined this consequence occurred in approximately 1 in 1,000 women.[31] Daughters exposed to DES also experience anatomical changes to the reproductive tract, menstrual irregularities, and poorer pregnancy outcomes, including miscarriage, ectopic pregnancies, and premature delivery. Based on animal models, DES exposure may be associated with breast cancer, but evidence in humans is thus far lacking. In addition to its use during pregnancy, DES was mixed into the feed of cows and poultry to promote growth. An estimated 13 tons were added annually until 1980, when the U.S. Food and Drug Administration (FDA) prohibited its use in food-producing animals.[32] Excess contamination of food with DES has, in at least one episode, led to precocious puberty in young girls and boys.[33]

Research Advances

It was the pioneering research on DES that stimulated investigation of the entire field of environmental estrogens. Recognition that a synthetic compound might mimic the effect of estrogen in the body and cause harm has spawned many new areas of inquiry. Substances as unrelated as plant estrogens, pesticides, and plastics are now under scrutiny for estrogenic effects similar to those of DES.

DES is somewhat unusual because it is even more potent than the body's own estrogen, in contrast to most other estrogen-like substances, whose effects are weaker. The DES story was special as well because its deleterious effects were first discovered in humans. Because DES caused a rare form of vaginal cancer in young women—a population not considered at risk for cancer—tracing the cancer to its cause was relatively straightforward. In most epidemiological research, however, the difficulty of linking a chemical exposure to common cancers is stymied because many factors may be responsible. For example, it is difficult to know the nature and extent of the exposure, and often the biological mechanism is unknown.

DES research has burgeoned as a result of the development and re-finement of animal models. In fact, some of DES's effects in humans—anatomical abnormalities in boys exposed during gestation—were identified on the basis of predictions from research on rodents and mammals.[34] The confluence of epidemiology and animal research has estab-lished the DES story as a model for examining an environmental toxin.

Although the threat of widespread DES exposure has been elimi-nated, DES research will be exceedingly valuable in helping to deter-mine its role in causing disease later in life. For example, DES daughters have yet to reach menopause, when other cancers, such as those of the breast and endometrium, more typically occur. Because these cancers have been identified in animals after DES exposure, it is critical to de-termine whether daughters exposed to DES face higher risks than other older women. If DES produces heritable changes to DNA, then a third generation of offspring also may be at risk. Further research is needed, especially at the molecular level, to clarify the range of DES effects and to apply this knowledge to the study of other environmental estrogens.

Fertility Drugs

As increasing numbers of women postpone childbearing, more women rely on fertility drugs to counteract the current epidemic of infertility among the baby-boom generation, individuals born between 1946 and 1964. The most common fertility drugs are clomiphene and human menopausal gonadotropin drugs that stimulate the development of eggs in the ovaries.

Case reports have suggested the possibility that these agents cause ovarian cancer, but it was not until the publication of recent epide-miological studies that the association became somewhat firmer. Al-though ovarian cancer is rare—an estimated 26,700 women will be given this diagnosis in 1996—it is the leading cause of death from a gynecological malignancy; the American Cancer Society estimates that 14,800 women will die from this disease in 1996. Among the few established risk factors are family history and not having children.

Because there are no early symptoms, diagnosis is often too late for effective treatment.[35]

Research Advances

The largest and most recent study of the impact of fertility drugs was conducted on 4,000 infertile women living in the state of Washington.[36] The study found women who had used clomiphene *for more than a year* had 11 times the risk of developing ovarian cancer than infertile women who did not use the drug. Neither clomiphene use for less than 1 year nor any use of human menopausal gonadotropin elevated the risk of ovarian cancer. It is fortunate that almost 80% of the women taking clomiphene in the study used it for less than 1 year. Because the study was limited in size, with only 11 documented ovarian tumors, the National Institute of Child Health and Human Development is underwriting a much larger study; results will be available in 1998. This new study of 12,000 women will examine the effects of fertility drugs on the development of ovarian cancer, breast cancer, and fetal malformations, among other serious effects.

Lead

Lead is a well-recognized environmental health hazard. Young children are most sensitive to lead's harmful, often irreversible, consequences. Even low exposure levels cause intellectual and behavioral deficits in youngsters, who are more vulnerable to the effects of this metal because their nervous systems are still developing. Adults, with their fully developed nervous systems, are less susceptible because they absorb and retain less lead than children do. However, with sufficient exposure that results in high blood lead levels, adults can experience ill effects. At the highest blood levels, now exceedingly rare, individuals can experience coma and seizures, whereas moderate to high levels can cause lethargy, fatigue, irritability, kidney damage, hypertension, and impaired fertility. Low-level effects are less noticeable in adults. In short, the higher the blood level of lead, the more damage occurs. There is no "safe" dose for adults or children.[37]

Bone is the largest repository for lead in the body, containing more than 95% of the cumulative lifetime environmental lead exposure.[38] Hormonal changes during pregnancy, lactation, and menopause appear to mobilize lead stored in the bone,[39] from which it can be released into blood. Thus, during these periods women can be at risk for the ill effects of lead, depending on the dose. Because lead crosses the placenta and is secreted in breast milk, the fetus and the nursing child also are vulnerable.

Banning lead from gasoline, paint, and plumbing has been one of the premier public health achievements of the past two decades. With less lead in the air and in drinking water, the average blood level in the population now is about 3 micrograms per deciliter, a 78% decline since 1976. Nevertheless, the Centers for Disease Control and Prevention estimates that there are still 1.7 million young children with elevated lead levels, defined as more than 10 micrograms per deciliter of blood. About 2% of reproductive-age women and 6% of elderly persons have elevated blood lead levels, but only a small fraction of each group has significantly elevated levels of 25 micrograms per deciliter or more. Blood lead levels follow a pattern over the life span: they are highest in childhood, lowest in adolescence, and then rise again with age.

Lead persists in the environment because it neither decays nor disintegrates. Thus, although it was eliminated from paint in 1978, lead is still present in older buildings in which lead-based paint was used. When lead-based paint deteriorates, as it does in poorly maintained older housing, it presents the gravest threat to children. This is because the flaking paint chips eventually crumble into a fine layer of dust that can be inhaled or ingested. The soil in urban and some rural areas also is contaminated by past deposits of lead from gasoline combustion. Poor nutrition—mostly deficiencies in calcium and iron—increases lead absorption. Despite progress in reducing new deposits of lead in the environment, earlier sources of lead remain and enter the body through different pathways. All of this explains why lead poisoning is a continuing threat to the poor, particularly in the inner cities.

In addition to lead exposure at home, women and men face further lead exposure in the workplace, particularly in smelting, battery manufacturing, and typesetting. Occupational exposure to lead also occurs in the production of art supplies, ceramics, textiles, and inks.

Research Advances

Scientists used to think that once lead accumulated in the bone it was inert and immobile. New research indicates, however, that there is a dynamic turnover of minerals in the bone, allowing the slow release of lead into the blood throughout life,[40] which can be accelerated with the explosive hormonal increases during pregnancy and lactation or their decrease during menopause. Scientists think that lead acts like, and even replaces, calcium. For example, when a woman needs extra calcium during pregnancy and lactation to sustain the growth and nourishment of her fetus, and she does not consume enough calcium in her diet, her body will compensate by drawing on calcium stored in her skeleton and teeth. Because lead can replace calcium in the bone, she may summon lead instead.[41] Lead stores mobilized from bone can be redistributed by the blood to lead's target organs, especially in the brain, heart, and kidney. Lead remaining in the bone is unlikely to be innocuous, possibly impairing bone function and contributing to disorders such as osteoporosis.[42]

The evidence for lead mobilization in humans comes from case studies and population-based research. In one case study, a woman and her fetus sustained serious lead toxicity during pregnancy despite the absence of current lead exposure. Researchers traced the lead toxicity to the mother's elevated lead exposure 30 years before. Scientists conducting a new study of more than 100 pregnant women living in Mexico City sampled their blood throughout their pregnancies.[43] Although lead levels in the women's blood declined somewhat during the early months, most likely the result of increased blood volume, lead levels increased predictably from the 20th week to delivery. The investigators attributed the rise to mobilization of bone lead and to increased absorption of dietary lead, which is still a problem in developing countries.

The mobilization of bone lead after menopause also has been inferred from population-based studies. Postmenopausal women have higher levels of lead in their blood than do premenopausal women. Childbearing has some protective effect because postmenopausal women who have had children have lower blood lead levels than postmenopausal women who have not.[44] These findings suggest that prior pregnancies deplete some of the bone lead deposits, leaving less reserve to be remobilized at or after menopause. A recently published study of white women older than 65 found the highest blood lead levels in the oldest women and in the women who lived in urban areas. Older women who had ever breast-fed their babies or who were taking ERT, which inhibits bone loss, had the lowest lead levels.[45]

Although public health measures have been successful at reducing lead exposure, children, pregnant and lactating women, and the elderly are still at risk. The mobilization of lead stores during pregnancy and lactation is especially worrisome because lead's adverse effects affect intelligence and behavior in children receiving lead in utero or through breast milk. Pregnant, lactating, and older women should be educated about the enhanced need for dietary calcium, which prevents both the greater absorption of environmental lead and the higher release of lead from bone. Steps to avoid lead exposure include testing for lead in drinking water and maintaining older housing with lead-based paint in good repair.

Smoking

The health consequences of cigarette smoking cannot be overstated. Smoking is responsible for about 30% of all cancers and approximately 90% of lung cancers. Lung cancer is now the leading cause of cancer deaths in both men and women; it surpassed breast cancer as the primary cause of cancer mortality in women for the first time in 1987 (see Figure 8–2). In fact, between 1973 and 1991, the death rate for lung cancer in women surged by more than 100%, rising more quickly than any other type of cancer death. Women accounted for 78,100 of the 177,000 cases of lung cancer diagnosed in 1996 and for 64,300 of the 158,700 deaths from this disease. These statistics are particularly horrendous in view of the fact that smoking-related cancers are preventable.

In 1991, about 23% of women in the United States smoked, a 30% decrease from female smoking prevalence in 1960. However, there was a whopping 46% decline among men during the same period, which went from 52% who smoked in 1960 to only 28% in 1991. Most alarmingly, the prevalence of women smokers increased from 1990 to 1991 by 0.7%, the first increase in 10 years.[46]

Smoking begins in adolescence: teenagers account for more than 90% of new smokers. This is why the tobacco industry, which spends

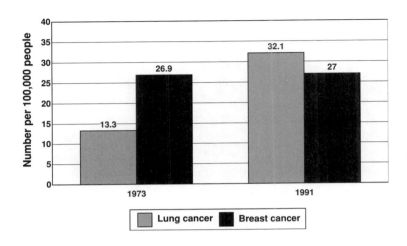

Figure 8–2.   Growth in lung and breast cancer deaths in women, 1973–1991. *Source.* National Cancer Institute Surveillance, Epidemiology, and End Results Program.

billions of dollars on advertising and promotional activities, targets adolescents, particularly at sporting events. Throughout the 1980s, more female than male high school seniors smoked, but by 1993, the rates for male and female smokers in this age group were the same, stabilizing at between 18% and 19% of all high school seniors. To combat this regular and potentially lethal use of tobacco, we need to implement policies aimed at decreasing or eliminating teenagers' access to tobacco products, self-service displays, and vending machines and to increase significantly the cost of tobacco products. Health education for adolescents and the elimination of seductive advertising are critically important measures to prevent smoking.

We know that smoking causes lung, esophageal, and bladder cancer, chronic obstructive pulmonary disease (COPD), and coronary heart disease (CHD). Less appreciated are the risks from smoking to women's reproductive health and the health of their children, which include reduced fertility, pregnancy complications, premature birth, low-birthweight infants, stillbirth, infant mortality, and increased childhood respiratory disease. Women smokers who use oral contraceptives face dramatically elevated risks of heart attack and stroke.

Research Advances

Researchers are exploring the reasons that young people, especially females, begin to smoke. Investigators estimate that the initiation of tobacco use takes about 3 years. Although starting to smoke is highly dependent on the accessibility of tobacco products and on tobacco advertising, the vulnerability of adolescents plays a large role. Studies have unveiled a host of personal risk factors, particularly low self-image, low self-esteem, and a lack of ability to refuse offers from peers.[47] Not surprisingly, the images from tobacco advertising present smokers as confident, attractive, and secure—images that are powerfully attractive to adolescents.

School-based health education programs are most effective when they cultivate self-esteem, promote assertiveness, and model refusal responses. Other effective strategies are raising the price of cigarettes, enforcing laws prohibiting the sale of tobacco to minors, and restricting smoking in schools, workplaces, and communities.

Women may be more susceptible than men to the deleterious effects of cigarette smoking, according to a recent epidemiological study of male and female smokers.[48] In comparison with nonsmokers, women with a history of 40 pack-years of smoking were found to be more likely to get lung cancer than men with the same smoking history. Researchers do not know the reason for the difference, although the finding that some lung tumors have estrogen and progesterone receptors is stimulating research on how female hormones contribute to tumor growth. Other research is exploring the role of women's smaller size and lung capacity.

Sunlight

Ultraviolet radiation from sunlight is a major culprit in skin cancer. The most common skin cancers, basal cell and squamous cell carcinoma, are directly linked to ultraviolet B radiation. Sunlight also is implicated in the development of melanoma, a skin cancer arising from the melanocytes, or pigment cells, in the skin. Scientists do not know which of the two types of ultraviolet radiation reaching the earth, ultraviolet A or B, is linked to melanoma.

Melanoma is rarer than other skin cancers but it is far more lethal, accounting for two-thirds of skin cancer deaths. Basal cell carcinomas are more common and less invasive than squamous cell carcinoma. These nonmelanoma skin cancers are usually found on the face, head, and neck—the parts of the body most likely to be exposed to sunlight. They accounted for an estimated 2,100 deaths in 1995.

Melanoma is growing at a striking rate, second only to increases in lung cancer. From 1973 to 1991, the incidence of melanoma skyrocketed by 75% in females (see Figure 8–3). Whites are at a much greater risk than African Americans: the incidence for whites is 13.2 per 100,000 compared with 0.8 per 100,000 in African Americans.[49] Surgical removal of melanoma is the standard therapy, and survival depends on how far the cancer has infiltrated. Superficial invasion carries a 75% to 100% 5-year survival rate, but when infiltration reaches greater depths, the survival rate plummets to about 20%.

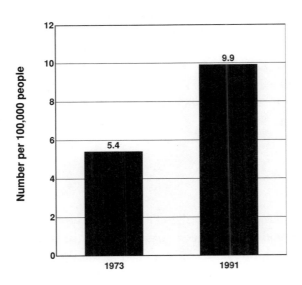

Figure 8–3.   Growth in melanoma incidence in women, 1973–1991. *Source.* National Cancer Institute Surveillance, Epidemiology, and End Results Program.

Research Advances

The mechanism by which sunlight causes or accelerates the development of skin cancer is somewhat uncertain, but, for melanoma in particular, molecular biologists have amassed increasing evidence of mutations in the genes that suppress tumors.[50] A mutation to a tumor suppressor gene can reduce the cell's ability to halt cell growth and division, thereby leaving it more vulnerable to cancer. Researchers have recently found that ultraviolet radiation of human skin cells leaves a distinct and reproducible mutation in a portion of a tumor suppressor gene called p53, and they have found mutations in other tumor suppressor genes.[51]

The incidence of basal cell and squamous cell carcinoma increases in proportion to total sunlight exposure. In contrast, melanoma is associated with intermittent rather than cumulative exposure to sunlight. A one-time event years earlier, which produced severe sunburn and blistering, can be enough to start the cancer process. People with fair skin who burn easily are at highest risk for melanoma.[52]

The greatest ultraviolet exposure occurs during the summer months between 11:00 A.M. and 1:00 P.M. Although latitude or distance from the equator primarily dictates the amount of radiation, altitude and ozone also play a role. The higher the altitude and the thinner the stratospheric ozone layer, the greater the exposure. Sunscreens that block ultraviolet radiation can reduce the incidence of skin tumors in animals. This has prompted public health authorities to recommend that people use sunscreens. It is also wise to avoid prolonged sunlight exposure to prevent future cases of skin cancer.

Electromagnetic Fields

The debate over whether electromagnetic fields (EMFs) cause cancer is one of the most polarized environmental controversies of the decade. Much is at stake because every segment of the population is exposed to EMFs, which come from power lines, home wiring, electrical appliances, video display terminals, and other sources. Even in the absence of scientific consensus, the economic implications are staggering: property values near existing power lines have already been devalued, the location of new power lines is being challenged, and the cost of electrical power may rise.[53]

The scientific community is profoundly divided because of a plethora of conflicting studies. Yet a mounting body of evidence exists tying EMFs to cancer—in children and adults, at home, and in the workplace. The first link in this chain was a landmark 1979 epidemiological study of EMF exposure in children living near power lines in Denver.[54] The weight of the research suggests, but does not confirm, a causal association between EMFs and leukemia, brain cancer, male breast cancer, and, possibly, breast cancer in women.[55] The link between EMFs and reproductive abnormalities is weak, although this also is an active area of research.[56]

EMFs linked to human disease are produced during the generation, distribution, and consumption of electrical power. Although EMFs have both electrical and magnetic components, scientists are now focusing primarily on the magnetic constituent, measured in milligauss, because it penetrates buildings without weakening, thereby creating the opportunity for exposure inside homes near power lines. The strength of the magnetic component of the field is related to the strength of the current but is inversely related to the distance. A high-current–carrying wire or appliance produces an elevated magnetic field right next to it, but the strength diminishes with distance. Although power lines produce high EMFs within about a 120-feet radius, electrical appliances—which are point sources rather than line sources—generate EMFs whose strength falls off rapidly with distance, usually within 1 to 5 feet.[57]

Much of the controversy surrounding EMFs stems from the difficulty of explaining how biological effects can occur. Critics contend that EMFs are too weak to break chemical bonds and damage DNA, the mechanism by which ionizing radiation, for example, causes cancer. EMFs are not ionizing. Proponents of the concept that EMFs can have adverse health effects point to more subtle biochemical changes that may lead to cancer. Biochemical alterations are produced by EMFs in the test tube and in animals, some of which are described later. Proponents point to the fact that the public health establishment concluded there was a causal relationship between smoking and cancer before they discovered a viable mechanism to explain how this happened.

Research Advances

Research is proceeding worldwide to determine whether EMFs cause cancer and adverse reproductive effects. Much of the epidemiological investigation has focused on residential exposures in children and occupational exposures in men. In some studies, exposures above 2 milligauss have been associated with a two- to fivefold increase in risk of cancer.[58] If research shows a possible association between EMFs and breast cancer, it would have enormous implications for women because breast cancer is so common, with a higher incidence than that of all the other cancers—leukemia, brain cancer, and lymphoma—that may be related to EMF exposure.[59]

Several occupational studies of men have found that electrical workers face a higher risk of male breast cancer, a rare condition found in the same cell types that are cancerous in females.[60] But, until recently, there was little research on EMF-related breast cancer in women. A new study by researchers in North Carolina has found an increase in breast cancer mortality among women in electrical occupations: female engineers, electrical line workers, and telephone installers faced about a 40% increased risk of dying from breast cancer in comparison with women employed in other occupations.[61]

However provocative these findings are, even the authors of this study acknowledge its limitations, which include the lack of exposure information, the possibility of occupational exposures other than EMFs, and the fact that increased risks were not found among female workers in related occupations, such as computer operators and programmers. An earlier study of women who routinely used electrical blankets, which generate high fields, did not find a relationship between EMFs and breast cancer. New research under way in Seattle may shed light on this issue. The study compares women with breast cancer with a control group of women without the disease to determine whether their EMF exposure profiles are different. Investigators will measure EMF residential levels and use personal dosimeters, which document exposure both inside and outside the home. They also will measure the women's levels of the hormone melatonin, which is produced at night by the pineal gland in the brain. Scientists know that EMF exposure suppresses the production of melatonin in animals. Because one of melatonin's many actions in the body is to inhibit tumor formation, if EMF exposure also suppresses melatonin levels in women, it might promote cancer by counteracting the beneficial effects of this hormone.[62]

Research has confirmed that melatonin by itself curtails the high rate of growth of breast cancer cells in tissue culture. The cells continue to divide and increase in number, but at a slower pace. This favorable outcome is blocked when the culture dishes are then bathed in EMFs: the breast cancer cells continue to proliferate at their normally high rate as if no melatonin were present. In contrast, when the breast cancer cells are exposed only to EMFs, there is no effect on their high rate of growth. The conclusion is that EMFs' deleterious action on breast cancer cells operates through melatonin.[63] A related but preliminary study in culture has shown that EMFs negate the beneficial, growth-inhibiting actions of tamoxifen on breast cancer cells.[64] Tamoxifen is the most widely used hormonal treatment for breast cancer.

Given the dearth of regulatory guidance from the federal government, and the possible relationship between EMF and cancer, individuals might adopt a policy of "prudent avoidance" of EMF exposure. Women and men should take reasonable action to prevent unnecessary exposure, such as moving a clock radio away from the head at night, stepping back from heavy appliances while in use, and testing areas of the home, school, and work environment where prolonged EMF exposure might occur.

Occupational Hazards

Women experience myriad injuries and disorders in the workplace, among them musculoskeletal injuries and reproductive disorders. This section highlights several workplace hazards that are responsible for these common conditions.

Computer Keyboards

Extended use of the computer keyboard is one of the leading causes of carpal tunnel syndrome (CTS). The condition is characterized by tingling, pain, or numbness in the hands and wrist and may progress to loss of grip and other hand impairments. The underlying problem is compression of the median nerve supplying the hand, a result of highly repetitive hand-wrist movements, awkward wrist positions, and vibration. These movements inflame the ligaments and tendons in the wrist, causing pressure to build up in the small tunnel through which the median nerve passes en route to the hand. No nationwide data exist on the prevalence of CTS, but several studies suggest a higher prevalence among women and an overall incidence of 125 cases per 100,000 people.[65] One authority states that CTS affects three times as many women as men because women hold most of the jobs requiring repetitive motion.[66] The occurrence of CTS in the workplace appears to be skyrocketing as a result of growing reliance on computer keyboards. In addition to keyboard operators, other female-dominated occupations at risk are waitresses, textile workers, supermarket checkers, and dental hygienists. Assembly line workers also may be at risk.

Much of the research on CTS has focused on new treatments. Non-surgical therapies include rest, splinting the wrist, anti-inflammatory drugs, and steroid injections into the wrist. Steroid injections appear to provide complete relief for about 50% to 60% of patients for up to 6 months. Although patients with severe symptoms are the least likely to benefit from steroid injections, they are usually candidates for carpal tunnel release surgery, which is effective in about 80% of cases. A new type of surgery, using an endoscope, a device similar to that used in knee surgery, is less invasive than conventional surgery and may facilitate a quicker recovery. Although there has been marked improvement in awareness of CTS and in use of wrist rests next to keyboards to minimize awkward wrist positions that cause nerve compression, there have been virtually no carefully controlled studies of new, ergonomic keyboard designs to determine whether they can prevent or at least reduce the severity of CTS.

Anesthetic Gases

Anesthetic gases have long been suspected of causing spontaneous abortions and infertility in women. There is strong animal and some human evidence of reproductive impairment following administration of nitrous oxide, one of the most common anesthetic gases. Other anesthetic gases include halothane, enflurane, and cyclopropane. An estimated 214,000 health care workers are at risk, including nurse anesthetists, anesthesiologists, surgeons, operating room nurses, dentists, dental assistants, and other health care personnel. The degree of exposure depends on the frequency of use, anesthetic technique, scavenging devices, and ventilation systems. A 1992 study of dental assistants found that those exposed to nitrous oxide for more than 5 hours a week were less than half as likely as unexposed women to become pregnant during each menstrual cycle.[67]

The chemical sterilizer, ethylene oxide, is used in medical settings to disinfect instruments and other equipment. An estimated 139,000 hospital and industrial workers may be exposed, according to estimates prepared by the National Institute of Occupational Safety and Health. Like anesthetic gases, the degree of exposure will depend on the design of equipment in which the sterilization is conducted and the type of ventilation system. Ethylene oxide causes cancer in animals, but evidence for human carcinogenicity is limited. One study found that exposed female hospital workers faced an increase in spontaneous abortions.[68]

For all these workplace hazards, a vigorous commitment to research is essential. Prevention should be a key priority. In the realm of computer technology, we need to know much more about the possible benefits of ergonomic seating, good posture, supported wrist position, and well-designed keyboards and what part each would play in reducing the chance of developing CTS. Similarly, improved ventilation and scavenging systems can reduce occupational exposure to anesthetic gases and chemical sterilizers in medical settings.

Nutrition

Despite a wholesome and copious food supply and an awareness of good nutritional habits, women's nutrition is out of kilter—too many calories, too much fat, and too little calcium and iron. These excesses and imbalances place women, especially poor women, at risk for a litany of disorders. Elevated fat intake is associated with high blood pressure, coronary artery disease, diabetes, and colon cancer. Inadequate calcium intake, particularly before age 25 when the body is best able to absorb it, is associated with a greater risk of osteoporosis later in life. Insufficient iron intake can lead to anemia, but this is a rare condition in the United States, affecting only 3.5% of the population. During pregnancy, women need to supplement their diets with iron, usually 30 to 60 milligrams a day, and vegetarians may have to do so because plant iron is less absorbable by the body than iron from animal sources. Insufficient quantities of calcium and iron also contribute to increased absorption of environmental lead, especially during pregnancy and lactation.

Obesity—excess body fat—is generally defined as being 20% above one's ideal weight. It affects about one-fourth of the population and is more common in women than men. Obesity's prevalence and trends are best gauged by the National Health and Nutrition Examination Surveys. Performed periodically since 1960, these surveys have revealed the percentage of overweight women to have increased from 26% to 35%. Increases were observed in all age categories, especially ages 50 to 59. The prevalence is highest among African American women, 50% of whom were overweight in 1991[69] (see Chapter 7).

A societal preoccupation with thinness and dieting has contributed to the eating disorders, such as anorexia nervosa and bulimia, which disproportionately afflict female adolescents. Estimates for anorexia nervosa from hospitalized cases and psychiatric registers in the United States and western Europe are 15 per 100,000 women and, among the most susceptible age group of 15- to 25-year-olds, 76 per 100,000 women. Ninety-five percent of patients with anorexia are women. The incidence of bulimia is 1% of adolescent and young women in the United States and 4.5% of college freshmen.[70]

The hallmarks of anorexia nervosa are extreme weight loss, electrolyte imbalance, and, in severe cases, the possibility of death by starvation. Anorexia nervosa's mortality rate of 15% to 21% is among the highest for any psychiatric disorder.[71] Bulimia occurs in half of the patients with anorexia nervosa and is marked by recurrent episodes of binge eating, only to be terminated by abdominal pain and self-induced vomiting. Apart from nutritional deficiencies, dieting can serve to mobilize environmental contaminants stored in body fat.

Research Advances

Research has demonstrated that even a modest weight loss in obese people lowers their risk of hypertension, cardiovascular disease, and diabetes and improves their self-esteem.[72] Body weight, a highly heritable characteristic, appears to be more influenced by genetics than by diet and exercise, but they also play important roles. After years of searching for the genes governing obesity, scientists have recently cloned and sequenced in mice at least one such gene,[73] which is nearly identical to its human analogue. Called *ob* for obesity, the gene codes for a protein released by fat tissue. Scientists postulate that this protein regulates fat storage by signaling the brain's hypothalamus to suppress appetite. Extremely obese mice have a mutation in the *ob* gene that inactivates the gene's protein product. Without the active protein, researchers think the message to the brain is lost, inducing the animal to eat to excess. Much work remains to be done on this gene and related genes, but this line of research offers the tantalizing prospect of treating obesity with the protein product of the *ob* gene (see Chapter 7).

Obesity is a remarkably stubborn condition and does not yield easily to conventional weight loss programs. People do lose weight with weight-management programs, but more than 90% usually regain the lost weight within 1 to 5 years. Some drug treatments on the market have shown promise in clinical trials. Long-term treatment for more 6 months with several agents, including phentermine, mazindol, fenfluramine, dexfenfluramine, and fluoxetine, has allowed obese individuals to reduce weight by more than 5%, with little weight regained.[74] None of these drugs is addictive, in contrast to earlier drug therapies. Physicians are encouraging the FDA to permit long-term use of these drugs in light of their effectiveness and few side effects. Currently, their use to treat obesity is limited by the FDA to 3 months.

Because poor nutrition contributes to preventable illness and premature death, women should try to follow the recommended dietary allowances (RDAs) of the National Research Council. To achieve and maintain weight loss, women should exercise regularly, reduce the number of daily calories consumed, reduce fat intake to no more than 30% of total calories, increase the amount of calcium in their diets, and, if their bodies' iron stores are deficient, raise their iron intake. Further research is needed to expand understanding of the role of genetics and diet in obesity and other eating disorders.

Substance Abuse

Substance abuse exacts a greater toll on society than any other health problem. The medical, productivity, and crime-related costs of alcohol and illicit drug abuse reached $160 billion in 1990, overshadowing cancer, respiratory disease, and heart disease.[75] About one-third of the expense of the criminal justice system—police protection, drug traffic control, and judicial services—is attributed to substance abuse. Alcohol abuse accounts for 50% of all homicides, 30% of suicides, and 30% of accidental deaths. Substance abuse is both a cause and an effect of homelessness.

The use of illicit drugs (cocaine, marijuana, opiates) affects an estimated 11.4 million people, and another 10 million have an alcohol-related problem. Women constitute about 1.5 million of those using illicit drugs and 4.4 million of problem drinkers. Women between ages 18 and 25 years have the highest rates of substance abuse.[76]

Although women's use of alcohol and drugs is not as great as men's, the health consequences can be more severe: women using intravenous drugs or prostituting themselves to purchase drugs can, and do, contract the human immunodeficiency virus (HIV) and transmit it to their fetuses and sexual partners. Drinking during pregnancy can cause fetal alcohol syndrome in infants, resulting in physical abnormalities and mental retardation, and using drugs during pregnancy can result in babies born with behavioral and neurological abnormalities.

Research Advances

Studies have repeatedly shown that treatment, including counseling and pharmacological therapies, not only is effective but also saves money. Every dollar invested in drug abuse treatment, for example, yields $4, and sometimes more, in societal benefits, such as reduced crime, enhanced productivity, and lower health care costs.[77] Despite the resounding effectiveness of drug and alcohol treatment programs, women are reluctant to enter treatment. Because of significant barriers, when they do enter treatment they have more serious disabilities.[78] One barrier is the threat of potential or imminent loss of child custody. Other impediments are stigma, perception of sexual promiscuity, and lack of transportation and child care.[79]

Research on the physiological, behavioral, and social factors involved in female substance abuse and willingness to seek treatment is in its infancy. Much of the investigation conducted thus far has come from studies of alcoholism. For instance, women have higher blood alcohol concentrations than men after consuming comparable amounts of alcohol, and women are more prone to alcohol-related liver damage. Although some of the gender difference is attributed to women's smaller body size, other factors may be involved. Women have a lower activity of the enzyme alcohol dehydrogenase, which is responsible for alcohol metabolism in the stomach. This means that women have higher blood alcohol levels because they cannot eliminate alcohol as quickly as men can.[80]

Social and behavioral factors contribute to the severity of the consequences of substance abuse. Women substance abusers are more likely to lose their jobs, probably as a result of their lower status. Women with alcoholism are more often abandoned by their spouses. Studies have identified female alcoholic patients as more susceptible to depression, lower self-esteem, and sexual abuse. They frequently encounter opposition from family and friends when they seek treatment.

Efforts must be intensified to educate the public about the serious consequences of substance abuse and the compelling need for treatment. More research is crucial for understanding the barriers that prevent women from entering and remaining in treatment. Studies should be undertaken on the redesign of treatment programs that are tailored to the needs of female substance abusers.

Conclusion

Environmental hazards abound, placing women at risk for a host of health problems, from cancer to reproductive irregularities. Women are usually more vulnerable than men because of their smaller body size, different hormone levels and reproductive organs, and greater percentage of body fat in which toxins can accumulate. Exposures to toxic substances can be harmful to women and to the unborn, who may bear the burden of exposure for their entire lives.

Too little attention has been paid to understanding and preventing the harmful effects of environmental hazards on women. Breast cancer, already the most frequently diagnosed reproductive cancer in women, is growing at an intolerable rate. Between 1962 and 1992, there was a 4% increase in breast cancer mortality.[81] Genetic and hormonal factors play a role, but other factors that have caused the increase remain a mystery. In fact, most women with breast cancer have no known risk factors. It is no wonder that women across the nation ask each day how they can protect themselves from this dreaded disease. Some of their questions include "What should I eat? Are pesticides, even on fruit and vegetables, a problem? Should I avoid EMFs? Is my workplace safe?" The answers are few and far between.

More research is needed, yet it is clear that breast cancer and many conditions afflicting women have environmental links. As research progresses, we should avoid complacence even though we do not have all the answers. Policy makers must act resolutely to assess the risks to women, design and fund environmental studies that will identify hazardous substances, establish safe exposure levels, and remove from our workplaces and neighborhoods those agents that clearly cause disease.

Endnotes

[1]Flynn J, Slovic P, Mertz CK: Gender, race, and perception of environmental health risks. *Risk Analysis* 14(6):1101–1108, 1994

[2]Davis DL, Bradlow HL, Wolff M, et al: Medical hypothesis: xenoestrogens as preventable causes of breast cancer. *Environmental Health Perspectives* 101:373–378, 1993

[3]U.S. Department of Health and Human Services: *Sixth Annual Report on Carcinogens* (U.S. GPO 306-499/50557), 1991; Henderson BE, Ross RK, Pike MC: Toward the primary prevention of cancer. *Science* 254:1131–1138, 1991

[4]Spicer DV, Pike MC: Hormonal manipulation to prevent breast cancer. *Science and Medicine*, July/August, 1995

[5]Colditz GA, Hankinson SE, Hunter DJ, et al: The use of estrogens and progestins and the risk of breast cancer in postmenopausal women. *New England Journal of Medicine* 332:1589–1593, 1995

[6]Kolata G: "Cancer link contradicted by new hormone study." *New York Times*, July 12, 1995

[7]Madigan MP, Ziegler RG, Benichou J, et al: Proportion of breast cancer cases in the United States explained by well-established risk factors. *Journal of the National Cancer Institute* 87:1681, 1995

[8]U.S. Department of Health and Human Services, op. cit.

[9]Soto AM, Chung KL, Sonnenschein C: The pesticides endosulfan, toxaphene, and dieldrin have estrogenic effects on human estrogen-sensitive cells. *Environmental Health Perspectives* 102:380–383, 1994

[10]Birnbaum LS: Endocrine effects of prenatal exposure to PCBs, dioxins, and other xenobiotics: implications for policy and future research. *Environmental Health Perspectives* 102:676–679, 1994; Safe SH: Environmental and dietary estrogens and human health: is there a problem? *Environmental Health Perspectives* 103:346–351, 1995

[11]Spicer DV, Pike MC, op. cit.

[12]McLachlan JA, Newbold RR, Teng CT, et al: Environmental estrogens: orphan receptors and genetic imprinting, in *Advances in Modern Environmental Toxicology*, Vol 21. Edited by Lolborn T, Clements C. Princeton, NJ, Scientific, 1992, pp 107–112

[13]Cook LS, Weiss NS, Schwartz SM, et al: Population-based study of tamoxifen therapy and subsequent ovarian, endometrial and breast cancers. *Journal of the National Cancer Institute* 87:1359–1363, 1995

[14]Soto AM, Chung KL, Sonnenschein C, op. cit.

[15]Guillette LJ, Gross TS, Masson GR, et al: Developmental abnormalities of the gonad and abnormal sex hormone concentrations in juvenile alligators from contaminated and control lakes in Florida. *Environmental Health Perspectives* 102:680–688, 1994

[16]Birnbaum LS, op. cit.

[17]Wolff M, Toniolo PG, Lee EW: Blood levels of organochlorine residues and risk of breast cancer. *Journal of the National Cancer Institute* 85:648–652, 1993

[18]Krieger N, Wolff MS, Hiatt RA, et al: Breast cancer and serum organochlorines: a prospective study among white, black, and Asian women. *Journal of the National Cancer Institute* 86:589–607, 1994

[19]Safe SH, op. cit.

[20]Soto AM, Chung KL, Sonnenschein C, op. cit.

[21]Fingerhut M, Halperin WE, Marlow DA, et al: Cancer mortality in workers exposed to 2,3,7,8-tetrachlorodibenzo-p-dioxin. *New England Journal of Medicine* 324:212–218, 1991

[22]U.S. Department of Health and Human Services, op. cit.

[23]DeVito MJ, Birnbaum L, Farland WH, et al: Comparisons of estimated human body burdens of dioxinlike chemicals and TCDD body burdens in experimentally exposed animals. *Environmental Health Perspectives* 103: 820–831, 1995

[24]Birnbaum L: Evidence for the role of the Ah receptor in response to dioxin, in *Receptor-Mediated Biological Processes: Implications for Evaluating Carcinogens. Progress in Clinical and Biological Research*, 387. Edited by Spitzer HL, Slaga TL, Greelee WF, et al. New York, Wiley Liss, 1994, pp 139–154

[25]U.S. Environmental Protection Agency: *Health Assessment Document for 2,3,7,8-Tetrachlorodibenzo-p-Dioxin (TCDD) and Related Compounds*, Review Draft (EPA/600/BP-92/001c), 1994

[26]Safe S, Astroff B, Harris M, et al: 2,3,7,8,-tetrachlorodibenzo-p-dioxin (TCDD) and related compounds as antiestrogens: characterization and mechanism of action. *Pharmacology and Toxicology* 69:400–409, 1993

[27]Kociba RJ, Keyes D, Beyer J, et al: Results of a two-year chronic toxicity and oncogenicity study of 2, 3, 7, 8-tetrachlorodibenzo-p-dioxin in rats. *Toxicology and Applied Pharmacology* 46:279–303, 1978

[28]Rier SE, Martin DC, Bowman RE, et al: Endometriosis in rhesus monkeys (macaca mulatta) following chronic exposure to 2, 3, 7, 8-tetrachlorodibenzo-p-dioxin. *Fundamental and Applied Toxicology* 21:433–441, 1993

[29]U.S. Environmental Protection Agency, op. cit.

[30]Newbold R: Gender related behavior in women exposed prenatally to diethylstilbestrol. *Environmental Health Perspectives* 101:208–213, 1993

[31]Ibid.

[32]U.S. Department of Health and Human Services, op. cit.

[33]McLachlan JA, Newbold RR, Teng CT, et al., op. cit.

[34]Newbold R, op. cit.

[35]King T: Ovarian cancer and fertility drugs. *The Cancer Bulletin* 46(2):181–184, 1994

[36]Rossing MA, Daling JR, Weiss N, et al: Ovarian tumors in a cohort of infertile women. *New England Journal of Medicine* 331:771–776, 1994

[37]Centers for Disease Control: *Preventing Lead Poisoning in Young Children*. U.S. Public Health Service, Department of Health and Human Services, 1991

[38]Mushak P: New directions in the toxicokinetics of human lead exposure. *Neurotoxicology* 14(2–3):9–42, 1993

[39]Silbergeld EK, Sauk J, Somerman M, et al: Lead in bone: storage site, exposure source, and target organ. *Neurotoxicology* 14(2–3):225–236, 1993

[40]Mushak P, op. cit.

[41]Silbergeld EK: Lead in bone: implications for toxicology during pregnancy and lactation. *Environmental Health Perspectives* 91:63–70, 1991

[42]Goyer RA, Epstein S, Bhattacharyya M, et al: Environmental risk factors for osteoporosis. *Environmental Health Perspectives* 102:390–394, 1994

[43]Rothenberg SJ, Karchmer S, Schnaas L, et al: Changes in serial blood lead levels during pregnancy. *Environmental Health Perspectives* 102:876–880, 1994

[44]Silbergeld EK, op. cit.

[45]Muldoon SB, Cauley JA, Kuller LH, et al: Lifestyle and sociodemographic factors as determinants of blood lead levels in elderly women. *American Journal of Epidemiology* 139:599–608, 1994

[46]Centers for Disease Control and Prevention: *Morbidity and Mortality Weekly Report CDC Surveillance Summaries.* 43(SS-3), November 18, 1994

[47]U.S. Department of Health and Human Services: *Preventing Tobacco Use Among Young People: A Report of the Surgeon General.* Atlanta, GA, U.S. Public Health Service, Department of Health and Human Services, Centers for Disease Control and Prevention, National Center for Chronic Disease Prevention and Health Promotion, Office on Smoking and Health, 1994

[48]Risch HA, Howe GR, Jain M, et al: Are female smokers at higher risk for lung cancer than male smokers? A case-control analysis by histologic type. *American Journal of Epidemiology* 138(5):281–293, 1993

[49]Ries LAG, Miller BA, Hankey BF, et al (eds): *SEER Cancer Statistics Review, 1973–1991: Tables and Graphs, National Cancer Institute* (NIH Publ No 94–2789). Bethesda, MD, 1994

[50]Coleman A, Robertson G, Lugo TG: Growth control by tumor suppressors in malignant melanoma. *Receptor* 5(1):9–19, 1995

[51]Pollock PM, Yu F, Qiu L, et al: Evidence for U.V. induction of CDKN2 mutations in melanoma cell lines. *Oncogene* 11(4):663–668, 1995

[52]Kricker A, Armstrong BK, English DR: Sun exposure and non-melanocytic skin cancer. *Cancer Causes Control* 5(4):367–392, 1994

[53]Florig HK: Containing the costs of the EMF problem. *Science* 257:468–492, 1992

[54]Wertheimer N, Leeper E: Electrical wiring configurations and childhood cancer. *American Journal of Epidemiology* 109:273–284, 1979

[55]Carpenter DO: Epidemiological evidence for an association between exposure to 50 and 60 Hz magnetic fields and cancer, in *Hydro-Electric Development: Environmental Impacts—Paper No 6.* James Bay Publication Series, 1994

[56]Shaw GM, Croen LA: Human adverse reproductive outcomes and electromagnetic field exposures: review of epidemiologic studies. *Environmental Health Perspectives* 101(suppl 4):107–119, 1993

[57]Oak Ridge Associated Universities: *Health Effects of Low-Frequency Electric and Magnetic Fields.* Prepared by Oak Ridge Associated Universities Panel for the Committee on Interagency Radiation Research and Policy Coordination (ORAU 92/F8). Oak Ridge, TN, 1992

[58]Savitz DA: Overview of epidemiologic research on electric and magnetic fields and cancer. *American Industrial Hygiene Association Journal* 54(4):197–204, 1993

[59]Ries LAG, Miller BA, Hankey BF, et al., op. cit.

[60]Savitz DA, op. cit.

[61]Loomis DP, Savitz DA, Ananth CV: Breast cancer mortality among female electrical workers in the United States. *Journal of the National Cancer Institute* 86:921–926, 1994

[62]Stevens RG, Davis S, Thomas DR, et al: Electrical power, pineal function, and the risk of breast cancer. *FASEB Journal* 6:853–860, 1992

[63]Liburdy RP, Sloma TR, Sokolic R, et al: EMF magnetic fields, breast cancer, and melatonin: 60 Hz fields block melatonin's oncostatic action on ER+ breast cancer cell proliferation. *Journal of Pineal Research* 14:89–97, 1993

[64]Liburdy RP, Harland JD, Hefferman C, et al: *ELF inhibition of melatonin's natural oncostatic action on MCF-7 cells: 60 HZ dose threshold determination.* Abstract for Bio-Electromagnetic Society, Sixteenth Annual Meeting, Copenhagen, Denmark, June 12–17, 1994

[65]Dawson DM: Entrapment neuropathies of the upper extremities. *New England Journal of Medicine* 329:2013–2018, 1993

[66]Rogers B: Women in the workplace, in *Women's Health Care*. Edited by Fogel CI, Woods NF. Thousand Oaks, CA, Sage, 1995, p 372

[67]Roland AS, Baird DD, Weinberg CR, et al: Reduced fertility among women employed as dental assistants exposed to high levels of nitrous oxide. *New England Journal of Medicine* 327:993–997, 1992

[68]Hemminki K, Mutanen P, Saloniemi I, et al: Spontaneous abortions in hospital staff engaged in sterilising instruments with chemical agents. *British Medical Journal* 285:1461–1463, 1982

[69]Kuczmarski RJ, Flegal KM, Campbell SM, et al: Increasing prevalence of overweight among U.S. adults: the National Health and Nutrition Examination Surveys, 1960 to 1991. *Journal of the American Medical Association* 272:205–211, 1994

[70]Fogel CI, Woods NF (eds): *Women's Health Care*. Thousand Oaks, CA, Sage, 1995

[71]U.S. Department of Health and Human Services: *The Surgeon General's Report on Nutrition and Health* (DHHS Publ No PHS 88-50210), 1988

[72]Institute of Medicine, Thomas PR (ed): *Weighing the Options: Criteria for Evaluating Weight-Management Programs*. Washington, DC, National Academy Press, 1995

[73]Zhang Y, Proenca R, Maffei M, et al: Positional cloning of the mouse obese gene and its human homologue. *Nature* 372:425–432, 1994

[74]Goldstein DJ, Potvin JH: Long-term weight loss: the effect of pharmacologic agents. *American Journal of Clinical Nutrition* 60:647–657, 1994

[75]Rice DP, Kelman S, Miller LS, et al: *The Economic Cost of Alcohol and Drug Abuse and Mental Illness: 1985* (DHHS Publ No ADM 90-1694). San Francisco, University of California, Institute for Health and Aging, 1990 (The figures in this publication were updated for 1990 in a personal communication to the Institute of Medicine publication *The Development of Medications for the Treatment of Opiate and Cocaine Addictions*. Washington, DC, National Academy Press, 1995.)

[76]Substance Abuse and Mental Health Services Administration: *Preliminary Estimates From the 1993 National Household Survey on Drug Abuse* (Advance Rep No 7), 1994

[77]Hubbard RL, Marsden ME, Rachal JV, et al: *Drug Abuse Treatment: A National Study of Effectiveness*. Chapel Hill, The University of North Carolina Press, 1989

[78]Weisner C, Schmidt L: Gender disparities in treatment for alcohol problems. *Journal of the American Medical Association* 268:1872–1876, 1992

[79]Beckman LJ: Treatment needs of women with alcohol problems. *Alcohol Health & Research World* 18(3):206–211, 1994

[80]Tivis LJ, Gavaler JS: Alcohol, hormones, and health in postmenopausal women. *Alcohol Health & Research World* 18(3):185–191, 1994

[81]American Cancer Society: *Cancer Facts & Figures—1996*. Atlanta, GA, American Cancer Society, 1996

Part 3

Women as Researchers and Participants

9

Formula for Change: Examining the Glass Ceiling

Florence P. Haseltine, Ph.D., M.D.

Numerous discussions about promoting women and minorities on university faculties have been happening recently. Obviously, the advancement of a group of individuals depends on the number of available positions and the size of the pool for a specific group of people. It is quite apparent that there has not been a large influx of women or minorities into higher positions within the greater academic community. The absence of women on university faculties means that women's health research tends to languish, because women researchers are more likely not only to investigate women's diseases than are men, but also to ask different scientific questions than male scientists do.

Pressure to promote women started in the early 1970s when an increase occurred in the number of women entering medical schools, as well as agitation from affirmative action programs. Laws were passed, committees were established, and universities started to maintain that they were affirmative action advocates. Many people thought that these attempts would be enough. However, 20 years later, we do not see a substantive difference.

Issues in the micromanagement of promotions and recruitment have been studied. New terms have entered our vocabulary. "Highlighting" is one such word. This refers to the observation that women and minorities are so few in number that, whenever an application for employment from a member of either group occurs, that person is limited by the fact that everyone in the field knows her and therefore knows every mistake she has made. Many faculties are so small that the same women can be named repeatedly when a group tries to enumerate its female faculty. These women have acquired the tremendous burden of representing the interests of all women, when many would prefer simply to do their work.

The interest in affirmative action came when the tenure system was strained. There were too many applicants, not enough turnover in tenure ranks, experimentation with nontenured tracks, and change in the law in 1978 that eliminated mandatory retirement. The assumption that academics would proceed through the ranks at a consistent and predictable pace was being challenged.

We need to examine some basic ideas to determine whether it is possible to model a system that could incorporate new people into it. Basically the equation will look something like this:

$$P_{full} = P_{ofull} + P_{assoc}(dF_{full}/dt)*t - dG_{full}/dt$$

P_{full} = full professor
P_{assoc} = Pool size of associate professors that are the group under consideration
P_{ofull} = the percentage of professors in the faculty at time
dF/dt = turnover rate for the entire faculty
dG/dt = the turnover rate of the minority group
t = time

This should equal the same turnover rate as other faculty multiplied by the number of minority individuals in that group.

Total turnover rate for the minority group can be expressed as:

$$dG_{full}/dt = (dF_{full}/dt)*P_{full}$$

However, this number is subject to great fluctuations because the group is usually so small that it is hard to approximate. It can increase dramatically with a specific donation or a set aside of chairs and it can increase by extensive recruitment.

Change in associate professors and assistant professors can be calculated in a similar manner:

$$P_{assoc} = P_{oassoc} + P_{assist}(dF_{assoc}/dt) * t - dG_{assoc}/dt$$
$$P_{assist} = P_{oassist} + P_{residents}(dF_{assist}/dt*) t - dG_{assist}/dt$$

To do the calculations, values can be found for the baseline P_o points; these are the number of individual members in the group at the beginning of the calculations. Faculty turnover will be estimated at average turnover rates; that is, the number of years a person is in each position. These values are from the American Association of Medical Colleges data.[1]

From the model, it is possible to determine whether a group can advance. It allows an organization to determine whether it is living up to its own standards. If the number of recruitments and advancements is below the predicted level, the reasons for the falloff should be investigated. If more progress is needed, then the turnover rate for that group will have to be changed. Better retention and better recruitment will be needed.

Nine percent of the full professors at the standard university are women, and professors stay in that rank for 25 years.

		Percentage at rank	Turnover		1/Average years in rank
P_{ofull}	=	9	dF_{full}/dt	=	1/20
P_{oassoc}	=	18	dF_{assoc}/dt	=	1/7
$P_{oassist}$	=	24	dF_{assist}/dt	=	1/5
$P_{residents}$	=	37			
$P_{medical\ students}$	=	39.4%			

(See Figures 9–1 and 9–2.)

The curves in the figures show that it will take a long time to fill the ranks. Assistant professors should be filled within 10 years, associate professors at about 13 years, but, for full professors, it will not happen in our lifetime.

Clearly, we need to work on the two areas that are flexible. One is pool size, and the other is the targeted change in numbers. It is imperative that

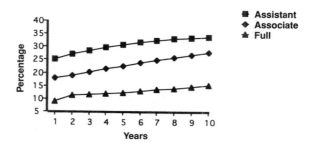

Figure 9–1. Prediction of faculty change at different ranks based on present American Association of Medical Colleges numbers for faculty in 1993.

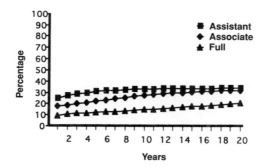

Figure 9–2. An expanded illustration of faculty promotion expectation with present faculty numbers.

qualified candidates be identified and pursued. Chairs need to be created, and good retention programs should be developed. Funds are needed to establish a data center for individuals looking for qualified female applicants.

Using these models, a medical school can determine whether it is making progress through the normal process or whether the number of people recruited will have to exceed the pool size. The model makes some assumptions that clearly are not true in every case. For example, the turnover rates are underestimated because forced retirement is no longer an option. Many senior faculty stay at their rank for more than 20 years, and we do not have those turnover numbers. Also, this model only deals with a limited group of positions. The associate and full professor ranks are changing because fragmentation of these ranks is occurring. For example, there are now clinical ranks with the same title but not the same tenure. These individuals may have a higher turnover because they are not as secure. Many women may be pushed into these ranks. Any attempt to make a perfect model is thwarted by human ingenuity to manipulate the system.

We can hope that there will be a continuing push to open the doors of medical schools to women faculty and that they can expect to have a fair chance of being promoted. But whenever an affirmative action program is attempted, it is important to develop a set of criteria that the program expects to accomplish and then to model the system. The model presented here is a model only for an equitable distribution of resources and fairness in promotion.

Although most people do not move to new jobs but either rise or fall at their own institutions, a great deal of attention needs to be paid to the women at the lower ranks, who should receive regular feedback on their progress.

It is important to admit that the present programs have not had a noticeable effect. It is useful to look at the few places that have recruited women successfully and ask how they did it. Was it a dean who would not take no for an answer? Was it an effective ombudsman from the faculty who sat in at search meetings? Was it an attempt to make sure that the women at a university knew the unwritten rules and understood the written ones? Wishful thinking does not help.

Endnote

[1]American Association of Medical Colleges: Number of physicians in training and percentages of women at different levels, in *Women in Academic Medicine Statistics*. Edited by Bickel J, Galbraith A, Quinnier R. Washington, DC, American Association of Medical Colleges, 1993

10

Funding for Research and Training

Donna L. Vogel, M.D., Ph.D.

A number of sources for research and training support, both public and private, exist. Although this chapter emphasizes National Institutes of Health (NIH) grants, it also covers other funding sources and mechanisms available to "young" investigators who are new to research.

The young investigator seeking support from NIH can survey a variety of options. Depending on the stage of his or her career and the type of previous education and training, these options generally fall into the areas of fellowships, career development awards, and certain types of research grants. Before getting into the specifics of these mechanisms, it is worth pointing out that different parts of NIH handle support of various areas. Most of the time, the applicant does not have to direct the application to a specific institute/center/division (ICD) within NIH. Applications are sent to the Division of Research Grants, an "umbrella" department whose scientists, known as the referral staff, decide which review group or study section will conduct initial peer review. Independently, they also decide which ICD will subsequently administer the application after the initial review. Applicants may request a particular assignment to a study section or an ICD, but it is not necessary to do so. In any event, the referral staff makes assignments in accordance with the established referral guidelines for the Public Health Service.

Distinct from the ICDs, the NIH Office for Research on Women's Health (ORWH) has a threefold mission: to increase research on topics important to the health of women, to boost the number of women included in clinical research, and to expand opportunities for women in biomedical careers through the recruitment, reentry, retention, support, and advancement of women scientists. Although the ORWH does not itself award grants, it provides substantial resources through the ICDs to co-fund and supplement grants, as well as to support conferences and workshops in its mission areas.

Specific NIH Mechanisms

Training

National Research Service Awards.   Most NIH research training is supported by National Research Service Awards (NRSAs) administered by the NRSA Program. The major NRSAs are individual postdoctoral fellowships (F32) and institutional training awards (T32). Most ICDs do not make individual predoctoral awards. Support is available for postdoctoral fellows; the full-time stipend depends on the candidate's level of experience. Applications include information about the candidate's previous education and training, the present research proposal, a statement from the applicant's mentor, and letters of reference.

Institutional training awards are made to entities, such as universities and freestanding research institutes, which have a proven record of successful training, qualified faculty, and suitable resources and environment to advance the education of predoctoral and/or postdoctoral fellows. Each program recruits and selects its fellows locally; they frequently advertise the awards in scientific journals and circulate letters to directors of graduate programs.

Other mechanisms exist to fund short-term training experiences for students in the health professions and senior fellowships for scientists who are seeking training to enhance their research capabilities.

NRSAs are made to citizens of the United States, noncitizen nationals, or those admitted to the United States for permanent residence. They are subject to certain reporting and career commitment provisions, known as "payback." These commitments—required of postdoctoral trainees only—refer to a specific period of time, usually 20 hours a week, devoted to research or teaching, for a period determined by the length of training. Recent changes allow recipients to count the second year of training as payback for the first year—an incentive to stay in the laboratory for at least 2 years. If the trainee does not perform the payback service, he or she must reimburse the NRSA Program financially.

Career development awards. These grants, also known as "K" awards, are directed toward the individual who has research potential but needs additional training and experience to become, or make progress as, an independent investigator. Applications are made by the institution, which nominates the candidate. The series of career awards, previously 14 different types, have recently been consolidated into six. Anyone considering applying should contact staff in the ICD that supports the relevant science area to check which K grants are available from that ICD and whether specific modifications or special instructions exist for that program.

Many ICDs use the following:

- *The Mentored Research Scientist Development Award (K01):* These grants support a supervised research experience of 3 to 5 years for scientists who are changing their research direction after a hiatus in their careers. In addition, they are used to support faculty at a minority institution who wish to enhance their independent research skills at a nearby institution.
- *The Mentored Clinical Scientist Development Award (K08):* This award is designed to facilitate the transition from a postdoctoral position to independent status for the clinically trained individual who has had more or less postdoctoral experience. A qualified sponsor provides guidance during the investigation of a well-defined problem in biomedical research. Awards may be requested for 3 to 5 years.
- *The Independent Scientist Award (K02):* This grant is for newly independent scientists who already hold a research grant, demonstrate outstanding research potential, and can establish the

need for a period of intensive, focused research to enhance their careers. Typically, the award provides salary support that relieves the investigator of institutional obligations, so that she or he can devote more effort to research.

Some ICDs use the following:

- *The Senior Scientist Award (K05):* This award supports the research of leaders in their fields and is used by the National Institute on Drug Abuse, the National Institute of Mental Health, and the National Institute on Alcohol Abuse and Alcoholism.
- *The Academic Career Award (K07):* This award promotes the development of expertise in a specific academic area or the advancement of a curricula and research capacity at an academic institution.
- *The Mentored Clinical Scientist Development Program Award (K12):* This award, an institutional version of the K08, is used exclusively by the National Institute on Aging and the National Institute of Dental Research.

The National Institute of Child Health and Human Development (NICHHD) also participates in several private sector research career development programs for physicians in pediatrics, obstetrics/gynecology, and rehabilitation medicine. These programs, which independently recruit and select their own candidates, have two phases: 1) a research experience for participants under a basic science mentor and 2) an independent research program at the sponsoring institution.

Research Grants

The backbone of NIH-supported research is the traditional R01 Research Project Grant, usually lasting 3 to 5 years, with recipients able to compete for a renewal of their grants. Most R01s are investigator-initiated; that is, the scientist himself or herself poses the question, decides on the topic, and plans the proposed research on which the application is based. Other forms of research support may be directed or solicited by NIH. These include contracts, in which the government purchases the research as a product; cooperative agreements, a type of government-awardee partnership; and grants that are invited under a request for applications

(RFA). RFAs are published in the *NIH Guide to Grants and Contracts* and are used when there is a need for research in a defined area that is not being met by the usual investigator-initiated process or when a special mechanism is to be used that is not available for investigator-initiated use.

In addition to the R01, other less well-known funding sources are available in certain situations. They include the following:

- *First Independent Research Support and Transition (FIRST) Award (R29)*: This is similar to a regular R01, given for a term of 5 years, and targeted to the new investigator. Applications are reviewed by the regular NIH study sections; less is expected in terms of preliminary data, but there are budget limitations.
- *Small Grant Awards (R03)*: These awards are used by some but not all ICDs and are generally accepted only when specifically invited in an RFA for specific topics or circumstances. These typically support pilot projects or feasibility studies of innovative, high-risk research.
- *Academic Research Enhancement Award (AREA; R15)*: These awards are made to small, 4-year colleges and universities that, to be eligible, must not have a major NIH-supported research base. They provide 3 years of support for small-scale projects.
- *Small Business Innovative Research (SBIR; R43, R44) and Small Business Technology Transfer Research (STTR; R41, R42)*: These grants finance research by small business concerns to establish feasibility and develop products with commercial potential in the mission areas of the various federal funding agencies. The STTR requires a partnership between the small business and an academic institution; the SBIR permits such a collaboration to a limited degree.

Larger or supplemental award.   Other opportunities for training or development exist within a larger award or as a supplement to an existing award. For example, certain large mechanisms have a component built in for young investigators. Program Project (P01) Grants often include research led by promising new investigators. In NICHHD, new or competing renewal applications for P30 centers may request limited funds for new project development support.

NIH may target specific populations to increase its participation in research at several levels. Although these announcements, published in the NIH guide, have not specifically targeted women, they have certainly been used to benefit women entering research careers.

Research supplements have been used to target underrepresented minorities. For example, scientists holding funded research grants may, in accord with published announcements, apply for supplemental funds to add to their projects students, fellows, or young investigators from particular ethnic or racial groups who have been underrepresented in biomedical and behavioral research. The university or other applicant institution determines which racial and ethnic groups are underrepresented. Research supplements also have been used

- To recruit individuals with disabilities into biomedical research careers. These supplements are designed to add students, fellows, or young investigators to existing projects supported by research grants.
- To promote reentry into biomedical and behavioral research careers. These supplements are designed to support scientists who had demonstrated excellent research potential but interrupted their careers for family care responsibilities and now need additional laboratory experience. Such grants allow reentry candidates to update their skills and advance toward becoming independent investigators.

Individuals who believe they may qualify for one of these categories may wish to seek out a funded investigator in the area of their interest and discuss the option of the investigator applying for this type of supplement to the existing NIH grant.

Investigators may be contacted by NIH staff if they are eligible to compete for certain other supplemental funding opportunities. These include supplements in targeted areas from ORWH and the new Office of Behavioral and Social Sciences Research.

NIH Information

The NIH scientific staff are available for consultation and administrative guidance about the application process, appropriate mechanisms,

ICD program areas, and so on, but the investigator needs to make the initial contact. Many people do not realize this. Such contacts certainly can help trainees and/or mentors in seeking support for the early stages of a career, as well as later in their development.

Some of the best sources for information are

- The *NIH Guide to Grants and Contracts*, the official source of announcements of initiatives, new and ongoing programs, and updated guidelines for specific mechanisms. It is available at the sponsored research office of most institutions that have grants or can be obtained electronically through the NIH Gopher or on the Internet (NIH Grant Line: 301-594-7270).
- The NIH Office of Grants Information has published guidelines and application materials. (Call 301-435-0714 for single copies or 301-435-1099 for multiple copies; fax request to 301-594-7384; or mail to 6701 Rockledge Drive, Room 1040, Bethesda, MD 20892.) For those new to the process, some of the more useful documents are
  - "Grants and Awards"
  - "NIH Extramural Programs—Funding for Research and Research Training"
  - "Helpful Hints on Preparing a Research Grant Application to NIH"
  - "Helpful Hints on Preparing a Fellowship Application to NIH"

Women Holding NIH Grants

The most recent data for fiscal year 1993 (1992 for trainees) indicate that, overall, the success rate for competing research project grants (R01 and FIRST awards) has been declining. The success rate for new grants for both women and men was 18%, although for renewal applications it was 40.2% for men and 38.4% for women. In fiscal year 1993, 16.4% of research grant dollars went to women, compared with 10.2% in 1984. In dollar terms, funding for men doubled and funding for women tripled during that interval. The 1993 success rates for women were a few points higher than for men in FIRST awards (28.5 versus 26.7), K awards (42.5 versus 38.9), AREA grants (29.0 versus 23.5), and Small Research grants (25.0 versus 21.9).

The percentage of women for trainee appointments to institutional training grants reached a record 45.5% in 1992. This has increased steadily since 1984, when it was 38.3%. The percentage of individual fellowships made to women was 32.8% in 1993, up from 28.7 in 1984, although the peak was 39.6% in 1991. Women received 33.8% of competing K awards in 1993 compared with 19.6% in 1984. These statistics are from the NIH publication 95-3876, "Women in NIH Extramural Grant Programs." This document, which contains many more details, is produced annually by the Statistics, Analysis and Evaluation Section, Information Systems Branch, Division of Research Grants. (Call 301-435-0650, or write to SAES/ISB/DRG, 6701 Rockledge Drive, MSC 7772, Bethesda, MD 20892 for copies.)

Other Public Health Service Agencies

The research programs previously in the Alcohol, Drug Abuse and Mental Health Administration have been brought into NIH and are now considered along with the other ICDs.

The Agency for Health Care Policy Research (AHCPR) supports and conducts research on quality, cost, and availability of health services. Its purview includes health care delivery, medical effectiveness, and translating new knowledge into clinical practice. AHCPR is located at 2101 East Jefferson Street, Rockville, MD 20852; the communications division can be reached at 301-594-1364.

The U.S. Food and Drug Administration (301-443-6170) and the National Institute for Occupational Safety and Health, a component of the Centers for Disease Control and Prevention (404-639-3343), also have grant programs. Grant applications for these three agencies are submitted to, and referred for review by, the NIH Division of Research Grants.

Highlights of National Science Foundation Programs

The National Science Foundation (NSF) supports research in biological, physical, and social sciences but specifically excludes those areas that are directly related to human disease. The Directorate for Biological Science includes Environmental Biology, Molecular and Cellular Biosciences, Biological Instrumentation and Resources, and Integrative Biology and Neuroscience. Other directorates relevant to women's health are Education and Human Resources, and Social, Behavioral, and Economic Sciences. For a comprehensive view of NSF programs, consult the *Annual NSF Guide to Programs* (NSF publication 94-91 and its annual successors).

NSF does have some special programs for women scientists and engineers. Visiting professorships for women enable independent women investigators to serve as visiting professors at domestic academic institutions in a 6- to 36-month period during which they do research and teach (see NSF 94-68).

The Research Planning Grant is a small, limited-term award, for individuals with no prior independent federal support, to be used to develop a project. The career advancement award can support a 1-year enhancement project to increase the woman investigator's research capability and productivity. These are announced in NSF publication 93-130.

Not specifically for women, but useful, is the faculty early career development program (NSF 94-101) for support of junior faculty who are planning a career involving both research and education.

For information on these special programs, contact the senior staff associate for cross-directorate programs, telephone 703-306-1603, or write to NSF, 4201 Wilson Boulevard, Arlington, VA 22230. To order NSF publications, call 202-357-7861 or 703-306-1130; fax 703-644-4278; Internet address: pubs@nsf.gov.

Other Sources

Professional societies, voluntary health agencies, and industry provide funding for research. A few nonprofit organizations particularly germane to women's health issues include

American Cancer Society
1599 Clifton Road, N.E.
Atlanta, GA 30329
404-320-3333

American Heart Association
7272 Greenville Avenue
Dallas, TX 75231-4599
214-373-6300

March of Dimes Birth Defects Foundation
1275 Mamaroneck Avenue
White Plains, NY 10605
914-428-7100

Arthritis Foundation
Research Department
1314 Spring Street, NW
Atlanta, GA 30309
404-872-7100

The pharmaceutical industry supports a great deal of research related to drug development. Grants for young investigators are usually
channeled through professional societies in specific fields. Often, the
office of sponsored research at an institution has information about private sources of funding.

This summary is an introduction to some different sources of research funding and types of assistance available from federal and other
sources, with a particular emphasis on women scientists, research in
women's health, and beginning investigators. More information about
the content of programs and use of mechanisms is available from staff
contacts at the relevant institute, directorate, office, or association.

11

Needed: A Women's Health Curriculum and Program

Janet B. Henrich, M.D.

N ew perceptions about women's health have led to a re-examination of the training of health professionals. The current concern reflects three factors that are changing the way we regard women's health. They are

1. An acceptance of the fact that the biological differences between the sexes are important and play a major role both in the incidence and progression of disease and response to interventions
2. An awareness of the psychosocial and environmental factors that particularly affect women's health
3. Research results from emerging clinical studies of women that are slowly adding to our knowledge base[1]

In fact, in 1993, Congress requested that the Office for Research on Women's Health (ORWH) at the National Institutes of Health (NIH), in cooperation with the Health Resources and Services Administration, the Public Health Service Office on Women's Health, and other organizations, survey the status of women's health education and training in medical school curricula to determine whether women's health issues are covered adequately and to make recommendations for a core curriculum on women's health.[2] The Council on Graduate Medical Education

(COGME) established an Advisory Group on Women in Medicine. Although its original mandate included establishing minimum competencies expected from physicians to provide general health care to women, the advisory group believed it was premature to establish *definitive* competencies because of the fragmentary knowledge regarding women's health. The group believed it was equally important to develop a "conceptual framework" that would allow the necessary curricular and program changes to promote a women's health agenda at all levels of medical education—not only for medical school but also for residency training, fellowships, and continuing medical education (CME) programs for practicing physicians.

United States Patient Profile in the Twenty-First Century

Before we can establish competencies for physicians who treat women, we have to know what the patient profile in the United States will look like in the coming years. Current data tell us that

- Continued increases in life expectancy and the baby-boom generation's arrival at retirement age will cause a population explosion among older age groups early in the next century.[3]
- By the year 2000 or shortly thereafter, women older than 65 will outnumber men of the same age by two to one and, for those older than 85, by three to one.[4]
- Three-quarters of 1.5 million nursing home residents are women, and estimates are that one-half of all women now 65 years old will spend some time in a nursing home in the coming years.[5]
- Of the 7 million women older than 75, 2 million are chronically ill and unable to carry on major activities or are limited in their ability.[6]
- Ethnic population shifts in the United States will cause a decline in the number of non-Hispanic whites from its current high of 74% of the total population to 60% in 2030 and 53% in 2050. Conversely, the present African American population will double by 2050, and, by 2030, the number of Hispanic Americans will increase from 10% to 18% of the population in the

United States, and the number of Asians and Pacific Islanders will increase from 3% to 8%.[7]

These facts and statistics mean that medical school education and postgraduate training will have to prepare physicians to treat large numbers of chronically ill older people, most of them women. Physicians also will face the serious health problems experienced in greater degree by minority women. Among these problems are high infant mortality rates; more diabetes, hypertension, cardiovascular disease, stroke, and cervical and stomach cancer (particularly high among Hispanic women); and an epidemic of human immunodeficiency virus (HIV) infection and acquired immunodeficiency syndrome (AIDS).[8] Moreover, the unacceptably high incidence of teenage pregnancy presents a challenge to medical caregivers, particularly because many of these young women have no health insurance. A recent article in the *Journal of the American Medical Association* found that 14 million women of childbearing age do not have health insurance and, for those who do have coverage, 5 million receive no prenatal care and delivery benefits.[9] A 1993 Lou Harris survey reported that 22% of Hispanic women and 16% of African American women lack health insurance compared with 13% of white women.[10]

Female victims of domestic violence present particular challenges to medical caregivers, who have to recognize and treat injuries without adding to the burden abused women face from the legal system and their abusers (see Chapter 4).

In addition, physicians and other caregivers may face an increasingly disaffected female patient population. The same Lou Harris survey of 2,500 women from all levels of society found that two of five women had switched physicians because they were dissatisfied with the care they received. One-third of those women who switched said their decision was caused by "communication problems," whereas 25% said the physicians either "talked down" to them or treated them like children. Another 17% complained that they were told their medical complaint was "all in their head," and 5% reported that the physician had made a distasteful sexual remark or an improper advance.[11]

Complicating the women's health care picture further is the change in women's work status. By 2000, estimates are that more than 80% of women will work outside the home.[12] As a society, we do not know how burdens placed on women by the multiple roles of mother and worker, as well as the impact of stress and environmental exposures at work, will affect women's health, but certainly this is one area of needed research. (See Chapter 8 for more on environmental issues.)

Women's Mortality

Specific statistics regarding women's health give us a profile of the diseases women face—and will face in greater degree in the next century. Heart disease is still the number one killer of women and, despite dramatic declines in the past two decades, is responsible for one-third of all female deaths.[13] Before age 75, mortality from heart disease is higher for African American women; after age 75, death rates are higher in white women. Interestingly, and for unknown reasons, Hispanic and Native American women have significantly lower heart disease death rates. Research is needed to find out why.

Cancer is second as a cause of death in women. Increased mortality from lung and breast cancer has offset gains made against cervical and uterine cancer, leaving overall death rates unchanged in the last half of the 20th century. Although breast cancer is still the most common female cancer, lung cancer has become the major cancer killer of women.[14] Because lung cancer is caused by smoking and is therefore preventable, this statistic presents a major challenge to the medical system—how best to convince women to stop smoking, and how to educate adolescent girls not to start in the first place, in a society in which tobacco companies specifically target young women in their advertising campaigns. Preventing smoking in women is particularly important because they have more difficulty stopping than do men[15] and because smoking has a clearly negative effect on the fetus during pregnancy. Along with the increase in lung cancer fatalities in women, death rates from chronic lung disease, also caused and exacerbated by smoking, have increased over the past 25 years, more so for women than for men.

Breast cancer mortality presents a different challenge to medical caregivers. Although mortality rates have remained stable, incidence has increased sharply, a function, in part, of better and more widely used screening mammography, which can detect cancers while they are small and outcomes are more favorable. But, although breast cancer rates among African American women are 20% lower than for white women, death rates are 15% higher, which may reflect significant diagnostic and treatment barriers for African American women, such as lack of health insurance; inadequate knowledge about, or trust in, the benefits of screening and the efficacy of the medical system in general; and biological factors. Another area in which race plays a role is stroke, which ranks third as a killer of women, and from which twice as many African American women die as white women.[16] Other conditions women face that contribute to their mortality are injury from automobile accidents, homicide, suicide, diabetes, and HIV infection.[17]

Women's Morbidity

It is well established that women go to a physician more than men do. A 1991 survey found that women made 60% of all office visits to physicians, primarily for general medical examinations, upper respiratory illnesses, rashes, stomach pain, headache, and injuries to muscles or bones. Another survey found that more women than men have chronic conditions, such as arthritis, thyroid disease, migraine headaches, urinary tract disorders, gastritis, colitis, and chronic constipation.[18] Although neither of these surveys reported on mental health, other studies have identified major depression and anxiety disorders as much more prevalent in women than men. One recent poll found that 40% of women had symptoms of severe depression in the week before the poll was taken, compared with 26% of men. Depression was most prevalent among minority and younger women.[19]

Women's Life Span and Disease

To develop an integrated concept of women's health, it is instructive to look at diseases prevalent among women across the life span.

Conception to Age 15

From fetal life to age 15, one major issue is the hormonal-related variations in brain development between males and females, which may be partially responsible for differences in verbal and mathematical ability between boys and girls and may contribute to disparate patterns of socialization. The major cause of death and illness among the young is injury, both intentional and unintentional, which causes half of all deaths in this age group. Chronic illness is rare in girls, but, when it does appear, it is usually related to the increase in sex hormones during puberty. Most of these conditions are autoimmune diseases, such as systemic lupus erythematosus (SLE), juvenile rheumatoid arthritis, and thyroid disease.[20]

Ages 16 to 44

From ages 16 to 44, injuries, cancers of the reproductive tract, HIV infection, sexually transmitted diseases (STDs), eating disorders, autoimmune diseases, alcohol and tobacco use, reproductive disorders, psychiatric conditions, and sexual abuse and assault are the most frequent causes of death and ill health among women.[21] Particularly challenging to physicians, and an important aspect of their training, are the following possible interventions that may mitigate or prevent serious illness and death:

- Most fatal and nonfatal injuries in young women are caused by motor vehicle accidents (43%), violence that ends in homicide (23%), or suicide (19%). Many are alcohol related. Thus, physicians and other health care providers need training in the best methods of recognizing women at risk and discouraging alcohol abuse.
- Among African American women, HIV infection is the fifth cause of death between ages 15 and 24 and the second cause of mortality for 25- to 44-year-olds. Because HIV can be transmitted from mother to fetus during pregnancy, HIV infection is the fifth cause of death among Hispanic and African American children younger than 14 years (phone call by B. Jacobson, National Center for Health Statistics, September 29, 1995; these

statistics are for 1992). Although research on HIV in women is just beginning, there is some evidence pointing to an interrelationship among HIV disease, infection by the human papillomavirus, and cervical cancer or precancer. Evidence also suggests that HIV in women may present differently and have a different clinical course and a worse prognosis than it does in men. Moreover, recent questions about the accuracy of the Pap test in HIV-infected women has led the Centers for Disease Control and Prevention to revise its guidelines with respect to this test. The spread of HIV infection is rapid, and its consequences are devastating. The challenge to physicians—helping to control HIV transmission through patient education—is a crucial part of the national effort at prevention.[22] Equally vital is the ongoing scientific effort to find better treatment and an effective and safe vaccine.

- Young people are risk takers. Physicians can help reduce risky behavior by counseling young women about the dangers of premature and unprotected sexual activity and its possible consequences—unwanted pregnancy, STDs (including AIDS), and reproductive disorders, such as pelvic inflammatory disease (PID), ectopic pregnancy, and infertility. Counseling about harmful substances, such as alcohol and tobacco, is particularly important because the death rate for women from alcohol abuse is higher than in men, and, as noted earlier, smoking has such long-term deleterious and lethal effects.

- Anorexia nervosa and bulimia are two eating disorders specific to young women, with a conservative estimate that 5% of adolescent girls and young women experience these afflictions. Difficult to treat, anorexia particularly can be life threatening because it has one of the highest morbidity and mortality rates of any psychiatric disorder.[23] The challenging role for physicians here is to recognize this condition early enough to prevent the consequences of starvation and to counsel family members or refer them for help.

- Because autoimmune diseases are prevalent among women in this age group, physicians must diagnose and treat conditions such as rheumatoid arthritis, SLE, scleroderma, Graves' disease, and Hashimoto's thyroiditis, all of which have female-to-male ratios that range from 3 to 1 to 15 to 1. (See Chapter 13 for a discussion of scleroderma.) Additional autoimmune diseases that affect women disproportionately are type I diabetes, multiple sclerosis (MS), idiopathic adrenal failure, and myasthenia gravis. In addition to more research on why autoimmune diseases are more prevalent in women in general, and on these illnesses in particular, we need to know much more about the role of autoimmunity in recurrent pregnancy loss and infertility.[24]

- Reproductive health and disease are primary concerns for women in this age group. Because success in achieving career goals depends on a woman's ability to control her fertility and plan her family, we need much more contraceptive research to provide American women with safer, more efficacious, and easier to use methods. Physicians need to understand the cultural mores that affect a woman's acceptance of different contraceptive methods so that they can prescribe suitable birth control. In addition, physicians must be aware that certain common disorders of reproductive function are not exclusively gynecological in nature. For example, the association of polycystic ovary disease (PCO) with insulin resistance and the hyperandrogenic state, the long-term effect of endometriosis on bone mass, and the nonreproductive causes of chronic pelvic pain demonstrate the medical nature of these disorders.[25]

- Physicians need training in the two emotional disorders— depression and anxiety—that affect women disproportionately. But they also must be aware of the mood, cognitive, and behavioral alterations in response to hormonal changes that affect some women, such as premenstrual syndrome and postpartum depression, to recognize and treat them sensitively.[26]

- Physical assault and sexual abuse have become watchwords as a major cause of injury and death among American women. The numbers are staggering. An article in the *Journal of the American Medical Association* reported that 20% of adult women, 15% of college-age women, and 12% of adolescent girls have experienced incidents of sexual abuse and assault, and one in eight women in a continuing relationship with a man has been assaulted by her partner.[27] (See Chapter 4 for more on domestic violence.) Physicians are in a unique position to recognize abuse and assault because women come to them for treatment of their injuries. Physicians need training to identify and treat the physical and emotional injuries that result from abuse, or to refer patients for additional therapy, but most physicians have little information about what their role should be in this area. Recognizing the problem, the American Medical Association (AMA) has published guidelines regarding the physician's ethical responsibility to diagnose and treat victims of domestic violence, and the organization is developing protocols to help physicians manage abuse.[28]

Ages 45 to 64

It is between ages 45 and 64 that chronic illness strikes women. The harmful effects of obesity—a major risk factor for diabetes, heart disease, stroke, gallbladder disease, and some cancers, and a possible factor in osteoarthritis—place weight control for women high on the list of medical priorities. Obesity is a particular problem for minority women; 44% of African American women and 32% of Hispanic women are overweight, compared with 24% of white women.[29]

Physicians have been historically undertrained in nutrition. Although some physicians in practice recognize this lack and refer patients in need of nutritional counseling to registered dietitians (RDs) or hire these professionals as part of their health care team, recent efforts to include nutrition in medical school curricula have not been successful. Despite a 1990 law passed by Congress requiring *all* medical schools in the United States to add nutrition to the curricula, a 1993 hearing before a subcommittee of the House Committee on Agriculture found that only 25% of medical schools had complied—*fewer* than before the law was passed (phone interview by B. Jacobson with Dr. Eleanor Young, professor of nutrition, University of Texas Health Science Center, San Antonio, and chair of the Nutrition Education Committee of the American Society of Clinical Nutrition, May 9, 1995). But it is not just lack of physician training in nutrition that contributes to the problem of overweight and obese patients. A readily available food supply, sedentary lifestyle, and failure of most weight control programs to maintain weight loss may help to explain why, according to recent government health surveys, Americans are becoming overweight despite a media barrage on dieting. Therefore, incorporating nutrition education into medical school curricula and CME courses is essential if physicians are to help women (and men) overcome the epidemic of overweight and obesity that is negatively affecting their health (see Chapter 7 for more on obesity).

The drop in estrogen levels at menopause is a factor in the rising incidence of heart disease among postmenopausal women and in osteoporosis, a condition causing disabling fractures in large numbers of older women. In fact, whether women should begin hormone replacement therapy (HRT) at menopause, and for how long they should continue it, is a major unanswered question and is one of the issues being studied by the Women's Health Initiative (WHI), the largest and most expensive clinical trial ever conducted.[30] Because HRT protects against cardiovascular disease and osteoporosis but may increase the risk of uterine and breast cancer, more research is needed to enable physicians and health care providers to advise women so that they can make wise decisions based on family history, individual needs, and personal philosophy.

The postmenopausal years can be difficult ones for women as their roles change. Children leave home, many women are widowed or divorced, and elderly, sick parents sometimes need care. Three percent of women in this age group experience a major depressive episode at this time in life and, for many others, disabilities increase. Physicians must understand these psychosocial changes to give mature women sensitive and comprehensive care.

After Age 65

In the senior years, the major causes of death among women are heart disease, cancer, and stroke, in that order, followed by chronic obstructive pulmonary disease (COPD), pneumonia, and injury, usually from falls rather than automobile accidents. Older women experience many other chronic illnesses, including hypertension, diabetes, arthritis, digestive disorders, thyroid diseases, neurological degeneration and dementia, osteoporosis and its attendant spine and hip fractures, and incontinence. In addition, social isolation often occurs because loved ones die, children often live far away, and financial problems sometimes become worse. Mental health conditions may first appear at this time or become more serious. The task of physicians is to recognize and try to lessen the impact of multiple problems on older women so that they can continue to function and enjoy a decent quality of life.

The Competencies Physicians Need

COGME's final report defined competence in women's health as "the ability to provide compassionate, comprehensive care to women through the acquisition and application of the requisite knowledge; clinical skills; attitudes; and ethical, medical, and professional behaviors."[31] But the report went further, pointing out that beyond clinical and technical skill there is a need for communication and collaboration skills—that is, learning to listen and talk to women as equal partners in their own health care.

COGME recommended that *all* physicians need an understanding of basic female physiology and reproductive biology to provide appropriate care to women. Moreover, physicians have to appreciate the complex interaction among environmental, biological, and psychosocial factors that affect women's health. When treating those diseases that are not exclusive to women, physicians should be aware of how these conditions may be different in women or have significant gender implications. They have to find ways of communicating with their women patients, who may have different cultural orientations than they do.[32]

Physicians need to acquire this information at all levels of medical education and training, be it basic science, clinical courses and training, certification and licensing, or CME. Specifically this means knowing

- How women's physiology affects their biological and cognitive function, behavioral changes, and psychosocial development
- The major gender differences in health and disease across the life span of women, including recent findings in women's health research, with particular attention to emerging epidemiological data
- How drugs act in women's bodies over time (their pharmacokinetics) and the impact of hormonal status on drug metabolism

- Community health issues related to promoting health and pre-venting disease and socioeconomic factors—particularly access to medical care—that influence health
- The different ways that culturally diverse women and their fami-lies deal with illness, treatment, prevention, and advice from the medical system, including how women's social roles and life cycle events affect their health, what their patterns of obtain-ing health care and communicating and interacting with their health care providers are, and how gender influences decision making[33]

All this means that physicians must integrate information from bio-medical and biobehavioral sciences and apply it to women's health needs at all stages of their lives, that they must view women within the soci-etal context in which they live, and that they must develop the ability to collaborate with women and their family members as part of the health care team.

Primary Care

The three disciplines that provide most of the routine health care to women are family practice, internal medicine, and obstetrics and gyne-cology (ob-gyn). Because each offers a different spectrum of services, the COGME report found that women's health care has been fragmented between gynecological and obstetrical services on the one hand and general health services on the other hand. For example, whereas data showed that diagnoses by family practitioners and internists included common gynecological and nongynecological conditions, ob-gyns did more Pap tests and breast and pelvic examinations during physical ex-aminations than family practitioners and internists, and, surprisingly, they performed more than half (57%) of all general medical examina-tions. But internists ordered a higher percentage of mammography and were more likely to screen for nongynecological medical disorders during physical examinations than the other two specialties. Although family physicians appear to provide a wider spectrum of routine care to adult women than do either of the other two specialist groups, available data do not supply the percentage of physicians in each of the three specialties who offer across-the-board care. Thus, the report concluded that "variation in practice among the specialties and among individuals within the specialties regarding women's health may leave women with health care gaps, or the need to coordinate their own care as they see multiple providers."[34]

In addition, several studies have documented inconsistencies and inadequacies in preventive care for women. One-third of women do not receive necessary services to detect breast, cervical, and other treatable cancers. One study found that the sex of the physician was a factor because women internists and family practitioners did more Pap tests and mammograms than did male physicians in those specialties.[35] Another study of highly trained family physicians and internists who were part of a National Cancer Institute investigation of the early detection and prevention of cancer found that one-third of these physicians did not perform a breast examination unless the patient asked for it, more than 20% did not address smoking cessation in women who smoked, and fewer than 20% discussed nutritional issues. The absence of uniform standards of primary care may result in poorly coordinated and incomplete care. Until this situation is corrected, women must take increasing responsibility for directing and monitoring their health care.[36]

Current and Developing Programs in Women's Health

Residency training. Fortunately, perhaps because of the growing influence of managed care plans with their similar guidelines for general practice, the medical specialties that provide care to women—internal medicine, ob-gyn, pediatrics, and family practice—are moving toward a common vision of the competencies residency training should provide. For example, although ob-gyn has long been seen as a surgical discipline, the Residency Review Committee for Obstetrics-Gynecology has shifted this focus and expanded its program requirements to give residents a much broader set of generalist skills. These include serving as the primary care physician to female patients for one-half a day a week during the 3 or 4 years of residency training, receiving instruction and clinical experience in managing the medical problems of women past reproductive age, and completing a 4-month rotation in either internal medicine or family practice, a 1-month rotation in emergency medicine, and a 1-month rotation in geriatric medicine.[37]

In internal medicine, which has been highly specialized in the past because of the development of subspecialization (for example, cardiology or gerontology), the shift for the past decade has been away from hospital-based training to outpatient settings, which has allowed for the reemergence of general internists qualified to provide primary care. This has led to an emphasis on community-based primary care training and practice. Concurrently, internal medicine has recognized the need for competence in gynecological care for women, which is now required as part of residency training.[38]

Similarly, residents in family medicine must be trained to manage the common gynecological conditions that occur throughout a woman's life, which include providing prenatal, delivery, and postpartum care. In addition, core educational guidelines in women's health and ob-gyn have been added to the formal training requirements. Pediatric residency programs have changed as well and now require training to provide comprehensive care to girls from infancy through adolescence, with increased time for education in behavioral, developmental, and adolescent medicine and in reproductive health.[39]

In addition, a new spirit of collaboration across specialties is taking place at many institutions, with departments of internal medicine and ob-gyn coordinating curricula and clinical training for residents. The American Academy of Family Practice (AAFP) and the American College of Obstetricians and Gynecologists (ACOG) have worked together to produce training guidelines in women's health.[40]

Although these are helpful changes, they will take time to implement fully. Those in charge of training programs, women's health advocates, and policy makers should monitor their progress so that an attainable standard of comprehensive care for women emerges as soon as possible.

Undergraduate medical education.   A radical change will be needed to train physicians in women's health because it will be necessary to cross traditional departmental boundaries. What is needed is a new way to develop curricula and establish collaborative relationships and interdisciplinary clinical models. One major problem is the difficulty of evaluating the women's health content of existing medical curricula in the preclinical and clinical years. Although many schools have interdisciplinary curriculum committees, not all have a central review and planning process that is separate from the individual departments. Thus, faculty and administrators often are unaware of what each department offers in its courses. At the clinical level, knowledge and skills acquired in clinical clerkships may overlap, conflict, or leave gaps in a student's preparation for practice.[41] A recent study found that fewer than one-fourth of medical schools in the United States offer an elective in women's health.[42] Few of the courses that did exist appeared to provide a comprehensive approach to women's health; rather, they were on specific topics, such as eating disorders or violence against women. To correct this situation, in 1993 Congress directed the ORWH at NIH and the Health Resources and Services Administration, along with the Public Health Service Office on Women's Health and other government agencies, to evaluate the extent to which medical school curricula address women's health. The results of the survey, which was coordinated by the Association of American Medical Colleges, and specific recommendations for a core curriculum on women's health should be submitted to Congress shortly.[43]

Continuing medical education.   Physicians are expected to maintain and upgrade their knowledge and skills after completing their formal training. Some disciplines require that physicians take a minimum number of CME hours and pass an examination to be recertified. Moreover, the rapid development of new technology makes continuing education imperative, and the information revolution allows easy and rapid access to new developments. With the increasing information on women's health, all physicians who treat women must increase their skills and knowledge.[44]

Curriculum content and structure.   The COGME report recommended that

> the educational philosophy, scope, and content of a comprehensive women's health curriculum needs to be developed. A core curriculum in women's health will help define the qualifications that physicians need to care for women as well as serve as a conceptual framework for medical institutions interested in restructuring medical school curricula,

developing or enhancing residency and fellowship training programs, or planning research initiatives in women's health. The goal is to incorporate gender related women's health education and information into medical education at all levels—undergraduate, graduate, and postgraduate—and thereby improve women's health. Curriculum objectives should be multidisciplinary and include psychosocial and behavioral components, emphasize health education and prevention, and be based on a life span approach.[45]

Clinical models for training.   In addition, new clinical models are needed to provide training in the comprehensive care of women. These models should be based on the collaboration of various disciplines so that resources and knowledge are pooled and innovations in education, clinical care, and research are developed.[46]

Faculty development.   Finally, it is necessary to recruit faculty with a broad view of women's health, able to integrate content from several disciplines, develop successful interdisciplinary relationships, and serve as role models for students and residents. Unfortunately, there are no government or foundation initiatives for fellowship programs and faculty development in women's health, and this remains a substantial barrier to change.

Achieving Competency in Women's Health: Changes Needed

COGME's report concluded that physicians in the past have not been adequately prepared to care for women and that *fundamental* changes in the education of physicians are needed to deliver comprehensive care to women. This means not only curricular reform at all levels of training but also establishing innovative academic programs that have broad institutional support.

These changes will not be attained easily because of significant barriers that still exist for women in medicine. The COGME report found that although many more women are now in medicine than in the past, a trend that is expected to continue into the next century, women are still underrepresented among leaders in medicine. Because women tend to cluster in five disciplines—family practice, internal medicine, ob-gyn, pediatrics, and psychiatry—they are at a particular disadvantage in other fields. But the major barrier is still gender bias. According to the COGME report, it "remains the single greatest deterrent to women achieving their full potential in every aspect of the medical profession and is a barrier throughout the professional life cycle."[47]

COGME made the following recommendations to improve the medical education of physicians in women's health:

1. Changes in physician education and training should reflect the altering demographics of the population and recognize the special needs of economically, socially, and culturally excluded population groups.

2. Institutions should ensure that women are full participants in the institutional, community, regional, and national changes that are occurring in health care. Institutions should foster collaboration between existing community and national health care groups and student and faculty organizations to achieve this goal.

3. Primary care physicians need a broad understanding of, competency in, and continuing education about women's health.

4. Academic health centers should evaluate the knowledge base in the basic and clinical science disciplines to determine what is being taught about gender issues and how new information is being incorporated. These centers should use the information to identify deficiencies in the understanding and teaching of women's health and make recommendations for change.

5. Evaluation of student performance in women's health should include assessment criteria to identify and correct deficiencies in knowledge, clinical management, and behavior toward and communication with women patients.

6. Medical school faculties should develop clinical simulations of the health problems most critical to the comprehensive care of women in all age, racial, and ethnic groups. Students should be expected to manage these simulations according to a faculty-accepted standard to receive a medical or osteopathy degree.

7. The National Board of Medical Examiners should review its three examinations to ensure adequate assessment of competency in

the knowledge and skills needed to provide comprehensive care for women. A subsequent nationwide assessment of knowledge and problem-solving abilities would help medical educators to identify the clinical simulations that should be included in undergraduate medical education.

8. The education of physicians should prepare them to recognize and respond appropriately to the effects of women's changing roles in their relationships to the medical system, patterns of acquiring health care, access to care, methods of communication, and compliance with treatment and medical advice.

9. Accreditation bodies—such as the Liaison Committee on Medical Education, the Accreditation Council for Graduate Medical Education, the American Osteopathic Association, and other national organizations involved in undergraduate, graduate, and CME, such as AMA, the Association of American Medical Colleges, the Association of American Colleges of Osteopathic Medicine, the National Board of Medical Specialties, the National Board of Medical Examiners, the Federation of State Medical Boards, and the Council of Medical Specialty Societies—should collaborate to increase the development of educational programs that address women's health issues at all educational levels.

10. CME should provide opportunities for practicing physicians to remedy any deficiencies in their knowledge and practices in the area of women's health.

11. Fundamental changes that cross traditional departmental boundaries in medical school and postgraduate curricula are needed. Such changes would be facilitated by collaborative centers or programs in women's health within academic health centers.

12. In addition to developing innovative approaches to medical education and training in women's health that cross traditional boundaries, medical schools and other teaching institutions should develop integrated curricula, interdisciplinary research, and more responsive clinical models and should support the development of expert faculty committed to advancing women's health at all levels.

13. Congress should provide funding for competitive grants to support and stimulate women's health initiatives within academic

institutions. The programs could include interdisciplinary educational offerings, research, health promotion and disease prevention, and patient care. Such grants should acknowledge programs on the basis of their innovation, their potential to be models for new programs, and their cost-effectiveness.

14. Congress should establish academic awards in women's health. Such grants should provide support to individual faculty members for their professional development and for the implementation of innovative programs in women's health. Congress should provide funding for competitive grants to support and stimulate academic institutions' efforts at improving women's health.

15. Interdisciplinary fellowship programs in women's health should be established to allow physicians to acquire additional skills and training in the comprehensive care of women and gender-relevant research. Although the programs would vary in emphasis and design, depending on the characteristics of the participating institutions, each would have a core program that would introduce fellows to basic principles and knowledge essential to an integrated understanding of women's health and to the scientific methods used in women's health research.

16. Current and expanded efforts to promote research in women's health should be supported.[48]

Implementing these recommendations would go a long way toward ensuring that the nation attains the highest standard of education, training, practice, and research in women's health.

Endnotes

[1] A good example of emerging information is the Postmenopausal Estrogen/Progestin Interventions (PEPI) Trial. A report in the *Journal of the American Medical Association* on January 18, 1995, of a 3-year study of HRT found that estrogen alone or in combination with progestin improved lipoprotein and lowered fibrinogen levels "without detectable effects on postchallenge insulin or blood pressure." The study found unopposed estrogen raises HDL (good) cholesterol levels the most, but, because it increases the incidence of uterine cancer, it should be used only by women without a uterus. Estrogen with progestin added also raised HDL cholesterol levels.

[2]Senate Report #102-397 & House Report #103-156, 1993

[3]National Institutes of Health: *Opportunities for Research on Women's Health.* Hunt Valley, MD, September 4–6, 1991 (hereafter called Hunt Valley)

[4]Day JC: Population projections of the United States, by age, race, and Hispanic origin: 1993 to 2050, in *U.S. Bureau of the Census, Current Population Reports* (P25-1104). Washington, DC, U.S. Government Printing Office, 1993

[5]Blumenthal SJ, Johnson T: *Women's Health Research: Perspectives and Priorities in the 1990s: Facts and Research Needs.* Washington, DC, Society for the Advancement of Women's Health Research, 1993

[6]Ibid.

[7]Day JC, op. cit.

[8]Hunt Valley, op. cit.

[9]Clancy CM, Massion CT: American women's health: a patchwork quilt with gaps. *Journal of the American Medical Association* 268:1918–1919, 1992

[10]Louis Harris and Associates for The Commonwealth Fund: Survey of Women's Health, July 1993 (hereafter called Harris L, op. cit.)

[11]Ibid.

[12]Rodin J, Ickovics JR: Women's health: review and research agenda as we approach the 21st century. *American Journal of Psychology* 45:1018–1034, 1990

[13]National Center for Health Statistics: *Advance Report of Final Mortality Statistics—1991*, August 1993

[14]Marshall E: Incidence rates and trends for the ten leading women's cancers. *Science* 259:618–621, 1993

[15]Gray MJ, Haseltine F, Love S, et al: *The Woman's Guide to Good Health.* Yonkers, NY, Consumer Reports Books, 1991

[16]Henrich JB: *Academic and Clinical Programs in Women's Health.* Paper submitted to the Council on Graduate Medical Education, April 1, 1994

[17]Ibid.

[18]Centers for Disease Control, National Center for Health Statistics: *Vital and Health Statistics: Current Estimates From the National Health Interview Survey, 1991* (DHHS Publ No PHS 93-1512). U.S. Department of Health & Human Services, December 1992

[19]Harris L, op. cit.

[20]Henrich JB, op. cit.

[21]Ibid.

[22]Ibid.

[23]Ibid.

[24]Ibid.

[25]Ibid.

[26]Ibid.

[27]Council on Scientific Affairs, American Medical Association: Violence against women: relevance for medical practitioners. *Journal of the American Medical Association* 267:3184–3189, 1992

[28]Council on Ethical and Judicial Affairs, American Medical Association: Physicians and domestic violence: ethical considerations. *Journal of the American Medical Association* 267:3190–3193, 1992

[29]Henrich JB, op. cit.

[30]Healy B: Women's health, public welfare. *Journal of the American Medical Association* 266:566–568, 1991

[31]Council on Graduate Medical Education: *Fifth Report: Women & Medicine* (DHHS Publ No HRSA-P-DM-95). U.S. Department of Health & Human Services, July 1, 1995

[32]Ibid.

[33]Ibid.

[34]Ibid.

[35]Lurie N, Slater J, McGovern P, et al: Preventive care for women: does the sex of the physician matter? *New England Journal of Medicine* 329:478–482, 1993

[36]Council on Graduate Medical Education, op. cit.

[37]Ibid.

[38]Ibid.

[39]Ibid.

[40]*ACOG-AAFP Recommended Core Curriculum and Hospital Practice Privileges in Obstetrics-Gynecology for Family Physicians* (AAFP Reprint No 261). Joint Ad Hoc Committee of the American Academy of Family Physicians, the American College of Obstetricians and Gynecologists, the Council on Resident Education in Obstetrics and Gynecology, and the Association of Professors of Gynecology and Obstetrics

[41]Ibid.

[42]Montgomery K, Moulton AW: Medical education in women's health. *Journal of Women's Health* 1:253–254, 1992

[43]Council on Graduate Medical Education, op. cit.

[44]Ibid.

[45]Ibid.

[46]Ibid.

[47]Ibid.

[48]Ibid.

Part 4

The Political Agenda and Priorities

12

Including Women in Clinical Trials: Policy Changes at the Food and Drug Administration

Ruth B. Merkatz, Ph.D., R.N., F.A.A.N.
Elyse I. Summers, J.D.

At the U.S. Food and Drug Administration (FDA), 1993 was a pivotal year for women's health. A new guideline was published that articulated two important, but slightly different, agency policies.[1] First, the FDA reversed a 16-year-old policy that had virtually banned participation of women with childbearing potential from entry into the early phases of clinical trials. Second, the guideline called for an analysis by gender of the safety and efficacy of all new drug applications (NDAs). Women, therefore, would have to be represented in clinical studies in sufficient numbers for such analyses to be possible. As part of the analysis, the guideline described sex-specific factors that should be examined in relation to the response of drugs in women. These factors included the female hormonal environment as well as body size, body fat content and distribution, and metabolic phenotype.

Events Leading up to the FDA's 1993 Policy Changes

The 1993 guideline for the study and evaluation of gender differences in the clinical evaluation of drugs represented a shift in both scientific and ethical thinking about whether women with childbearing potential could or should participate in the earliest phases of clinical trials, specifically Phases 1 and 2. To understand the impact of this new policy and its potential to contribute to the health and well-being of women, it is useful first to examine how drugs are developed in the United States and then to consider earlier policies regarding the participation of women in the drug development process and analysis of data.

Drug Development Process

Most drugs are developed by pharmaceutical and biotechnology companies that conduct clinical trials to determine whether new therapies are safe and effective. The various steps for proceeding with these trials are codified in regulations that are subject to a formalized rule-making process.[2] They are delineated further through guidelines or guidance documents that are written periodically as new scientific information becomes available or as situations arise that affect the conduct of clinical trials, such as the need to speed delivery of new products to market in the face of novel health crises (for example, the acquired immunodeficiency syndrome [AIDS] epidemic).

In accordance with federal regulations, before a company may begin testing in humans, it must submit an investigational new drug (IND) application to the FDA.[3] This application must include results of preclinical trials (testing conducted in the laboratory and with animal species) to provide relative assurances of safety and some promise of effectiveness. The IND application also must describe the design of the protocol(s) that will be followed in conducting human studies.

Premarket trials in humans consist of three phases (see Figure 12–1). Phase 1 trials are the initial studies in humans and generally involve small numbers of healthy volunteers or patients treated over a short period of time. These studies assess the most common acute adverse

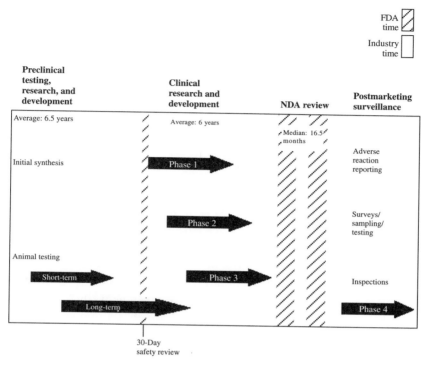

Figure 12–1. New drug development timeline.

effects and examine the size of doses that patients can take safely without a high incidence of side effects. Initial clinical studies also begin to clarify what happens to a drug in the body—whether it is changed (metabolized), how much of the drug or metabolite gets into the blood (the pharmacokinetics of the drug), and how much accumulates in tissues or target organs for which the drug is to be prescribed (the drug's pharmacodynamics). Phase 2 studies normally involve a few hundred patients who have the condition that the drug is intended to treat. These are the earliest controlled trials designed to demonstrate preliminary effectiveness and relative safety. Phase 2 trials also involve dose-ranging studies to test various doses for safety and efficacy. In the final phase of drug development, Phase 3, large randomized clinical trials are conducted to provide more information about safety, effectiveness, and dosages of a drug. It is important to note that although the three phases of drug trials appear to occur in essentially a chronological sequence, generally there is a certain degree of overlap between the phases and the work being done in each. For example, a Phase 2 trial may begin while certain work is still ongoing with Phase 1 trials.

Before Phase 1 studies can begin, certain preclinical studies conducted in animal species (generally the mouse and the rabbit) must be completed. These studies are aimed at demonstrating that a drug shows promise of being effective and assessing relative safety and effects on vital organs. Because of the length of time it takes to develop drugs, the associated costs, and the likelihood that only a relatively small percentage of drugs will complete the development phases, not all segments of the preclinical studies are completed before the Phase 1 studies begin in humans. Specifically, the preclinical reproductive toxicology studies to determine effects on male and female fertility and the potential of a drug to be teratogenic or cause malformations in a developing fetus are usually not done until Phase 2 of the clinical studies are under way.

Reproductive toxicology studies take approximately 15 months to complete.[4] It also has been noted that if these segments had to be completed in all cases before initiating Phase 1 studies in humans and early Phase 2 studies, preclinical studies would have to be started approximately 1 year before filing an IND. Such a requirement would add time and cost to the development of drugs.

Reproductive toxicity testing of new drugs is done in three segments, as shown in Table 12–1.[5] Segment 1, a study of fertility and reproductive performance, is usually conducted in rats and provides an overall view of drug toxicity. The entire reproductive process, including the effect of a drug on gonadal function, estrous cycles, mating behavior, conception rate, organ development (organogenesis), duration of gestation, nature of birth (parturition), lactation, growth, and postnatal development of the offspring, is evaluated. Postnatal evaluation includes physical development and general fertility of the offspring. Although in this segment both parents are given the drug, no distinction between effects on the male or the female is made. However, if an adverse effect is observed, the treated animals are then mated with the control animals of the opposite sex.

Segment 2, a teratological evaluation, is conducted in two species, the rat and the rabbit. The main purpose of this segment is to determine whether a drug given to a pregnant animal during organogenesis has

Table 12–1. Reproductive toxicity testing of new drugs

Segment 1	Segment 2	Segment 3
Drug effects on entire reproductive process	Teratological evaluation of drug during organogenesis	Perinatal and postnatal testing
Gonadal function		Day 16 of gestation
Estrous cycles		Until weaned
Mating behavior	Embryotoxicity	
Conception rate	Teratogenic effects	
Organogenesis	Maternal toxicity	
Duration of gestation	Offspring toxicity	
Nature of parturition		
Lactation		
Growth		
Postnatal development: physical; offspring fertility		

potential for being toxic to the embryo and causing deforming (teratogenic) effects. An attempt is made to distinguish between maternal toxicity and toxic effects directly on the offspring.

Segment 3, a perinatal and postnatal study, is usually done in rats treated during the last trimester of gestation (beginning on day 16) and continued until the animals are weaned (see Table 12–1).

On completion of all clinical studies, data are presented to the FDA in the form of an NDA. The FDA conducts an initial review of the NDA within 45 days of receiving the application to determine whether the application is complete relative to the data elements required for a full review. If accepted, the application is then filed and will undergo a total review pertaining to the safety and efficacy of the drug. As noted in Figure 12–1, this review can take from 2 months to 7 years. In 1994, the median review time was 20.8 months. However, as implementation of the Prescription Drugs User Fees Act of 1992[6] has progressed, many important new drugs are being reviewed and approved in less than a year; in 1994, 14 NDA or PLAs (product licensing application, for biological products) were approved in less than 12 months. Recently, an important new osteoporosis drug, alendronate, was reviewed and approved by the FDA in just 6 months. In 1996, the median total time for approval of priority drugs (for example, protease inhibitors for the treatment of human immunodeficiency virus [HIV] and drugs for cancer) was 7.8 months. Beyond the review and approval of new products, before a new drug or device can be released to the market, the FDA and the pharmaceutical company also must agree on information that will be included in the product's label. Often, FDA convenes an advisory committee of outside experts and consumer representatives to make recommendations about the approval of new drugs and labeling issues.

Selection of Subjects for Clinical Trials—1977 Guideline

In terms of appropriate subjects for sponsors to select for entry into clinical trials, a guideline issued by the FDA in 1977 stated that drugs should be studied in the population that will receive them.[7] This guideline specifically stated that all age groups should be included, but it was not explicit about the need to study both sexes. It did contain a prohibition on the participation of women of childbearing potential in Phase 1 and early Phase 2 trials, except when the drug being tested was for the treatment of a serious or life-threatening illness. Specifically, the 1977 guideline stated that "a woman of childbearing potential is defined as a premenopausal female capable of becoming pregnant. This includes women on oral, injectable, or mechanical contraception; women who are single; women whose husbands have been vasectomized or whose husbands have received or are using mechanical contraceptive devices. . . . In general, women of childbearing potential should be excluded from the earliest. . . studies." Wide participation for women with childbearing potential was permitted after the results from segments 1 and 2 of the reproductive toxicology studies were available.

Protection of human subjects.   It is not surprising that in the 1990s, as issues of women's health gained national attention, the 1977 FDA restrictions for women in clinical trials began to be debated and criticized. However, this restriction is best understood when viewed in the context of the larger issue of protection of human subjects. Historically, the need to protect human subjects grew out of abuses in human experimentation that were visited on defenseless populations.

    In the early 19th century, for example, while Europeans were denouncing American surgical practices as barbaric and cruel, American physicians viewed their considerable advances as proof of a dynamic culture characterized by mechanical ingenuity and frontier resourcefulness. Often, the subjects in this preanesthetic era were American slave women who were exposed to extreme pain and suffering inflicted during experimental procedures. Most notable were the experiments conducted by Dr. J. Marion Sims, who was developing techniques to correct openings between the bladder and vagina (vesicovaginal fistulas). As one surgical pioneer put it, "Even the most severe pain should never be an obstacle to the performance of life-saving operations."[8]

From the beginning of the post–Civil War period through the end of the 19th century, there was a general downturn in medical experimentation. When it picked up again, in the early 20th century, institutionalized populations were frequently used as research subjects. Joseph Goldberger, the Public Health Service (PHS) investigator who proved that pellagra was a nutritional deficiency disease—caused by inadequate nicotinic acid in the diet—and not a communicable illness as previously thought, did his experiments on Mississippi convicts and Georgia mental patients.[9] In this instance, however, the subjects benefited by getting a better diet than normally provided in these institutions. During World War II, prisoners volunteered to test drugs used to fight tropical diseases. The use of prisoners to conduct clinical trials continued well into the 1960s, when serious questions arose regarding this population of subjects. In 1965, a deadly blood plasma epidemic was traced to an Alabama prison in which a private firm had not only conducted nearly 25% of the entire United States' Phase 1 drug trials but also sold prisoners' plasma, for which the inmates were given a token payment. Until 1972, 90% of all investigational drugs were first evaluated in prison populations. By the time Jessica Mitford wrote a provocative chapter titled "Cheaper than Chimpanzees" in a popular 1973 book on prison conditions, prisoner testing in the United States had virtually disappeared.[10]

However, it was not until the abuses of the infamous Tuskegee syphilis study were revealed in the early 1970s that there was a widespread recognition that human research subjects in the United States were not being adequately protected and that more formal regulations were needed. The Tuskegee observational study began in 1932 and lasted 40 years, into the early 1970s. It involved approximately 400 African

American men, many of whom were allowed to remain untreated for their disease even after antibiotic treatment became widely available and the standard of care for the treatment of syphilis.[11]

It is notable that the Tuskegee study began before the promulgation of the Nuremberg Code in 1947, the first internationally recognized standard for human research. This code was developed as a result of the Nazi atrocities of World War II, which included horrendous medical experimentation on concentration camp victims. It was drafted during the Nuremberg war crimes trial as a set of standards for judging physicians and scientists who had conducted biomedical experiments on concentration camp prisoners. The Nuremberg Code became the prototype of many later codes intended to ensure that research involving human subjects would be conducted in an ethical manner.

In 1953, flowing from the spirit of the Nuremberg Code, the National Institutes of Health (NIH) established its first panels of scientists to review research proposals involving human volunteers. Throughout the 1950s and 1960s, however, medical ethics generally supported the autonomy of individual researchers. It was not until 1974 that the U.S. Department of Health, Education and Welfare (the precursor to the Department of Health and Human Services) issued federal regulations for the protection of human subjects involved in federally funded research.[12]

With regard to the specific involvement of women in clinical research, it was the thalidomide disaster that changed the face of research permissiveness and fostered a belief in the need to protect women from the risks of research. Thalidomide, a hypnotic drug, was given to thousands of women in Europe and Australia during the 1950s and early 1960s. It caused an epidemic of babies with severely deformed limbs (phocomelia defects). This drug was never approved by the FDA in the United States, principally because of the work done at the FDA by Dr. Frances Kelsey, who, along with her fellow FDA reviewers, was most concerned that the application did not contain any information about the effects of the drug on a fetus. Dr. Kelsey refused to approve the application for thalidomide until she felt assured regarding the teratogenic effects of the drug.[13] For her work in reviewing the drug, she was awarded the Presidential Medal of Honor. Congress responded to this event, as well. They enacted the Kefauver Harris amendments[14] to the Pure Food and Drug Act of 1938,[15] which gave to the FDA the regulatory authority to require that new drugs be screened for efficacy as well as safety, that new investigational drugs be approved for studies in humans before trials could begin (the NDA process as described earlier), and that investigators obtain informed consent from research subjects.

The thalidomide tragedy led many to believe that women of reproductive age were a particularly vulnerable research population; the discovery in the early 1970s about adverse effects on offspring from diethylstilbestrol (DES) served to confirm this belief. DES had been prescribed to thousands of American women over a 30-year period in the mistaken belief that it prevented spontaneous abortion. In 1971, the first reports were published about reproductive abnormalities and cancer in young females who had been exposed in utero.[16] Based on these two major medical events, and the fact that in the 1970s there was little public discussion of possible medical benefits for including women in the early phases of drug trials, it is not surprising that the FDA, in researching and writing its 1977 guideline, determined an ethical need to restrict from the earliest clinical trials women who had the potential of becoming pregnant. Even though women were being excluded regardless of their pregnancy status, it was held that, as long as there existed the physiological possibility of a pregnancy, there was a potential risk to a fetus or putative fetus.

1977 Guideline Revisited

Beginning in the late 1980s and early 1990s, a growing awareness of research inequities gave rise to a desire by many within FDA and affected communities to revisit the 1977 guideline. As discussed earlier, the broad protectionist policy outlined in the 1977 guideline reflected a philosophy of zero-risk to a fetus, even to a potential fetus. Although protecting a fetus from unanticipated exposure to possibly harmful drugs was and obviously continues to be of paramount importance, banning from early drug trials all women who can conceive came to be seen as an unduly burdensome way to achieve the goal of fetal protection. The ban articulated in the 1977 guideline began to be viewed as problematic on two levels—ethical and scientific.

The ethical issues raised reflect a need to respect a woman's autonomy and ability to decide for herself whether to participate in clinical research. That is, women are capable of controlling their fertility so that they will not become pregnant while participating in a clinical trial. This right to choose whether to participate in a given activity was supported by the Supreme Court in the landmark case of *United Automobile Workers v. Johnson Controls*, which held that the Pregnancy Discrimination Act prohibits the blanket exclusion of pregnant women from jobs they are qualified to perform solely because working conditions pose potential risks to exposed fetuses.[17] Although there is a clear distinction between employment rights and participation in clinical trials, inherent in the court's decision is a woman's right to decide about fetal risk, which in turn supports the principles of autonomy and informed consent. Moreover, regarding clinical trials, it is now well established that the danger of fetal exposure can be reduced by protocol design. Because early clinical studies are short term, sometimes involving only a single dose of medication, it is possible to administer a drug to a woman immediately following a pregnancy test that has confirmed that she is not pregnant. With longer studies, the 1993 guideline clearly states that the FDA expects that women considering entry in a clinical trial will receive counseling, when necessary and appropriate, about the importance of using reliable contraception (or practicing abstinence). In addition, the FDA expects local institutional review boards (IRBs) to continue to review closely investigational protocols that may present potential risks to the fetus from known or probable teratogens before the trials are allowed to proceed. Finally, the FDA itself reviews the risk-benefit ratio of such protocols.

Regarding the scientific imperative to change the 1977 guideline, specific questions began to be asked about the drug development process for women; for example, was there adequate information about how drugs worked in women; were the unique physiological characteristics of women considered relative to dosage formulation and overall drug safety and efficacy? FDA surveys conducted in 1983 and 1988 found that both sexes generally had substantial representation in the later phases of clinical trials, usually in numbers that reflected the prevalence of the disease being studied,[1,18] but it was equally clear that gender analysis was not being done regularly. For example, although there were more women in studies of nonsteroidal anti-inflammatory drugs, there were few analyses to detect possible differences in safety and efficacy between women and men. This continued to be the case even after the FDA, in 1988, issued guidelines that called for analyses of whether safety and effectiveness were similar within various population subgroups defined by sex, age, and race. The General Accounting Office (GAO) reviewed the participation of women in Phase 2 and 3 clinical trials of drugs approved between 1988 and 1991 and reported that analysis by sex was done in approximately 50% of the trials.[19]

Because the GAO study included the review of many applications that had been submitted before the 1988 guidelines were published, FDA surveyed NDAs from June 1991 to July 1992. The agency found that gender analysis of safety data occurred 64% of the time, and effectiveness data were analyzed according to sex 54% of the time. By 1993, it had become obvious to observers both within and outside FDA that there would be a scientific benefit gained by obtaining information about how drugs behave in women.

1993 Guideline

Against this historical backdrop, the 1993 "Guideline for the Study and Evaluation of Gender Differences in the Clinical Evaluation of Drugs" was written by the FDA. As noted, the guideline accomplished two slightly different yet important policies: 1) the FDA reversed a 16-year-old policy that had virtually banned participation of women with childbearing potential from entry into the early phases of clinical trials, and 2) the guideline called for an analysis by gender of the safety and efficacy of all NDAs. We have discussed the important ethical implications of removing the restriction against women's participation in the early phases of clinical trials in the foregoing pages. It is the second aspect of the 1993 guideline—the issue of good science—that warrants further examination.

Drug Response and Sex-Related Factors

The way a drug responds in the body is influenced by many factors. Gender is one, but age, ethnic background, body size, body-fat content and distribution, the degree of metabolic activity, the presence of diseases other than the one for which a study drug is being tested, and the use of other therapies at the same time as the test drug (concomitant therapies) all play a role in the way a drug behaves. These variables affect both the pharmacokinetics (the amount of the drug in the blood) and the pharmacodynamics (the accumulation of the drug in targeted tissues or organs) of a substance. By recognizing such differences, physicians can adjust the size and/or interval of the dose or the way the drug is monitored; they also can select another drug that may improve patient outcome.

Researchers have identified several drugs that display sex differences in pharmacokinetics. For example, women metabolize propranolol, used to treat cardiac arrhythmias, more slowly than men; sex hormones may regulate some of the enzymes that break down this drug.[20] Theophylline, a widely used therapy in emphysema and other congestive lung diseases, stays in the body for a significantly shorter time in females than in males—both in smokers and nonsmokers—presumably because of gender differences in liver metabolism.[21] Other drugs that display lower rates of clearance in women include acetaminophen and aspirin (pain killers), several benzodiazepines (used to treat anxiety), lidocaine (topical anesthetic, treatment for ventricular arrhythmias), ondansetron (an antiemetic), and mephobarbital (anticonvulsant, sedative).[22] Recent research has shown a dramatic excess risk of torsade de pointes (a potentially fatal form of ventricular tachycardia) with the use of drugs that block cardiac potassium channels in women compared with men.[23]

Variations in body size and composition and the metabolic effects of enzymes and hormones are likely causes of some sex-related differences in drug response. With respect to enzymes, metabolism of drugs through the liver and variations in the concentration of hepatic enzymes such as cytochrome P-450 may influence sex-related differences of drugs. Women's normally smaller body size and higher body-fat content may influence the level of a drug in the blood or other tissues. For example, even though men and women produce the same enzyme to break down alcohol—alcohol dehydrogenase—women experience relatively higher blood alcohol concentrations from the same amount of alcohol consumed because they are usually smaller in body size and have more fat and less water in their bodies. Scientists have recently demonstrated that, in women, the lining of the stomach produces less alcohol dehydrogenase than it does in men.[24]

Women's hormonal cycling may, in addition, affect both the pharmacokinetics and pharmacodynamics of drugs in various ways. Important considerations include 1) the varying levels of sex hormones during the menstrual cycle, 2) the effects of significantly higher hormone levels during pregnancy and the metabolic consequences of pregnancy itself, and 3) the effect of oral contraceptives on the metabolism of concomitant therapies and the effect of other drugs on the efficacy of contraceptives. In addition, hormonal differences between pre- and postmenopausal women may play a role in drug reactions. For example, the varying levels of female sex hormones (estrogen and progesterone) affect the way insulin binds to blood cells. One study showed insulin binding to red and white blood cells was higher in the follicular phase of the cycle (when ovulation occurs) than in the luteal phase just before menstruation. This correlation may exacerbate high blood sugar levels during the luteal phase in some women with insulin-dependent diabetes mellitus because of this lower blood level of insulin.[25]

The differences in hormonal patterns between pre- and postmenopausal women and the use of hormone replacement therapy after menopause may affect pharmacokinetics. For example, the half-life of prednisolone (an anti-inflammatory and antiallergic agent) is significantly longer in women using female hormones than in those who do not. Young women taking oral contraceptives and postmenopausal women taking conjugated estrogens both experience this extended drug presence.[26]

Other drugs that have an effect on contraceptives by lowering their levels in the blood are the antibiotics griseofulvin and tetracycline, the antitubercular agent rifampin, and some anticonvulsant drugs, such as carbamazepine and phenytoin (personal communication to R. Merkatz, by R. Temple, FDA). Because approximately 10 million women in the United States use oral contraceptives, the possibility that concomitant therapies may decrease their effectiveness is a serious concern. Susceptible women may experience breakthrough bleeding or even become pregnant when they take these agents in conjunction with oral contraceptives, especially the low-estrogen oral contraceptives currently available.

Women and Clinical Trials: Looking to the Future

The publication of the 1993 guideline served as a call to both drug sponsors and FDA reviewers to recognize the scientific importance of gender analysis and to perform it on data gathered during clinical trials. FDA now reviews all NDAs shortly after submission to make certain that they include appropriate gender analyses. If FDA receives an NDA that does not contain gender analysis where it reasonably should be included, the agency works with sponsors to develop their plans for analyzing sex-response differences and may consider refusing to start a review of the application unless sex-specific analyses are provided within a reasonable time (personal communication to R. Merkatz, by R. Temple, FDA).

In addition, the 1993 guideline calls for including women in the earliest phases of human drug testing so that the information gathered can guide the design of later trials.[27] The guideline emphasizes that "reasonable numbers" of women be included in the studies of new drugs without precisely defining reasonable numbers. The agency expects, however, enough representation of both sexes to detect possible differences, particularly pharmacokinetic differences, using either formal studies or pharmacokinetic screening.

Pharmacokinetic screening assesses a full range of factors, such as demographic characteristics of study subjects, underlying diseases they may have, and other drugs they are taking that can change a drug's level in the blood or other tissues.[28] It requires obtaining a small number of steady-state blood concentration measurements in most subjects in Phase 2 and 3 trials and then analyzing them to detect the relationship between the drug's pharmacokinetics and particular characteristics of the subgroup, such as sex, age, kidney and liver function, body size, muscle mass, and concomitant therapy. If results suggest significant gender differences, more formal pharmacokinetic studies can begin.

Because few clinically important sex-related differences in the way the body responds to a given concentration of a drug have been documented to date, the guideline does not require separate clinical or pharmacodynamic studies in women in most cases. Instead, FDA relies on the substantial representation of both sexes in studies of safety and efficacy and the examination of data for sex differences in effectiveness, rates of adverse effects, and responses to specific doses of a drug. If these analyses suggest gender differences, or if such differences could be especially important, as with drugs that have a narrow therapeutic range (a small margin between efficacy and toxicity), more formal studies may be needed.

FDA recognizes that implementation of the 1993 guideline has not always been easy. Indeed, many of the comments that FDA received in response to the 1993 guideline sought clarification and further guidance on how to implement it. To be responsive to the questions, the agency has pursued both regulatory and educational activities. On September 8, 1995, the FDA proposed a regulation to define clearly in the NDA format and content requirements the need to present effectiveness and safety data for important demographic subgroups, specifically gender, age, and racial subgroups.[29] The rule codifies the expectations that FDA described in the 1993 guideline. The proposed regulation, which will be published as a final rule early in 1997, also requires IND sponsors of drugs—including biological products—to characterize, in their annual reports, the number of subjects in a clinical study according to gender, age group, and race.

On the educational front, in November 1995, FDA sponsored a 2-day scientific workshop to examine issues related to gender analysis and identify significant areas for further policy development and clarification. More than 600 people from industry, academia, government, and consumer groups attended this conference designed to answer key questions on how to design trials and conduct gender analysis. Some questions raised included

1. How can clinical trials be designed to detect clinically relevant factors in drug response between men and women and other patient groups?
2. When during the medical product review processes does it become essential to identify gender effects?
3. What key factors are important to determine whether an observed difference is of sufficient magnitude to warrant further study?

4. Under what circumstances are dosing regimens apt to be different for men and women and how can this be determined?

In addition, as a "next step" taken from the information presented at the conference, and to implement the recommendations of the conference, FDA has convened an internal gender analysis working group.

Human Immunodeficiency Virus/ Acquired Immunodeficiency Syndrome

The issue of women's access to clinical trials is nowhere more important than in trials to test products for the prevention, diagnosis, and treatment of HIV/AIDS. Even though, as previously discussed briefly, FDA has never restricted women from entering clinical trials of drugs intended to treat serious or life-threatening illnesses, only 5% of those enrolled in the expanded access trials for didanosine (ddI) and stavudine (d4T) were women, despite the absence of gender-based restrictions— except pregnancy and lactation—in any part of the drug development program. Clearly, other factors beyond exclusion criteria have an impact on whether HIV-infected women enroll in trials. FDA is committed to identifying aspects of clinical trial programs that pose barriers to women's participation. In addition, FDA works closely with sponsors of HIV/AIDS drugs to ensure that they make appropriate efforts to recruit HIV-infected women.[30]

Actual stories from women about difficulties they have had in entering trials have served to further energize FDA to increase its efforts to educate pharmaceutical sponsors, IRBs, and FDA staff to ensure that decisions are not made that explicitly or implicitly exclude women with HIV/AIDS from participating in trials. The agency has worked hard to form meaningful partnerships with women with HIV/AIDS.

Testing Drugs in Pregnant Women

FDA and the scientific community recognize the difficulty of testing drugs and biological agents (e.g., vaccines) in pregnant women. Prudent concerns over protecting the fetus, an understandable fear of liability by drug developers, and the lack of systematic procedures for assessing the effects of postmarketing exposure on pregnant women have all combined to allow many drugs to be used during pregnancy without reliable data on their maternal and fetal effects. An unfortunate example of how this happens is the recent postmarket discovery of sometimes fatal kidney problems in newborns exposed to angiotensin converting enzyme (ACE) inhibitors prescribed to mothers during the second and third trimesters of pregnancy to treat hypertension.[31] Serendipity was involved in gaining this knowledge, which emerged from scattered clinical reports and the experience of a particular physician. It is clear that a more formal method of studying drugs likely to be used in pregnancy before they are approved is needed, as well as systematic data collection of adverse effects after marketing.

When a clinical trial is the only source of a promising experimental therapy for a life-threatening illness, it becomes even more important to include pregnant women. FDA has advocated including HIV-infected pregnant women in the early testing of new therapies for AIDS. In addition, even in conditions that are not life threatening, if it is likely that drugs being tested will be used during pregnancy, the participation of pregnant women in formal studies may be appropriate. In a public conference held in November 1994, FDA explored some of the complex issues of including pregnant women in clinical trials of new drugs and biological agents and of improving collection of postmarketing data. (An executive summary of the conference has been published.[32]) Throughout the 2-day conference, speakers underscored the need for more data about the safety and efficacy of drugs used in pregnancy. The best way to achieve the twin goals of maximizing the therapeutic benefit of pharmaceutical products for pregnant women and minimizing risks to the fetuses was the subject of considerable discussion. Timing—when pregnant women enter a study—emerged as a particularly complex issue. The importance of a stronger science base for decision making also was emphasized throughout discussions about informed consent, the role of IRBs, FDA labeling, liability, and ethics. This conference began a process that FDA is continuing, in collaboration with other agencies of PHS, academia, industry, public health professionals, and consumers. An internal FDA working group has been formed and is considering the complex issues regarding the testing and use of FDA-regulated products in pregnant women.

Office of Women's Health

FDA's Office of Women's Health (OWH) was established in 1994 to focus agency-wide attention on women's health, particularly the issue of women and clinical trials; to ensure that women are appropriately represented in clinical trials of FDA-regulated products; to provide leadership and policy direction in women's health issues for the agency; to promote gender sensitivity in FDA's regulatory and oversight activities; and to seek to correct gender disparities in drugs, devices, and biologics testing policies.

In addition to its major responsibility of ensuring that women are included in clinical trials, that trials are properly designed to allow for meaningful gender analysis, and that gender analysis is actually conducted, OWH pursues other women's health initiatives. OWH's current activity includes initiatives on contraceptives and sexually transmitted diseases, breast implants, breast and other cancers, women's issues, women with HIV/AIDS, and pregnant women's issues.

Endnotes

[1] Guidelines for the study and evaluation of gender differences in prescription drug testing. *Federal Register* 58:39406–39416, July 22, 1993
[2] 21 CFR 310, March 29, 1974
[3] 21 CFR 312, March 19, 1987
[4] Goldman BJ: *Food and Drug Law Journal* 48(2):171, 1993
[5] Raheja KL, Jordan A, Fourcroy JL: Food and Drug Administration guidelines for reproductive toxicity testing. *Reproductive Toxicology* 2(3-4):291–293, 1988
[6] Prescription Drugs User Fees Act of 1992 (PL 102-571)
[7] Department of Health & Human Services, U.S. Food & Drug Administration: *General Considerations for the Clinical Evaluation of Drugs* (Publ No HEW FDA 88-3040). Washington, DC, U.S. Government Printing Office, 1977
[8] Pernick MS: The calculus of suffering in 19th century surgery, in *Sickness and Health in America*. Edited by Leavitt JW, Numbers RL. Madison, WI, University of Wisconsin Press, 1985, p 100
[9] Ethridge E: Pellagra: an unappreciated reminder of southern distinctiveness, in *Disease and Distinctiveness in the American South*. Edited by Savitt TL, Young JH. Knoxville, TN, University of Tennessee Press, 1988, pp 100–119; Roe DA: *A Plague of Corn: The Social History of Pellagra*. Ithaca, NY, Cornell University Press, 1973

[10]Mitford J: Cheaper than chimpanzees, in *Kind and Unusual Punishment: The Prison Business*. New York, Knopf, 1973

[11]Jones JH: *Bad Blood*. New York, Free Press, 1981; King PA: The dangers of difference. *Hastings Center Report* 22(6):35–38, 1992

[12]45 CFR 46, revised June 18, 1991

[13]Kelsey FO: *Problems Raised for the FDA by the Occurrence of Thalidomide Embryopathy in Germany 1960–1961*. Presented at the 91st annual meeting of the American Public Health Association, Kansas City, MO, November 14, 1963

[14]Drug Amendments of 1962 (PL 87-781)

[15]Pure Food and Drug Act of 1938 (21 USC 201)

[16]Herbst AL, Ulfelder H, Poskanzer DC: Adenocarcinoma of the vagina: association of maternal stilbestrol therapy with tumor appearance in young women. *New England Journal of Medicine* 284:878–881, 1971

[17]International Union, United Automobile, Aerospace and Agricultural Implement Workers of America, UAW, et al v Johnson Controls, Inc. 111 SCT 1196 (1991). Pregnancy Discrimination Act of 1978, 92 Stat 2076, 42 USC 2000e(k)

[18]Office of Legislative Affairs: Letter to Senator John Heinz. Survey of Recent New Drug Applications. Washington, DC, Food & Drug Administration, September 27, 1983 (also personal communication from R. Temple, FDA, to R. Merkatz)

[19]General Accounting Office, Women's Health: *FDA Needs to Ensure More Study of Gender Differences in Prescription Drug Testing*, 1992

[20]Walle T, Walle UK, Cowart TD, et al: Pathway-selective sex differences in the metabolic clearance of propranolol in human subjects. *Clinical Pharmacology and Therapeutics* 46:257–263, 1989

[21]Nafziger AN, Bertino JS Jr: Sex-related differences in theophylline pharmacokinetics. *European Journal of Clinical Pharmacology* 37:97–100, 1989

[22]Merkatz RB, Temple R, Sobel S, et al: Women in clinical trials of new drugs. *New England Journal of Medicine* 329:292–296, 1993

[23]Makkar RR, Fromm BS, Steinman RT, et al: Female gender as a risk factor for torsades des pointes associated with cardiovascular drugs. *Journal of the American Medical Association* 270:2590–2597, 1993

[24]Frezza M, di Padova C, Pozzato G, et al: High blood alcohol levels in women: the role of decreased gastric alcohol dehydrogenase activity and first-pass metabolism. *New England Journal of Medicine* 322:95–99, 1990

[25]Widom B, Diamond MP, Simonson DC: Alterations in glucose metabolism during menstrual cycle in women with IDDM. *Diabetes Care* 15:213–220, 1992

[26]Gustavson LE, Legler UF, Benet LZ: Impairment of prednisolone disposition in women taking oral contraceptives or conjugated estrogens. *Journal of Clinical Endocrinology Metabolism* 62:234–237, 1986

[27]Guidelines for the study and evaluation of gender differences in prescription drug testing. *Federal Register* 58:39406–39416, July 22, 1993

[28]Temple R: The clinical investigation of drugs for use by the elderly: Food and Drug Administration guidelines. *Clinical Pharmacology & Therapeutics* 42:681–685, 1987

[29]60 FR 46794, September 8, 1995

[30]FDA Response to a Citizens Petition from the AIDS Service Center HIV Law Project, the NOW Legal Defense and Education Fund, and the American Civil Liberties Union AIDS Project, October 27, 1994

[31]Piper JM, Ray WA, Rosa FW: Pregnancy outcome following exposure to angiotensin-converting enzyme inhibitors. *Obstetrics & Gynecology* 80: 429–432, 1992

[32]Food & Drug Administration: *Executive Summary: FDA Regulated Products & Pregnant Women*, September 1995

13

Scleroderma:
A Case Study of Policy

Sharon Monsky, M.B.A.

S haron Monsky was a fast-track business management consultant with McKinsey and Company, when in 1982, at age 28, she first noticed her health beginning to deteriorate. She became increasingly sensitive to cold temperatures and observed that the skin on her extremities, particularly her hands, would often blanch quickly from pink to blue. Her energy level, usually high, decreased markedly. Initial health examinations told her little. The physicians she consulted thought she simply needed rest from an admittedly draining lifestyle, but Sharon knew it had to be something more. It took 2 years of determined searching, and travel to more than a dozen physicians all over the United States, for Sharon to get an accurate diagnosis. In 1984, she was told she had scleroderma and that her internal organs were involved. She probably had 2 to 3 years to live.

Like most Americans, Sharon had never heard of scleroderma. She literally had no idea what was killing her or how she had contracted the disease. She never would have guessed that there are more people with scleroderma—a half million patients in the United States alone—than with muscular dystrophy (MD), multiple sclerosis (MS), or cystic fibrosis, diseases much more familiar to the American public.[1] Funding comparisons explain why few people were familiar with this disease before the Scleroderma Research Foundation came on the scene and why the cause of this condition is still a mystery (see Table 13–1).

Statistics on broader governmental disease spending available through advocacy organizations present an even starker contrast.[2] Per-patient research spending by the government is $1,000 for MD, $203 for cancer, $161 for MS, $130 for heart disease, and $.25 for scleroderma. There are many reasons why serious, often life-threatening, illnesses do not receive the attention they deserve. Scleroderma is an excellent case study for policy makers because the story of this disease happens to point out several critical flaws in the current system of medical research funding and decision making. In particular, it is important to anyone concerned about a women's health agenda because it is an amazing example of the factors that must be overcome to create change in the current set of research priorities. One other reason shows why scleroderma is an important issue for women's health research: more than 80% of patients with scleroderma are women, mostly of childbearing age.[3]

What Is Scleroderma?

Literally, scleroderma means "hard skin," but it is not actually a skin disease. It is a chronic, degenerative autoimmune disorder that leads to the overproduction of collagen in the body's connective tissue. The overabundance of collagen hardens the connective tissue and damages the organs involved. Scleroderma affects patients quite differently. In about half of those afflicted, only the skin is involved, and sometimes it is limited to the face and hands. In the other half, patients like Sharon are diagnosed with systemic sclerosis, in which internal organs are implicated as well. Because this disease causes extreme sensitivity in the tissues of vital organs, such as the heart, kidneys, and lungs, almost 70% of

Table 13–1. Comparative statistics

Disease	Numbers affected	Funding (millions)
Scleroderma	550,000	$3.3
Multiple sclerosis	333,000	$64.2
Muscular dystrophy	250,000	$78.3

patients with systemic sclerosis do not live more than 7 years after their initial diagnosis.[4]

Even in its most limited form, scleroderma is often quite disfiguring and debilitating. When skin around the mouth hardens, the size of the oral opening is reduced, significantly affecting speech, breathing, and swallowing. In many cases in which the hands are involved, dexterity is limited, and grasping is nearly impossible. Simple acts such as dressing oneself or holding a child's hand become arduous and painful.

There are those who believe that descriptions of people turning to stone in the Bible are actually references to the effects of scleroderma. It was first described in the medical literature as early as 1754, by Carlo Crusio in Naples, who treated a young woman, Patrizia Galiera, who had "an effective tension and hardness of her skin all over her body, by which she found herself so bound and straightened, that she could hardly move her limbs."[5] At the time, her physicians were proud to announce that they had in fact found a "cure" for the strange disease. This consisted of frequent vapor baths, an "emollient" diet consisting of foods considered to have a softening effect on body tissue, the ingestion of 12 grains of pure quicksilver followed by a half pint of sarsaparilla, and, of course, bloodletting.[6] It is easy to dismiss the crude medicine of the mid-18th century, but it would be difficult to argue that much direct therapeutic progress has been made since that time. Bloodletting may have disappeared in the treatment of scleroderma, but many physicians still prescribe treatments such as dipping affected limbs in hot wax to soften the skin.

The best treatments available for scleroderma patients now are organ-based therapies—that is, treatments that help to relieve some of the symptoms of the disease that occur in various sites. For example, kidney failure is one of the common consequences of the disease. Captopril, a drug that works for about 30% of patients, keeps many people with scleroderma alive. Other therapies rely on calcium channel blocking agents and vasodilators, which help alleviate symptoms in some patients. D-Penicillamine, a medication that occasionally acts to stop collagen proliferation and soften the skin, may slow the degenerative process down for some patients. But this drug is highly toxic, acting like radiation, so physicians have to "go low and slow" because it can cause serious complications.

Nothing is available to attack the disease itself or to prevent its onset. In fact, so little is known about the origin and natural progression of scleroderma that there is not even agreement on standards to judge the best available treatments. Patients are often left to make health decisions without the benefit of informed counsel because even the best clinicians do not know for sure what they are up against in this disease. Many scleroderma patients turn to nontraditional techniques with mixed results. In a climate rich in false hope, charlatans, and so-called wonder drugs, discerning a genuinely effective therapy from a wishful one is extremely difficult. The Scleroderma Research Foundation receives frequent claims of treatment efficacy from established nontraditional therapies, such as acupuncture and dietary regimens, to dubious approaches, including shock therapy, new age counseling, "miracle creams," and— my favorite—a simple tonsillectomy. Regardless of the veracity of these claims, it is undeniably true that scleroderma has been recognized for a long time as an "incurable" disease with no known cause and that it is seen around the world in roughly the same incidence across racial and ethnic lines.[7] Currently, there is no effective remedy either for the disease or its symptoms.

A New Approach

After her diagnosis, Sharon Monsky began doing what any patient with such a serious illness would do—investigating her disease. She quickly found out that there was not much to know. No U.S. Food and Drug Administration (FDA)–approved therapeutics existed for any aspect of the disease, and none was on the horizon. In fact, little research was being done on the condition.

With her condition worsening in 1985, Sharon Monsky became pregnant and, against the strongest medical advice, decided to have the child she and her husband had always wanted. Physicians were emphatic that the pregnancy would likely kill her. In doing her own investigation, however, Sharon questioned scleroderma experts and discovered that the possibility of a successful pregnancy was better than she had been led to believe. It was certainly true that some scleroderma patients had died during pregnancy, but nothing specifically implicated pregnancy itself as an independent factor. The lack of successful case studies demonstrated clearly just how little tracking information had been kept on these patients. The only thing that was clear regarding scleroderma was that pregnancy is an extremely taxing condition for the body. From this assumption, physicians had decided that patients with internal organ involvement could not handle the stress. Physicians had simply suggested the lowest-risk path—"we don't know, so don't do it." Sharon kept probing for specific reasons why she could not have the child she wanted so much. Once she got past the wall of initial resistance, she found that the medical reasoning was based on little hard substance. After careful deliberation with her husband, she decided to continue her pregnancy.

The pregnancy was extremely hard on Sharon's system. She almost died several times from complications associated with the disease. Again she was told she should end the pregnancy to save her life. She was determined to persevere. In the end everyone but Sharon was surprised when she successfully gave birth to her son, Max. She now sees that experience as a turning point in her life. It was then that she decided she no longer wanted to hear that nothing could be done about this disease.

The First Steps

McKinsey and Company, the consulting firm for which she had worked in San Francisco, had been extremely supportive of Sharon through her initial struggle with the disease and had helped her get in touch with many of the medical experts she consulted in her search for an accurate diagnosis. She left the firm in the fall of 1984 when it was clear she could no longer bear the work load. But she turned to her friends and former associates for advice, meeting with her prior contacts in medicine and biotechnology, as well as with business leaders, such as Bob Waterman, Jr., her mentor at McKinsey and author of *In Search of Excellence.*

Sharon began to outline an approach based on the business management principles she knew. After completing a nonprofit market analysis, she assembled a board of directors to guide a newly incorporated enterprise, the Scleroderma Research Foundation in Mill Valley, California, which she started in late 1986. Its purpose: to raise money to fund the most promising research on scleroderma.

By mobilizing everyone she knew for help and advice, within months Sharon organized a casino night fund-raiser and a benefit golf tournament. One of Sharon's dearest friends from college, the head chef at a trendy Los Angeles restaurant, offered to host an event attended by as many Hollywood stars as she and others could persuade to come. Robin Williams agreed to perform, which suddenly put this new nonprofit organization into the limelight. At the end of the first year, the foundation had raised $150,000. It was in the business of funding scientific research.

For 5 years, the foundation has selected the most promising research projects and funded them on a case-by-case basis. One of the most exciting was the development of the first accurate clinical diagnostic tool to identify the disease. Because of the foundation's work, physicians can now take a sample of skin from beneath the base of a fingernail and use it to diagnose most forms of the disease. But there was no progress in the search for a cure.

Cure Advocacy

By 1991, Sharon had discovered what many scientists have long known. In a climate of institutional competition, career pressure, publishing demands, and poor peer communication among researchers, progress is often slow or unrecognized, and the most important information regarding failures rarely comes to light. Her own business skills, as well as her close advisers, soon told her that the foundation needed a team approach, which would bring the best people from private industry, academia, and government together to pool knowledge and resources. Just as in the for-profit world, success depended on getting the right people to the table to focus on a common goal.

To address these issues, the foundation decided to use a new approach—"cure advocacy"—literally working backward from the information that would be needed to find a cure for scleroderma. For years, Sharon had asked her team of scientific advisers to review grant applications the foundation received and advise the board on what to fund, a standard operating method for foundations of all kinds. In 1991, foundation officials decided to turn that process on its head. Instead of being selectively reactive, the foundation would put together the top scleroderma researchers with experts from related fields and ask them to brainstorm the kind of research it would take to develop a fast-track search for a cure. The foundation would then assemble investigative teams that would focus on the areas highlighted by the advisers.

The genius of this approach lies in bringing together great business minds and top scientific and biomedical advisers to design a research center that features

- Elimination of duplicate efforts
- Exchange of ongoing results
- Collaboration between private and academic institutions
- Clinical application of conclusions
- Ongoing evaluation of research direction

With an initial grant of $450,000 from the Scleroderma Research Foundation, the Bay Area Scleroderma Research Center opened in 1992—the first collaborative scleroderma research center in the nation. Research teams from Stanford University, Genentech Inc., the San Francisco Veterans Hospital, and the University of California at San Francisco were selected by a scientific advisory committee, itself composed of top-level scientists. These teams were funded to work at three sites in this "center without walls." One condition was tied to every grant—that investigators would share findings continually and meet regularly with scientific advisory committee members to review progress and reevaluate the direction of the research. Getting investigators to agree to reveal their work before publication was no easy task. "We're so naturally competitive, we don't like to share," said Youn Kim, one of the lead investigators, in a September 1993 *Business Week* article. "But this way, we don't have to wait until one group presents [to collaborate]."

The scientific advisory committee has been instrumental in the success of the center. Committee members are all well-established experts who became interested in the foundation's efforts because of its innovative approach. Their preoccupation with helping people has been enhanced by the fact that each member has reached a point in his or her career at which it is possible to dedicate significant energy and resources to projects of personal importance. Committee members take an active role in working directly with research team members on an ongoing basis to advise and oversee the team's progress. Because scientific advisory committee members are some of the top research scientists in the United States, their insight has provided a tremendous resource for the investigative teams in their day-to-day operation. The entire advisory committee makes a formal site visit every 6 months, during which the research teams present their progress reports and research goals, and research directions are reassessed. This process is keeping the center on a fast track in the search for a cure for scleroderma.

The benefit of this approach has become clear as the researchers tried to create an animal model of the disease. The groups working with mouse models in particular have shared information about successes and failures, preventing duplication. As one investigator put it, "Normally, failures don't get published." Yet the cross-institutional nature of the center's operation allows researchers to communicate their failures, saving valuable time, money, and resources and permitting research to be directed to potentially more rewarding areas.

The foundation was surprised at the positive reception this "sharing" approach received, not only from research team members but also from others within the scientific community, who have been eager to lend their expertise. Outside research consultants, who are often world-recognized specialists, have been generous with their knowledge and have provided necessary blood and tissue samples to the center in appreciation of its innovative approach. These contributions have been invaluable, confirming the foundation's belief that progress is being followed by researchers not only in the scleroderma field but also in related autoimmune and skin diseases.

Because of this innovative approach, we can claim success in several key areas in a remarkably short time. For example:

- We have created a special clinical laboratory test that can diagnose several forms of the disease quickly. More important, we can now arrive at an accurate diagnosis early in the development of the disease.
- For the first time, we can announce significant progress in the development of tight-skinned (TSK) and severe combined immunodeficient (SCID) mouse models, an important step in

understanding the pathogenesis of the disease and developing potential therapeutics.

- We have established the importance of, and can understand better, the role of the endothelial cells that line the small blood vessels walls in the early onset of scleroderma.
- Specific research priorities have been established to guide investigation at two complementary research centers, one in the San Francisco Bay area and the other on the East Coast. The work of each center has been divided into key areas to keep it on the fast track to finding a cure.

Because of the positive evaluation of the foundation's research approach and the substantial progress the foundation has made in the first year of operation, a second research center opened in the Washington, DC–Baltimore corridor. In November 1993, a research symposium was held in Washington, DC, with scientific leaders from academia, government, and the private biomedical industry, including the Johns Hopkins University, the University of Maryland, the National Institutes of Health (NIH), Merck, Dupont, and representatives of the Baltimore biotechnology corridor. These leaders in scleroderma-related research reviewed the current work in the field and discussed important questions that should be pursued to complement the work already under way at the Bay Area Scleroderma Research Center. East Coast center research focuses on understanding the likely triggers of the disease and its development.

Why Has This Taken So Long?

An important question remains: why has so little scleroderma research been done until recently? Understanding why this disease remains unknown and unexplored may help to unravel some of the larger issues surrounding public health research.

Several important factors will determine which diseases get public attention and research funding. One is "celebrity power," the clout a well-known champion can bring to a cause. MD is just as difficult a phrase to understand and remember as scleroderma. But Jerry Lewis has given millions of Americans direct and personal knowledge of an illness they would be likely to understand only if they happened to be connected to one of the approximately 250,000 people affected by MD. His enormous power as a spokesperson has made the Muscular Dystrophy Association a major charity, bringing in about $100 million annually.

Scleroderma has never had such a champion; no famous person has appeared to lead the fund-raising and publicity effort. Without personalizing the illness, without giving it a face, it has been easy for scleroderma to remain just another Greek word that is hard to pronounce, leaving patients self-consciously hidden from view by a disfiguring disease.

Another key factor has to do with the population the disease afflicts—mostly women. It is no secret that research on women's health has long been ignored. One reason is that women have not been well represented in decision-making areas of government, academia, and the biotechnology industry. In addition, scleroderma patients have not been organized activists. It is easy to understand why. Scleroderma typically attacks women of childbearing age. Most of these women find themselves stricken with an unknown, ugly, debilitating illness while they are still the keystone of their families, usually responsible for their young children. Trying to hang on to whatever had constituted a "normal" life often becomes the central organizing principle of their existence as patients. The merest public appearance is difficult, let alone the idea of organizing with other patients to get needed research attention. Marching on Washington, DC, is out of the question.

Not to be overlooked as well is the role that prior research plays in later funding. NIH is the major arm of public research funding in the United States. Its mission is not to ensure that research funds are allocated equitably according to patient need or even public health impact. NIH focuses on funding the most potentially promising research across the board. What constitutes "promising" research depends, however, on the current state of knowledge in a given field. With so little known about a disease such as scleroderma, research funds tend to flow where there is "more bang for the buck," where the basic science of a particular disease is advanced enough to support many proposals with a high potential return.

It would be impossible to beat this standard if it were not for the fact that even relatively small research outlays support projects that generate many new questions, along with whatever answers appear. Indeed, if such small studies produce answers, it becomes apparent that additional progress is possible, stimulating investigatory interest and funding sources.

A second point is equally valid. Research is, of course, dependent on researchers. Few investigators are willing to work on an unknown disease. When little progress has been made in the basic science of a mysterious illness, few researchers will stake years of their life and a substantial part of their reputation doing the fundamental ground-work from which more promising investigation might unfold. This is especially true if there are higher profile areas of study that carry with them the guarantee of ample funding. It is not cynical to observe that researchers make the same decisions business professionals often do: they invest their lives and work in areas that promise substantial return on the risk they take by acquiring specific knowledge.

Nonetheless, Dr. Bruce Alberts, president of the National Academy of Sciences, believes that the approach the Scleroderma Research Foundation has brought to biomedical investigation "will serve as a model for future medical and scientific research, because of its unprecedented, unified plan of attack." Dr. Eugene Bauer, professor and dean of the School of Medicine at Stanford University, describes the collaborative, interdisciplinary work sponsored by the foundation as "both novel and daring." The foundation hopes that the research approach outlined and areas of investigation targeted will spur increased interest in the field of scleroderma research to overcome some of the obstacles mentioned earlier.

All of the work thus far has been done without a dollar of collaborative federal spending. Indeed, the sums of money involved are not significant even in the realm of private scientific research dollars—but the results have been important in the search for a cure for this disease. It is a true example of a high-yield investment. Success in scientific research has much less to do with how much money is allocated than with the scientists who are brought together to do the research and how the work is organized.

The Role of Government

Despite the achievements the foundation has demonstrated without government funding, it is important to note that government has several vital roles. One role is as a full partner in this and similar research approaches. More than 75% of the study proposals in this area of research submitted annually to NIH go unfunded because the institute responsible for scleroderma and other related disorders, the National Institute of Arthritis, Musculoskeletal and Skin Diseases (NIAMS), is underfunded in comparison with other arms of NIH.[8] In 1994, NIAMS received $223,280,000 compared with the largest institute, which receives almost $2 billion annually.[9] The allocated budget growth for NIAMS has been 7% annually, well below NIH's overall 10% annual growth rate. But the cost to society for medical care and lost wages because of the conditions for which NIAMS provides research funding (osteoporosis, other musculoskeletal illnesses, arthritis, and skin diseases) is an estimated $133 billion.[10]

The second aspect of government's role is less direct but perhaps even more important. Government must work to create a climate that supports and encourages private efforts. The FDA is crucial to this climate of research for any disease. FDA sets research standards to prove the efficacy of each drug or therapeutic regimen that comes before the agency for approval. Those standards control the likelihood of private industry investment. Biomedical research is by its nature a high-risk venture, and few companies have the resources to withstand years of delay and battles over new drug approval. FDA standards can quite literally strangle efforts to find effective therapies and, in some areas, can kill entire fields of investigation.

Scleroderma is a good example of this. The standards for scleroderma research have been set disturbingly high when one considers that the disease is still so mysterious. The problem here, of course, is that it is extremely difficult to determine the efficacy of a drug in relation to a disease if the natural history of that disease is not well understood. By raising the burden of proof to standards well beyond the level of research that exists in this field, FDA makes any research into even the most limited drug therapy prohibitive. For example, companies currently are asked not only to prove that scleroderma patients using their therapy do better than patients do without it but also are expected to establish the baseline natural history of the disease—that is, how it begins and its course over time—which even the best scleroderma experts are incapable of providing at present. In the case of systemic sclerosis, the most serious form of the disease, we believe these standards are absolutely immoral. To prove the efficacy of a drug used by these patients, FDA requires double-blind, placebo-controlled studies—that is, two groups of patients, one receiving the drug being tested, the other receiving a dummy medication, with neither the patients nor those giving the medicines knowing which patients are in each group. This mandate does two things. First, it prevents drug researchers from recruiting enough study participants to test a drug or therapy accurately because few patients with life-threatening diseases are willing to forgo all treatment to participate in such a trial. Second, it guarantees that people will die as a result of any study ostensibly designed to help them, if they are assigned to the placebo group and receive no medication. As mentioned at the beginning of this chapter, 70% of patients with systemic sclerosis are extremely ill within 2 years of diagnosis and die within 7 years. Forcing these patients to go without therapy so that the effect on other patients can be understood creates a legal and ethical dilemma that prevents all but the most determined companies from moving ahead.

Besides giving the message to the biotechnology community not to invest in research on this disease, FDA, by this requirement, is treating scleroderma differently from other life-threatening disease, such as acquired immunodeficiency syndrome (AIDS) and breast cancer, which have gotten fast-track approval for research studies or have obtained compassionate use waivers. The Scleroderma Research Foundation has asked the FDA to allow scleroderma patients the right to choose to use new drugs that have been proven nontoxic on animals, and it wants freedom to design controlled studies in which the effects of different agents on the progress of the disease are compared—with half of the study group getting one treatment and half getting another—so that no one must go without any treatment. Furthermore, the foundation maintains that it is impossible to follow the same rules with scleroderma as with AIDS and breast cancer because those diseases are definable, whereas scleroderma is a vascular connective tissue disease—less prevalent but not less life threatening—and care needs to be individualized to keep patients safe while trying to help them. Discussions between the foundation and the FDA have produced an agreement by the FDA not to mandate double-blind, placebo-controlled trials, although the agency may accept them. Currently the foundation is considering other alternative research procedures that can be used to achieve faster research progress.

Where Do We Go From Here?

The nature of this disease, the patient population it affects, and the lack of research attention it receives make scleroderma an excellent test case for anyone who wonders how women's health issues have been ignored for so long or what it will take to create a more equitable research agenda in the face of potentially declining federal health research dollars and significant new threats to public health, such as the reemergence of tuberculosis and the continuing AIDS epidemic. The lesson to be learned has less to do with why scleroderma deserves more attention than with how we may change the very paradigm of scientific and medical investigation that has overlooked this and many other serious illnesses.

The Scleroderma Research Foundation is the only organization dedicated solely to the goal of funding research on this illness. From the foundation's vantage point, the question is not how to compete with other worthwhile causes for dwindling funds but how to make every research dollar yield the best possible results by bringing the right people together with one goal in mind: finding a cure.

As a women's health research foundation, the scleroderma foundation realizes that its experience is similar to that of many other foundations for diseases that have not been considered important by the traditional, male-dominated investigative establishment. The foundation also knows that its job is to change that model. Accusations that it is only the interference of women that has politicized the nation's research agenda are flatly wrong. Health research allocation has always been a political process. Women just have not been the constituents served by that process. But it is not good enough simply to add a women's health research agenda to the overall investigatory mix to compete for an ever-shrinking pool of funds. A process must be implemented that looks more soberly at the true public health impact of any disease. Above and beyond that, we must ensure that we spend every dollar better. Daily we hear about Pentagon cost overruns and misspent social services funding, but we see few media reports about the amount of money that has been wasted on unfocused, redundant medical research.

It comes as no surprise to policy makers when the public observes that the loudest mouth often gets the most to eat. Until recently, women's voices were largely unheard in the health research field, leaving substantial areas of our health literally starved for attention. Our goal is not simply to raise our voices above the din and clamor for more research allocation. We are determined to lead by example, to make every resource as valuable as it can be in the search for a cure for scleroderma. We will not demand handouts; instead, we will look for a true partnership in the search for better health for all women.

What of Sharon Monsky herself? She and her husband, Mark Scher, have two daughters, Samantha and Montana, and one son, Max. They are perfectly healthy children and are "the joy of my life," says their mother. Because pregnancy softens collagen, Sharon experienced some benefit from her pregnancies with her daughters, but, on the whole, having children took a significant toll on her system. "My disease continues to progress; I am more crippled than I was 5 years ago, and my lung disease is worse. But Mark and the kids keep me alive," says Sharon. Then, quietly, she adds, "I'm going to beat this disease." If anyone can, it will be Sharon Monsky.

Endnotes

[1] The Foundation's estimate, based on published medical data, ranges from 20,000 to 1.2 million Americans with scleroderma, depending on whom the definition of the disease includes and how incidence and mortality rates are reported. Press estimates typically vary from 300,000 to 750,000 U.S. cases. We believe that the most accurate assumptions lead to a conservative estimate of more than 550,000, but all data are dependent on unsatisfactory study and analysis of the disease. By comparison, there are 333,000 patients with MS and 250,000 with MD.

[2] National Alliance for Research on Schizophrenia and Depression (NARSAD).

[3] Again, this estimate is compiled from available literature, although it is more firmly supported than overall incidence rates. Dr. Virginia Steen et al. reported in 1988 a varied rate of 76% diffuse scleroderma and 84% of limited scleroderma patients at their University of Pittsburgh clinic were women, based on 1972–1986 statistics. These figures are widely corroborated in available literature.

[4]Leroy EC, Leroy RL: The spectrum of scleroderma. *Hospital Practice* 24(10A):33–42, 1989

[5]*Philosophical Transactions Giving Some Account of the Present Undertakings, Studies and Labours, of the Ingenious in Many Considerable Parts of the World*, Vol XLVIII, Part II, Chapter LXXVII. London, C. Davis, Printer to the Royal Society, 1754

[6]Ibid., p 584: "As she was judg'd to be of too full a habit, and as she had not the regular menstrual discharge, she was ordered to lose twelve ounces of blood from the foot; and it was thought, that this evacuation might contribute to produce a general relaxation, and, by consequence, make the circulation of the blood, and other fluids, more free and easy through their respective canals. It was surprising to see what difficulty the surgeon found in opening the vein, on account of the hardness of the skin; insomuch that, in the operation, the lancet yielded, and bent. However, at last, it pierced the skin, and the vein, but not without a good deal of pain to the patient."

[7]LeRoy C: Scleroderma, in *Encyclopaedia Britannica*, 1988

[8]Coalition of Patient Advocates for Skin Disease Research Memo, NIAMS Level of Grant Funding Average 1987–1992 graph, January 26, 1994

[9]Ibid., NIAMS Funding Levels chart

[10]NIAMS Coalition Goal for FY 1995

14

Women's Health Research: Congressional Action and Legislative Gains: 1990–1994

Lesley Primmer, M.A.

Within days of her 1991 Senate confirmation, the first female director of the National Institutes of Health (NIH), Cleveland cardiologist Bernadine Healy, told a House of Representatives appropriations subcommittee about her plans to conduct the largest prevention study ever done in the United States. The more than 160,000 subjects for this comprehensive long-term study of cancer, heart disease, and osteoporosis prevention would all be women.

The subcommittee members—some of the most senior men in the House of Representatives whose legislative responsibilities included funding NIH—were not surprised by her emphasis on women's health. For nearly a year, they had heard from their female colleagues in the House that women's health was being neglected by the nation's premier medical research facility. Despite a tight budget that held little for new initiatives, Dr. Healy's bold proposal was warmly received by the all-male panel. Women's health research was an issue they knew could no longer be ignored. Over the next 5 years, the House Appropriations Subcommittee on Labor, Health and Human Services, and Education would appropriate several billion dollars for research on women's health issues at NIH,[1] as part of a larger campaign to ensure equitable treatment for women in the health care system.

Women's health has been the subject of intensive congressional activity since 1990. Hundreds of bills have been introduced, and scores of congressional hearings and investigations were held during this 5-year period. This effort has been driven in Congress by members of Congressional Caucus on Women's Issues (CCWI), backed up by women scientists, advocates, and voters. Armed with a highly publicized General Accounting Office (GAO) report documenting the exclusion of women from federally funded research, and a comprehensive legislative response to the issues the report raised, the caucus created a climate that led to the enactment of more than 25 pieces of legislation to improve the health of American women.

This chapter summarizes key congressional actions on women's health research over a 5-year period beginning in 1990. Although it is not a complete record on women's health legislation, it is intended to provide a comprehensive review of legislation to expand women's health research acted on by Congress from 1990 to 1994. The majority of these bills were initiated by members of CCWI.

Women's Health Emerges as a Congressional Priority

Two issues—increasing breast cancer rates and a decreasing commitment to contraceptive research—formed the backdrop for the caucus' early efforts to develop comprehensive women's health legislation. Galvanized by her sister's battle with breast cancer and concern about rising breast cancer rates, former Rep. Mary Rose Oakar (D-OH) used her position in the House to fight for coverage of mammography under Medicare. Rep. Oakar also worked to require physicians to provide information on treatment options to women with breast cancer. Her own sister had entered the operating room for a simple biopsy and left with a radical mastectomy. Rep. Oakar soon expanded her legislative efforts to seek additional funding for basic research to find a cure for this dreaded disease.

At the same time that Rep. Oakar was scrutinizing NIH's breast cancer research budget, CCWI co-chair Patricia Schroeder (D-CO) was alarmed by a more general disregard for women's health research that she believed was rooted in the antiabortion politics of the Reagan and Bush administrations. Together with her fellow caucus co-chair Olympia Snowe (R-ME), Schroeder introduced legislation to expand research on contraception and infertility at NIH. Ultimately, they hoped their efforts to help women prevent unintended pregnancies would build common ground among members of Congress on both sides of the abortion debate.

However, the spark that ignited the explosion of legislative action around women's health was a GAO report critical of NIH for excluding women from a number of large, federally funded clinical trials.[2] Among them was the Physicians Health Study of 22,000 male physicians that demonstrated the benefit of aspirin in preventing heart disease. Five years later, this GAO report is still cited as prima facie evidence of the medical establishment's disregard for women's health.

The women's health legislation considered since 1990 can be characterized in one of several ways. A number of the bills reflect the personal interests or experiences of the members of Congress who introduced them. The experience of Rep. Oakar with her sister's breast cancer is just one example. Other congresswomen also had known the tragedy of breast cancer in their families. Rep.—now Senator—Olympia Snowe lost her mother to breast cancer when she was young.

Several years after their women's health campaign got under way, caucus members were stunned and saddened to learn that a colleague—former Rep. Marilyn Lloyd (D-TN)—had just received a diagnosis of breast cancer. In fact, their colleague's personal experience influenced the views of some congresswomen on one women's health issue: silicone breast implants. Rep. Lloyd's breast cancer surgery coincided with the U.S. Food and Drug Administration's (FDA) decision to remove silicone breast implants from the market. Her anger at FDA's action muted what might otherwise have been an enthusiastic endorsement for its decision from the caucus. FDA action also transformed Rep. Lloyd's position on a more sweeping policy debate: the right to reproductive choice. Outraged that a federal agency would deny her the right to choose reconstructive surgery using a silicone implant, Rep.

Lloyd—up until then a staunch abortion opponent—announced on the House floor that she would no longer vote to deny a woman the right to choose an abortion.

Other congresswomen also shared stories of personal health crises when seeking colleagues' support for women's health legislation. Rep. Rosa DeLauro's (D-CT) personal battle with ovarian cancer and Rep. Patsy Mink's (D-HI) years of anguish over the effects the diethylstilbestrol (DES) she took decades before would have on her children argued the case for expanded research more effectively than any GAO report could.

The legislation introduced on women's health also reflected, to a certain extent, the committee assignments of the congresswomen. Reps. Schroeder and Lloyd sponsored legislation to improve women's health research and treatment in the military. Both women were senior members of the House Armed Services Committee to which the bill was referred. Rep. Barbara Kennelly (D-CT)—one of only two women on the House Ways and Means Committee—offered legislation to restore mammography coverage under Medicare, a program under her committee's jurisdiction.

Still, at the time the caucus introduced its omnibus women's health bill, only one woman—Rep. Cardiss Collins (D-IL)—served on the House Energy and Commerce Committee, which had jurisdiction over most health issues addressed by the legislation. Not a single woman served on the appropriations subcommittee, which controlled funding for NIH or other federal health programs of importance to women.

The minimal representation by women on key committees in the House improved somewhat after the 1992 congressional elections, which tripled the number of women in the Senate and increased by two-thirds the female representatives in the House. Four women were named to the Appropriations Subcommittee on Labor, Health and Human Services, and Education—which had not had a woman on it in more than 20 years. Three women were added to the Energy and Commerce Committee, although none was assigned to its health subcommittee. Many of the newly elected women had made women's health and reproductive choice priorities in their campaigns, and they came to Washington, DC, eager to act on those issues. Their sheer numbers and determination, along with improved representation of women on important committees, helped fuel the budding women's health movement already under way in Congress.

A third factor directly influenced both the women's health legislation that was introduced and, more importantly, which pieces ultimately became law. That factor was the overall congressional agenda. The need to reauthorize NIH in 1990 provided a prime opportunity to address the issue of research on women's health. In the jargon of Capitol Hill, it is known as "having a vehicle," and the NIH reauthorization bill provided the congresswomen with the vehicle they needed to move their legislation.

By 1993, the NIH bill was law, and health care reform dominated the congressional agenda. The congresswomen shifted their efforts accordingly to focus greater attention on access to health care services for women. They lobbied the president and White House staff to ensure that reproductive health services, including abortion, were covered under the Clinton health care reform plan. With several different plans pending in Congress, the caucus worked with the sponsors of each to ensure equitable coverage for health services important to women.

Along the way, the annual appropriations bills for the Departments of Labor, Health and Human Services, and Education, as well as periodic reauthorizations of existing programs within the Centers for Disease Control and Prevention (CDC) provided important opportunities for the congresswomen and others to address specific women's health issues.

However, most women's health legislation considered by Congress from 1990 to 1994 was first introduced by the congresswomen as part of an omnibus legislative package known as the Women's Health Equity Act (WHEA). The introduction of an omnibus legislative package was a strategy that had previously worked well for the congresswomen in pushing for greater economic equity for women. Beginning in 1981 and in every Congress through 1993, the caucus introduced its Economic Equity Act (EEA), a package of several dozen bills to improve the economic status of women in the United States. The acts addressed a number of issues, including workplace fairness, child care, retirement, and pay equity.

In fact, the congresswomen's first attempt to address women's health came as part of the EEA of 1989, which contained one title devoted to health care. The issues addressed included Medicare reimbursement for mammograms, increased funding for the maternal and child health block grant, the creation of public health clinics in public housing, and domestic violence. Although several of these measures became law, the effort was not successful in drawing attention to women's health in a broader sense.

Omnibus legislative packages such as the EEA fulfilled several important functions for the caucus. First, they served an educational purpose. Combining related bills together in one omnibus measure made it easier to demonstrate the relationship among different types of gender discrimination. A lifetime of low wages, for example, contributes directly to inadequate retirement income.

In addition, omnibus bills helped individual congresswomen broaden support for their projects. Many members of Congress who were reluctant to cosponsor individual pieces of legislation signed on as cosponsors of the entire package as a way of demonstrating support for women. Moreover, the legislative package provided a ready measuring stick at the end of each Congress to access its record on behalf of women. At a year-end press conference, caucus members would characterize a congressional session, in part, by the number of bills in the EEA that became law.

Because the EEA had been such an effective model, an omnibus package of women's health legislation was a natural companion to it and an effective way of expanding the caucus agenda to address an issue of concern to virtually every caucus member. As a result, the WHEA of 1990 was born.

Indeed, plans to introduce the WHEA were already under way when caucus co-chairs Schroeder and Snowe asked GAO to investigate the exclusion of women from clinical trials. They were joined in the request by Rep. Henry Waxman (D-CA), chair of the House Energy and Commerce Subcommittee on Health and the Environment. Not only do requests from subcommittee chairs take priority, but also Rep. Waxman asked GAO to complete its work in time for his subcommittee's upcoming hearings on NIH reauthorization legislation. This effectively put the project under a tight 6-month deadline, a key factor in maintaining the momentum on women's health.

The congressional request noted that in 1986 NIH had adopted a policy to encourage the inclusion of women in clinical research trials. The main question the members of Congress asked GAO to address was how well NIH had implemented its own policy. GAO's conclusion was that 4 years after its adoption, little progress had been made in expanding women's access to clinical trials.

The GAO report was released at a hearing before the Energy and Commerce Health Subcommittee on June 18, 1990. A month later, on

July 27, Reps. Schroeder and Snowe introduced the caucus' legislative response. The WHEA of 1990 consisted of 20 separate bills to improve women's health research, access to health care, and disease prevention services. A companion bill was introduced in the Senate on July 31. The following day, WHEA's chief Senate sponsor, Sen. Barbara Mikulski (D-MD), attached three provisions—creating an Office for Women's Health Research (ORWH) at NIH, requiring that women be included in clinical trials, and establishing five contraceptive and infertility research centers—to legislation reauthorizing NIH.

Faced with the prospect of swift congressional action, NIH officials announced on September 10, at a meeting with caucus members, that an ORWH would be created under the office of the NIH director. NIH officials also pointed out that a revised policy statement on the inclusion of women in clinical research studies had been published. The new policy *required* that adequate numbers of women be included in such studies, unless a compelling justification for their exclusion was provided. Grant proposals that did not comply with the new policy would not be funded.

In addition to the changes at NIH, the GAO report and the speedy legislative and administrative response to it created a climate in which other women's health legislation flourished. Hearings were held on a host of women's health issues, from the threat posed by dioxin in sanitary napkins to federal regulation of infertility clinics. The appropriations committees directed the National Cancer Institute (NCI) to make research on breast, cervical, and ovarian cancer its top priority. Health conditions more prevalent in women than men, such as lupus and interstitial cystitis, also received heightened attention, as did conditions such as heart disease and human immunodeficiency virus (HIV), which affect women differently than they do men. The flurry of attention to women's health even spawned new interest in men's health issues, particularly prostate cancer, which had recently afflicted several members of the House and Senate appropriations committees.

After decades of neglect, women's health research was in the congressional spotlight, a fact that was evident to officials at NIH, who quickly climbed on the bandwagon. By the time Dr. Healy unveiled plans for the initiative she described as equivalent to a "moon walk for women," the ground had already been tilled and the seeds planted for a fertile legislative response to the issue of women's health.

The following information is a summary of that legislative response, including brief descriptions of the three versions of WHEA, the health bills that served as vehicles for WHEA provisions, and an issue-by-issue review of action on a number of health issues.

Women's Health Equity Act

The WHEA was introduced on three separate occasions by CCWI co-chairs Schroeder and Snowe. These packages helped to establish an agenda for congressional action on women's health. Each of the bills in the package also was introduced separately by a caucus member. Whatever legislative action subsequently transpired was on the individual bill rather than on the package as a whole.

Women's Health Equity Act of 1990
(H.R. 5397/S. 2961)

The WHEA of 1990 was introduced in the House on July 27, 1990, and in the Senate on July 31. This first WHEA contained 20 bills divided into three titles: research, access to services, and prevention. The research title called for the establishment of a Center for Women's Health Research at NIH and contained the requirement that women and members of racial and ethnic minority groups be included in medical research, whenever appropriate. WHEA 1990 also increased funding for research on breast cancer, osteoporosis, contraception and infertility, and HIV infection in women. Other titles of the bill addressed the need for comprehensive health and social services for pregnant adolescents and parenting teens, better screening and treatment for the sexually transmitted disease chlamydia, reimbursement under Medicare for mammograms and bone scans that detect osteoporosis, and a new initiative at CDC to provide cancer screening services to low-income women.

Of all these proposals, only two WHEA 1990 provisions became law: the Breast and Cervical Cancer Mortality Prevention Act, a new program administered by CDC to provide mammograms and Pap smears to low-income women, and Medicare coverage for screening mammography. (Mammogram coverage had previously been approved by Congress as part of the Catastrophic Health Coverage Act of 1988, which was repealed the following year after intense opposition from senior citizens, making it necessary to pass separate legislation on mammography coverage.)

Women's Health Equity Act of 1991 (H.R. 1161/S. 513)

WHEA of 1991 contained all of the provisions of WHEA 1990 that were not enacted by the 101st Congress (1989–1990). It added several new provisions by establishing an Office for Women's Health Services at the Substance Abuse and Mental Health Services Administration (SAMHSA), increasing funding for research on ovarian cancer and alcohol abuse in women, and mandating federal standards for mammography screening facilities.

All or part of seven provisions of the WHEA's research title were incorporated into NIH Revitalization Act, which was approved overwhelmingly by Congress—only to be vetoed by then-President Bush.

WHEA 1991 provisions that became law during the 102nd Congress (1991–1992) included two provisions passed as part of legislation reorganizing the Alcohol, Drug Abuse, and Mental Health Administration. They included

- Establishing an associate administrator for women's health services at the newly created Substance Abuse and Mental Health Services Administration
- Requiring the NIH ORWH to monitor research on women's mental health and substance abuse

In addition, WHEA 1991 created

- An infertility prevention program at CDC to encourage more effective screening and treatment of sexually transmitted diseases in women
- New federal standards to regulate mammography screening facilities

Women's Health Equity Act of 1993 (H.R. 3075)

WHEA of 1993 comprised 32 bills (including 23 new initiatives) divided into two titles: one focusing on research needs and the other on health care services. Issues addressed by WHEA 1993 included acquired immunodeficiency syndrome (AIDS) research and prevention, review of federal environmental risk assessment policies with respect to women, expanded analysis of gender differences in new drugs approved by FDA, and increased research on the drug RU-486. Additional new initiatives were designed to improve medical school education on women's health issues, enhance federal smoking prevention efforts, and expand women's health research and services within the Armed Services and the Veterans Administration (VA).

Measures signed into law during the 103rd Congress (1993–1994) included legislation reauthorizing the Breast and Cervical Cancer Mortality Prevention Act, which contained new authority for several demonstration projects offering additional preventive services (such as hypertension screening) at program sites already providing mammograms and Pap smears to low-income women. The Defense Women's Health Act, which authorized primary and prevention services for women at military hospitals and clinics and separate funding for the Defense Women's Health Research Program, also was enacted.

A handful of other WHEA 1993 provisions nearly made it through the entire legislative labyrinth—only to die in the final days of the Congress. Four WHEA provisions were added to the Minority Health Initiative Act, which failed to pass after the Senate blocked action on the conference report, the final step in the legislative process. The WHEA provisions that failed to pass included

- Statutory authority for the Office of Women's Health within the Public Health Service (PHS)
- A requirement that NIH establish policies regarding the employment of women scientists with respect to tenure, family leave, and the recruitment of women of color
- A study of the adequacy of women's health curricula in medical schools
- A requirement that the Office of Minority Health and the Office of Women's Health investigate the number of women in the United States who have been subjected to female genital mutilation and conduct outreach activities to educate individuals about the physical and psychological health risks of female genital mutilation

Legislation to improve the health and services of women veterans met with mixed success in the 103rd Congress. Sections of the WHEA's Veterans Women's Health Amendments were added to a veterans' health bill moving through Congress and would have allowed eligible women veterans to receive primary and preventive services, such as mammograms and Pap smears, treatment of sexually transmitted diseases, and limited reproductive care. The bill also provided for expanded research on women's health, inclusion of women in VA clinical studies, and treatment for victims of sexual violence associated with military service. In the final days of the session, abortion opponents—fearful that VA hospitals would be required to provide abortion services—held up passage of the bill. Ultimately, the bill was stripped of the primary and preventive women's health services and passed, with the research and sexual trauma provisions becoming law.

NIH Reauthorization and Other Health Legislation

The primary vehicle for WHEA provisions from 1990 to 1994 was legislation to reauthorize NIH, which finally became law in 1993. A different bill that never made it through the legislative process—the Minority Health Initiative Act—also served as a vehicle for some WHEA provisions.

NIH Revitalization Act of 1990 (H.R. 5661/S. 2857)

The legislation to reauthorize programs at NIH also lifted the ban on fetal tissue research and contained major pieces of the research title of the WHEA of 1990. The House NIH bill would have

- Required the inclusion of women and minorities in research studies funded by NIH
- Established the ORWH and an intramural clinical program in obstetrics and gynecology at NIH
- Created five centers for research on contraception and infertility
- Increased funding for breast cancer and osteoporosis research

The women's health provisions in the Senate bill were similar to those in the House, with two exceptions. First, in addition to establishing an ORWH, the Senate bill also required NIH, within 3 years, to establish a Center for Women's Health Research to conduct research on women's health. Second, it omitted the specific authorizations for breast cancer and osteoporosis.

The 101st Congress adjourned without completing action on this legislation. The Senate passed its version by unanimous consent, after stripping out the contraceptive and infertility research provisions. The House Energy and Commerce Committee approved H.R. 5661, but the House took no further action on the bill.

NIH Revitalization Act of 1991 (H.R. 2507)

As approved by Congress, H.R. 2507 contained all or part of seven pieces of the WHEA of 1991, including the requirement that women and minorities be included in clinical trials, permanent authorization for offices for research on women's health at NIH and SAMHSA, and increased funding for research on important women's health issues. Specifically, the bill authorized an additional $225 million for basic research on breast cancer; $100 million for clinical research, including six multidisciplinary breast cancer research centers; $75 million for basic and clinical research on ovarian and other reproductive tract cancers; $20 million for contraceptive and infertility research; and $40 million for research on osteoporosis and related bone disorders. The bill also required NIH to establish a clinical research program in obstetrics and gynecology and directed the National Institute on Aging (NIA) to conduct research into the aging process in women. The National Center for Nursing Research was elevated to an institute.

The most controversial item in the bill was a provision lifting the ban on fetal tissue research. The Bush administration actively opposed a number of the bill's provisions, including those on women's health that were termed *unnecessary* in a letter from NIH Director Bernadine Healy to members of Congress. However, it was undoubtedly strong opposition from antiabortion groups to the fetal tissue provisions that produced President Bush's veto and resulted in the House voting narrowly to sustain it. The fetal tissue question lost its political potency in the Senate when Sen. Strom Thurmond (R-SC), a leading abortion opponent, took the Senate floor to express his support for overturning the ban on fetal tissue research. Citing his daughter's diabetes, the Senator expressed his hope that fetal tissue research might some day lead to a cure for this disease and others. This action had no effect on sustaining the veto, however, because action by either the House or the Senate is all that is needed to sustain a presidential veto.

NIH Revitalization Act of 1993 (H.R. 4/ S. 1)

Virtually identical to legislation that was vetoed by President Bush in 1992, the NIH Revitalization Act of 1993 won speedy approval from the 103rd Congress. Surrounded by congressional women's health advocates, President Clinton signed it into law on June 10, 1993. The most controversial aspect of the bill in previous Congresses—the ban on fetal tissue research—was scarcely mentioned in debate on the 1993 legislation. President Clinton had issued an executive order lifting the ban on his second day in office.

Minority Health Initiative Act (H.R. 3869/S. 1569)

The Minority Health Initiative Act—which failed to pass—would have reauthorized the Office of Minority Health at PHS and established offices of minority health at several PHS agencies. The Migrant and Community Health Center programs also would have been reauthorized and improved. The House version contained four provisions of the WHEA of 1993 that addressed the need for an Office of Women's Health at PHS, the treatment of women scientists at NIH, the adequacy of medical school curricula with respect to women's health, and public education about female genital mutilation. The Senate version did not include the women's health provisions, but they were adopted by House-Senate conferees on the bill. In the end, the Senate blocked final approval of the conference report, and the bill died.

Women's Health Research: Issue by Issue

The following is a summary of congressional action on women's health research from 1990 to 1994.

Inclusion of Women in Research

Congress' most direct response to the GAO findings that NIH had not implemented its own policy was to write into law a requirement that women and minorities be included in clinical trials when appropriate. (A parallel policy on the inclusion of minorities in clinical trials was authorized by NIH shortly after it issued the policy on women in 1986.) Enacted in June 1993, the NIH Revitalization Act finally put this requirement into law. There could be exceptions, however, based on the health of the subjects, the purpose of the research, or when substantial scientific data demonstrate that women and minorities will not be affected differently than white men in the study. The new law also permitted the secretary of health and human services to designate other circumstances in which the requirement would not be appropriate. However, Congress made clear in the law that the cost of including women and minorities in research is not an acceptable justification for exempting a researcher from this requirement. The law also required researchers to analyze what gender differences may exist. In other words, the mere inclusion of women in clinical research is not sufficient to satisfy the goals of the legislation. NIH issued new guidelines implementing these provisions in March 1994.

Office for Research on Women's Health

The NIH Revitalization Act of 1993 also gave statutory authority to the NIH ORWH, first established by NIH in September 1990. The legislation identified several primary goals for the office, including identifying projects and multidisciplinary research relating to women's health that should be supported or conducted by NIH, and monitoring the inclusion of women in clinical trials. The new law also established a coordinating committee, composed of institute directors and outside experts, to advise the office, and a data bank and clearinghouse to collect and disseminate information on women's health. The NIH office received $11 million in fiscal year (FY) 1994 and $16.7 million in FY 1995.

Clinical Research in Obstetrics and Gynecology

The dearth of gynecologists at NIH was cited frequently by women's health advocates as further evidence of the agency's disregard for women's health. The NIH Revitalization Act of 1993 required the National Institute of Child Health and Human Development to establish an intramural clinical research program in obstetrics and gynecology.

Treatment of Women Scientists

The NIH bill also gave ORWH responsibility for monitoring the status of women physicians and scientists at NIH and NIH-funded institutions and for initiating activities to increase the representation of women as senior scientists and physicians.

The WHEA of 1993 moved further to address the status of women scientists at NIH by requiring the agency to establish policies regarding the employment of women scientists (including tenure, family leave, and recruitment of women of color) and to conduct a study to identify any pay differences among male and female scientists, with recommendations for adjusting inequities. These provisions were incorporated into the Minority Health Initiative Act but failed to become law.

Women's Health Initiative

Since 1991, Congress has provided more than $191 million to fund the Women's Health Initiative (WHI), a long-term study of heart disease, breast cancer, and osteoporosis prevention in women—virtually the full amount requested by NIH for the study. WHI is expected to cost $625 million over its 14-year duration. In 1992, the House Appropriations Committee asked the Institute of Medicine (IOM) to weigh the financial costs and informational benefits expected from the study. Although critical of several aspects, the IOM report expressed support for the goals of the WHI and the need for increased research on women's health. The IOM's concerns ranged from the large number of questions the study is attempting to answer to the fact that it is tightly budgeted with little to no room for cost overruns.

Breast and Other Reproductive Tract Cancers

No single issue has benefited more from the surge of attention to women's health research than breast cancer. Although heart disease and lung cancer claim more lives each year, breast cancer holds a special terror for women. A seemingly random killer of women from early middle age on, its causes—although affected by genetics, environmental toxins, and poor diet—remain a mystery. According to NCI, a woman born today in the United States has a one in eight chance of having the disease in her lifetime.

In May 1990, Rep. Mary Rose Oakar, whose sister died in 1993 after a 12-year battle with breast cancer, convened a hearing of the House Select Committee on Aging's Subcommittee on Health and Long-Term Care to examine the need for increased research on the causes of the disease. The hearing was an opportunity to promote legislation she had introduced to authorize an additional $25 million for basic research into the causes of breast cancer. Of the $77 million budgeted by NCI for breast cancer research in 1989, only $17 million had been spent on basic research.

The timing of the Oakar hearing and legislation could not have been more opportune. A bill to reauthorize NIH, including NCI, would soon begin to wend its way through Congress. Health subcommittee chair Rep. Henry Waxman heeded Congresswoman Oakar's plea for more money for basic breast cancer research, directing NCI to allocate no less than $35 million for breast cancer research.

By the time the NIH Revitalization Act was signed into law by President Clinton in 1993, an additional $325 million had been authorized for breast cancer research at NCI, $225 million of it for basic research. Moreover, this was the first time Congress had set the funding level for research on a specific cancer in NCI's authorization. In one sense, the language was unnecessary. NCI had all the authority it needed to conduct research—basic or otherwise—on breast cancer. However,

Congress had found NCI's commitment to breast cancer research lacking and assumed a more directive role with the institute.

The pressure on Congress to make funding for breast cancer research an urgent priority came from several different sources. A number of prominent women who had battled breast cancer, including several former first ladies and Marilyn Quayle, wife of then-Vice President Dan Quayle, came forward to demand more money for research. In 1992, at the request of Vice President Quayle, NCI established a Special Commission on Breast Cancer to the president's cancer panel, which ultimately recommended that the federal government spend no less than $500 million per year until breast cancer can be prevented and cured.[3]

A growing number of members of Congress—female and male—also spoke out strongly in favor of additional research dollars. In addition to two congresswomen who were breast cancer survivors—Reps. Lloyd and Barbara Vucanovich (R-NV)—a number of congressmen had wives or other family members stricken with the disease.

A third important force critical to the successful effort was a scrappy coalition of breast cancer survivor groups who borrowed a chapter or two from the political playbooks of AIDS activists. In 1991, they showered Congress with 600,000 letters and came to Washington in force to lobby personally for research funds. In 1992, the Breast Cancer Coalition convened its own conference of breast cancer researchers to find out how much money it should ask Congress to allocate for FY 1993.[4] The researchers' answer was $300 million. The coalition appealed to Congress for the funds, over the objections of the medical research establishment, who charged the coalition with interfering in the setting of scientific priorities. By the time Congress adjourned that year, nearly $440 million had been approved under two appropriations bills.

During the 5-year period from 1990 to 1994, appropriations for breast cancer research increased more than fivefold, from approximately $90 million to more than $500 million, the majority of it at NCI. However, beginning in FY 1993, a significant amount of money also has come from the Department of Defense (DOD) budget for a peer-reviewed breast cancer research program conducted by the army.

Two other reproductive tract cancers—cervical and ovarian—received substantial increases in research dollars over the same period. The long-term survival rate for ovarian cancer has improved little in the past 30 years because, with no easy diagnostic test available, the disease is often advanced by the time it is detected. The NIH Revitalization Act of 1993 authorized $75 million for research on ovarian cancer and other cancers of the reproductive tract. In 1993, a panel of congresswomen asked a House appropriations subcommittee to increase its allocation for research on ovarian cancer. Seated on the dais was one of the subcommittee's four new female members—Rep. Rosa DeLauro (D-CT)—an ovarian cancer survivor who credits luck, rather than science, for her survival.

But the dramatic increase in research dollars for breast cancer and other reproductive tract cancers at NIH was not always spelled out by Congress, the way most other federal programs are given an annual appropriation to conduct their activities. Rather, funding increases for women's health research were often the result of congressional pressure, part of a complicated game in which—in the name of promoting science—members of Congress seek to influence but not dictate the research agendas of the various institutes.

NIH scientists and their defenders in Congress adamantly oppose the earmarking of funds for disease-specific research. The research agenda, they argue, should be determined by promising scientific leads, not political pressure from Congress or outside special interests. Yet, in reality, members of Congress often seek to play an active role in decisions about how federal research dollars are spent.

Typically, Congress provides a single line item in its annual appropriations bill for research at each of the 17 institutes that constitute NIH. A separate report spells out how the appropriations committee hopes the funds will be used. Several lines in an appropriations bill are typically accompanied by a dozen or more pages of directives and recommendations on how the funds should be spent.

Whether such report language carries the same weight as the provisions of a bill depends on whom you ask. In 1988, the director of the Office of Management and Budget (OMB) advised federal agencies that committee reports had "no force of law." He was quickly rebuked by the chairmen and ranking minority members of the House and Senate appropriations committees, who pointed out that the spending bills passed by Congress contain a provision stating that the funding provided "shall be in accordance with the reports accompanying the bills."

In reality, the weight accorded specific report language depends on a variety of factors. How strongly worded is the language? Does it "direct" or merely "encourage?" Does similar language exist in both the House and Senate reports? (In other words, will ignoring it risk alienating powerful members of Congress on both sides of the Capitol?) Is it mentioned again in the statement of the conferees appointed to resolve differences in the House and Senate bills? Each reference to a specific issue—by the House, the Senate, and the conference committee—strengthens the entreaty in the eyes of the federal agency in question.

Still, constrained by tight budgets and faced with more directives than money, agencies are often reluctant to treat committee report language as law. However, agency heads who disregard report language do so at their own risk because policy recommendations laid out in report language one year, if ignored, may become statutory mandates the next.

Dollar amounts for research on breast and other reproductive tract cancers have been spelled out in the committee reports, with varying levels of direction on the part of Congress. At times, the House and Senate reports have even contained different instructions and, absent a specific agreement by House-Senate conferees, NCI was left to split the difference between the funding levels ordered by the two bodies. The following descriptions of appropriations made from FY 1991 through FY 1995 demonstrate a number of the ways Congress has sought to pressure NCI to increase funding for breast and other reproductive tract cancer research.

FY 1991 appropriations.   Signed into law in 1990, the FY 1991 Labor, Health and Human Services, and Education appropriations bill increased funding for NCI by nearly $170 million, which was considered a substantial increase at the time. The House committee report urged that research on breast and cervical cancer be increased, whereas the House-Senate conference report recommended that a major study be undertaken to look at the use of tamoxifen to prevent breast cancer. Actual spending for breast cancer by NCI in FY 1991 totaled $92.7 million, up 14% from the previous year. NCI also spent $22.3 million for cervical cancer and $13.6 million for ovarian cancer in FY 1991. Although most cancer research is conducted by NCI, some research on reproductive tract cancers also is done by other institutes, primarily the National Institute of Child Health and Human Development.

FY 1992 appropriations.   By 1991 the campaign for increased funding for women's health research was fast gaining steam, leading both House and Senate appropriators to earmark specific funding levels in their FY 1992 appropriations committee reports. The House directed that an additional $30 million be spent for research on breast, ovarian, and prostate cancer research, telling NCI to redirect other funds for research on these cancers. Not to be outdone, the Senate directed that $40 million be spent on breast, ovarian, and cervical cancer research.

Rep. William Natcher (D-KY), chair of the House Appropriations Subcommittee on Labor, Health and Human Services, and Education, vehemently fought the earmarks for breast cancer and other disease-specific research in conference. Caucus members fought hard to maintain the earmarks, even storming the all-male conference meeting to demand that funding for breast cancer research be written into the bill. The conferees met for an unprecedented 3 weeks before an agreement was reached. In the end, the conferees gave NCI a hefty $275 million increase but declined to earmark specific funds for breast cancer research. The conference report, however, urged NCI "in the strongest way" to make research on breast cancer and other women's health issues a top priority and to provide significant increases as outlined in the House and Senate reports. Actual spending by NCI for breast cancer research in FY 1992 increased by 56% to $145 million. Funding for ovarian and cervical cancer increased by 52% and 38%, respectively. Also, 1992 was the first year in which an appropriation of $10 million for the NIH ORWH became a reality. The House report directed the office to give priority to research on various reproductive health problems, the relationship between breast cancer and oral contraceptives, women and AIDS, and DES-exposed women.

FY 1993 appropriations.   In 1992, the House Appropriations Committee again directed NIH to give women's health "highest priority," but it took a different tact in attempting to set funding levels for breast cancer research. In its report, the committee told NCI to increase funding for breast, cervical, ovarian, and prostate cancer by at least one-third over FY 1992 levels. (This translated to a $48 million increase for breast cancer research at NCI, for a total of $193 million.) The House report also expressed concern about a number of reproductive health disorders—including uterine fibroids, endometriosis, and pelvic inflammatory disease (PID)—and reallocated funds to ensure expanded research in these areas. The Senate went a step further, directing NCI to add $87 million to the breast cancer research effort for a total of $232 million. In the end, NCI said it would split the difference between the House and Senate, spending $211.5 million in FY 1993. Total funding for breast cancer research at all NIH institutes in FY 1993 was $228.9 million. Funding for ovarian cancer at NCI increased 57% to $32.5 million; cervical cancer research increased 37% to $42.2 million. The Senate report also directed that an additional $1 million be set aside for a study of states with elevated levels of breast cancer.

However, it was not only the 47% increase in funding at NIH that made 1992 the banner year it was for breast cancer research. Rather, it was approval of $210 million in funding for the army's research program, which brought total breast cancer research funding for the year to nearly $440 million, a 144% increase over the previous year. Frustrated by his inability to transfer money from defense to domestic accounts, Sen. Tom Harkin (D-IA)—who lost both of his sisters to breast cancer—succeeded in earmarking $210 million to be spent over 2 years for breast cancer research in the DOD appropriations bill. Although a number of Senators objected that the Harkin amendment breached the spirit of the 1990 budget agreement—which prohibited funds from being shifted between defense and domestic programs—in the end, it was approved by a vote of 89 to 4. When it was clear that the amendment would pass, several dozen Senators returned to the Senate chamber to switch their votes, fearful of coming down on the wrong side of what had become a potent political issue.

FY 1994 appropriations.   For the first time since their campaign got under way, women's health leaders in Congress were joined by the White House in requesting substantial increases for women's health research. In his FY 1994 budget request, President Clinton asked for a total of $1.6 billion for PHS programs to improve women's health, $394 million more than had been spent the previous year. Funding for breast cancer research in 1994 was set at $292 million in the president's budget. House and Senate appropriators simply ratified the president's budget request for NIH. Signaling a new harmony between the legislative and executive branches of government, the Labor–Health and Human Services–Education conference report said there would be no earmarking of research dollars for NIH to respond to the priorities in the NIH Revitalization Act, which President Clinton had signed earlier that year. An additional $25 million was provided in the DOD budget to continue the research effort begun the previous year.

The House Appropriations Committee did, however, take the opportunity to urge NCI to expand research on the relationship between nutrition and breast cancer and to encourage the National Institute of Environmental Health Services to continue its research on the relationship between substances in the environment and breast cancer. The House report also prodded NIH to conduct an aggressive research effort for ovarian and cervical cancers and gynecological problems associated with DES. The Senate committee report simply identified breast cancer as a high priority for research, along with a laundry list of other health issues that had collectively come to represent women's health, including DES, osteoporosis, interstitial cystitis, chronic fatigue syndrome, and the health problems of midlife women. The Senate report also instructed NIH to hold a conference on endometriosis and charged PHS with developing an action plan to reduce the number of unnecessary hysterectomies.

FY 1995 appropriations.   The funding push continued in FY 1995, with the president's budget calling for an increase of $84 million in breast cancer research at NCI for a total of $383 million. The House budget resolution went even further, recommending a $600 million increase for NIH research on diseases primarily affecting women, including $421 million for breast cancer research. The House Budget Resolution also recommended that a hiring freeze be waived for certain research areas, including breast and prostate cancer. In the end, faced with many competing priorities, Congress set breast cancer research at $350 million, a nearly 20% increase over the previous year but $33 million short of the president's request. An additional $150 million was approved for the army's breast cancer research program, with funding earmarked for the development of digital mammography technology. The navy also received $5 million to develop a Center of Excellence in

Breast Cancer at the National Naval Medical Center and $2 million for digital mammography technology. The army for the first time will receive $7.5 million for ovarian cancer research and $5 million for research on osteoporosis and related bone diseases. The Senate committee report expressed disappointment that Health and Human Services (HHS) had not submitted the action plan it requested the previous year on unnecessary hysterectomies.

Contraception and Infertility

The campaign to increase federal investment in contraceptive research got a big boost in 1990 when the National Research Council published a report criticizing the limited choices in contraceptive methods as poorly suited to the religious, social, economic, or health circumstances of many Americans.[5] Unless public policy with respect to contraceptive development changed, the report warned, contraceptive choice in the next century would not be appreciably different from what it is today.

By 1990, all but one major pharmaceutical company in the United States had withdrawn from the contraceptive research field. Federal support for contraceptive and infertility research was minimal. Throughout the 1980s, NIH received only about $8 million a year for applied research in contraceptive development.

Congress ultimately approved legislation authorizing $30 million for three contraceptive and two infertility research centers (as part of the NIH Revitalization Act of 1993); however, opposition from abortion opponents made it one of the more controversial items on the women's health research agenda. Senate approval of the NIH bill in 1990, for example, came only after an agreement was reached to remove the contraceptive research provisions. The NIH bill went no further in that Congress, and the provisions were restored when the bill was reintroduced in 1991.

As with research on breast cancer, congressional support for increased contraceptive and infertility research also came through the appropriations process. In FY 1992, the Senate appropriations committee report directed NIH to provide an additional $6 million to establish contraceptive and infertility research centers, a figure that has remained fairly constant over the years, despite the higher authorization approved by

Congress. The NIH reauthorization also directed NIH to establish a loan repayment program to encourage health professionals to enter this field of research.

Osteoporosis

Osteoporosis is an important cause of disability and death in older women, afflicting some 90% of women older than 75 years. Health costs associated with osteoporosis are estimated at $7 to $10 billion annually. The NIH Revitalization Act of 1993 authorized $40 million to expand research programs on osteoporosis and related bone disorders. The provision also authorized the creation of an information clearinghouse. That same year, the House FY 1994 appropriations report urged a number of NIH institutes to increase funding for osteoporosis, noting that current funding stood at $20 million, half the level recently authorized by Congress. In FY 1995, Congress approved $5 million for osteoporosis research under the army's medical research program.

Women and AIDS

Although they constitute a minority of AIDS cases in the United States, women make up the fastest growing group of new cases. Yet, until recently, what research there was on women and AIDS focused primarily on women as vectors of transmission to men and infants rather than on treatment and prevention of the disease in women themselves. Although the NIH Revitalization Act stopped short of authorizing a specific amount for research on women and AIDS, it mandated that HIV-infected women, including pregnant women, be included in appropriate studies on the safety and efficacy of HIV vaccines, when appropriate.

Congress also has sought to encourage expanded research on women and AIDS at NIH through the appropriations process. Beginning in FY 1992, the House appropriations report expressed concern that no research was being conducted on the development of the disease in women or on the development of physical and chemical barriers to HIV infection. The committee also urged CDC to convene a consensus conference to determine HIV-related symptoms specific to women. In FY 1993, the House provided NIH with funding for a natural history study of

HIV infection in women. Research on microbicides—substances that kill HIV and other microorganisms on contact—was identified as a high priority for investigation at the National Institute of Allergy and Infectious Diseases in the FY 1994 House appropriations report. The Senate report also identified the need for topical microbicides to protect women against HIV as vital. In FY 1995, the House again urged NIH to develop a safe, effective microbicide and to give priority to the Women's Interagency HIV study.

Diethylstilbestrol

In 1992, Congress approved legislation authorizing expanded research on DES, a drug given to about 5 million pregnant women between the 1940s and 1971. Prescribed to women in the mistaken belief that it prevented miscarriages, DES was later found to cause a rare form of cancer and other reproductive problems in some of the children exposed in utero. The new law created a research and education program to encourage studies and dissemination of health information on the side effects of DES, both for women who took the drug and for children who were exposed in utero. The same year, the Senate FY 1993 Labor–Health and Human Services–Education appropriations report earmarked $1.5 million for implementation of the new research and education program. The FY 1995 Labor–Health and Human Services–Education appropriations conference report strongly encouraged NCI to expand its support for DES research and education efforts.

Lupus

Congress also has indicated support for expanded research on systemic lupus erythematosus (SLE), an incurable autoimmune disease that affects primarily African American women between ages 15 and 65. Legislation to authorize $20 million for an expanded research effort on the causes, diagnosis, treatment, and prevention of lupus was considered by the Senate Labor and Human Resources Committee in August 1994. The committee approved the bill after deleting the specific funding authorization, noting that the Appropriations Committee consistently ignored specific authorization levels for disease research. No further action occurred on the legislation during the 103rd Congress. For FY 1994, the House Labor–Health and Human Services–Education appropriations report directed the National Institute of Arthritis and Musculoskeletal Diseases to spend $5 million over the president's request. In FY 1995, the House report again strongly encouraged NIH to support research aimed at understanding gender- and ethnic-related factors associated with the high prevalence of lupus in women and minorities.

Environmental Health Issues

A growing concern about the effects of the environment on women's health led to several hearings in 1992 and 1993. In June 1992, the House Government Operations Subcommittee on Human Resources and Intergovernmental Relations examined the potential contamination of consumer goods, particularly feminine hygiene products, by the chemical dioxin. Dioxin has been linked to cancer and birth defects in animal research.

In October 1993, the House Energy and Commerce Subcommittee on Health and the Environment heard testimony from scientists, environmental activists, and women's health advocates on the relationship between pesticides and breast cancer. Witnesses presented evidence that exposure to certain common pesticides is associated with rising breast cancer rates in the United States, a worldwide decline in sperm counts, and widespread reproductive failures in wildlife. Experts believe that pesticides may accumulate to a greater degree in women, who have a higher percentage of body fat than men. These toxins are potentially released during dieting and by the hormonal changes of pregnancy, lactation, and menopause.

The WHEA of 1993 contained two bills to increase understanding of environmental health issues in women. One of the bills would have required a full study of all federal exposure and risk assessment techniques and policies relating to women's health; the other would have authorized the National Institute on Environmental Health Sciences (NIEHS) to study the impact of environmental factors on women's health. Although neither bill was considered by the 103rd Congress, the FY 1994 House Labor–Health and Human Services–Education appropriations report urged

NIEHS to continue research on how substances in the environment may lead to breast cancer. However, Congress appropriated no money for this purpose (see Chapter 8 for more on environmental issues).

Menopause

The dearth of research on menopause has been a particular concern of many congresswomen. Not only was it an issue of personal interest for some, but also there was growing frustration over a spate of conflicting studies that emphasized either the risks or benefits of postmenopausal hormone replacement therapy. No sooner did one study find that hormone therapy offered significant benefits in terms of reduced coronary artery disease and osteoporosis than another study would be released suggesting increased breast cancer rates in the women who used it.

At the request of CCWI, the U.S. Office of Technology Assessment (OTA) prepared a report titled, "Menopause, Hormone Therapy, and Women's Health."[6] Published in 1992, the report confirmed what many women already suspected: there is a great deal of uncertainty surrounding our understanding of menopause and the treatment of related symptoms. According to OTA, physicians prescribe hormone treatment guessing at what is best, and women take it hoping it will help without adequate knowledge of the potential risks and benefits for them as individuals. The report recommended expanded research on hormone therapy and its alternatives.

The NIH Revitalization Act of 1993 required NIA to conduct research into the aging process in women, with particular emphasis given to the effects of menopause and the physiological and behavioral changes occurring during the transition from pre- to postmenopause. The act also directed NIA to conduct research into the diagnosis, disorders, and complications of aging and into the effect of the loss of ovarian hormones on older women.

Military Women's Health Research

The mammoth defense budget increasingly has been recognized as a potentially abundant source of funding for women's health research. In addition to the appropriation of more than $400 million to date for the army's breast cancer research effort, Congress has approved substantial funding for a Defense Women's Health Research Program. The FY 1994 DOD authorization bill included provisions from WHEA's Defense Women's Health Improvement Act, which authorized primary and preventive health services for women at military hospitals and clinics. Although the House also approved $40 million to establish a Defense Women's Health Research Center, the conference agreement left the decision up to the secretary of defense, who was authorized to spend $20 million toward the establishment of a center. The FY 1994 DOD authorization bill also directed the army to continue its breast cancer research program and instructed the Uniformed Services University of the Health Services to promote the inclusion of women's health in medical school curriculum. FY 1994 appropriations for DOD actually provided $40 million for the Defense Women's Health Research Program, the amount originally approved by the House.

In FY 1995, Congress authorized the full $40 million for the Defense Women's Health Research Program. DOD abandoned the idea of creating a research center, choosing instead to use its existing medical infrastructure to establish an information clearinghouse and coordinate research on the health care needs of military women and their patterns of illness and injury. The program also planned to examine how DOD policies affect women's health and identify areas for improvement.

Epilogue

In 1995, Republicans assumed leadership in both the House and the Senate. One of the first actions of the new Republican-led House was to eliminate legislative service organizations, including the CCWI. Although a bipartisan group of congresswomen—co-chaired in the 104th Congress by Reps. Nita Lowey (D-NY) and Constance Morella (R-MD)—continue to meet under the same name to advocate on behalf of women, the House action deprived CCWI of its office, six-member staff, and $250,000 annual budget.

The rise to power of a new leadership with a different set of legislative priorities—as spelled out in the campaign-driven "Contract With America"—dampened congressional fervor around women's health.

Deficit reduction dominated the annual budget and appropriations processes, bringing an end to sharp funding increases for women's health research.

Still, funding for women's health fared better than many other domestic programs during the 104th Congress. Funding for the Breast and Cervical Cancer Mortality Prevention Program at CDC increased $40 million over 2 years. Congress boosted funding for NIH by 5.7% in FY 1996 and 6.9% in FY 1997, although the Appropriations Committees refused to earmark funding for any specific areas of women's health research. It was a different story for the DOD's more sizeable budget. Congress earmarked a total of $237 million over 2 years for breast cancer activities within DOD, including $187 million for research. Congress also earmarked funds in the DOD budget for research on ovarian cancer and osteoporosis.

Why has funding for women's health continued to fare better than other federal programs? In part, women's health advocates can thank two moderate Republicans—Rep. John Porter (R-IL) and Sen. Arlen Specter (R-PA)—the chairmen of the House and Senate appropriations subcommittees that oversee NIH funding. Both men are strong supporters of medical research in general and women's health in particular.

However, more important than the efforts of any one person or group is the issue itself: women's health research has proven to be an enduring legislative concern capable of winning broad bipartisan support. In policy terms, women's health is an issue that resonates, transcending virtually every demographic division—race, class, age, and to a certain extent, even gender. As one mammogram public service announcement intones, "They are our mothers, sisters, daughters. . . ."

The period between 1990 and 1995 witnessed the growth of a tremendous federal investment in women's health research, with the 103rd Congress (1993–1994) lauded as the most productive Congress ever on women's health issues. The challenge in the 104th Congress was to maintain these gains in the face of a new set of congressional priorities, a goal that was largely achieved.

Women recently celebrated the 75th anniversary of winning the right to vote. In November 1996, the power of the women's vote was clearly demonstrated when women cast ballots in greater numbers than men and were the deciding factor in both the presidential race and a number of key congressional races. However, the so-called gender gap had far less to do with an allegiance to any one political party than it did with women voters bringing a different set of policy priorities to the voting booth, including their health and that of their families.

Congress and the medical establishment ignored women's health once, and a new women's health movement was born. They will do so again at their own peril.

Endnotes

[1]Stith-Coleman I, Johnson JA: *CRS Report for Congress: Women's Health Research:1.* Washington, DC, Congressional Research Service of the Library of Congress, June 1994

[2]Testimony of Mark Nadel before the House Energy and Commerce Subcommittee on Health and the Environment, "National Institutes of Health: Problems in Implementing Policy on Women in Study Populations." U.S. General Accounting Office, June 18, 1990

[3]Johnson JA: *CRS Report for Congress: Breast Cancer.* Washington, DC, Congressional Research Service of the Library of Congress, March 1994

[4]*Congressional Quarterly Almanac, 1993* (Vol XLIX). Washington, DC, Congressional Quarterly, 1994

[5]National Research Council: *Developing New Contraceptives: Obstacles & Opportunities.* Washington, DC, National Academy Press, 1990

[6]*Menopause, Hormone Therapy, & Women's Health.* Washington, DC, U.S. Office of Technology Assessment, 1992

15

Conclusion

Florence P. Haseltine, Ph.D., M.D.
President, Society for the Advancement of
Women's Health Research

I n the foreword, I described how research on women's health evolved from a single issue concept (reproduction) to a multi-faceted inquiry. Now I believe we are ready for the next great leap. We have to start looking at the differences between women and men in terms of "gender-based biology."

Gender-based biology examines the differences between the genders in a cell, an organ, or an individual to discover what these differences tell us about the system in which they function. This approach makes real the concept that women's health research is truly interdisciplinary, embracing topics that range from bench science through the clinical identification and treatment of disease. The field can thus be looked at systematically by using a model composed of three main elements:

1.   The multidisciplinary perspective involves training people from various backgrounds to approach problems in an organized fashion.
2.   The diagnostic perspective uses a standardized approach to solving problems.
3.   The triage perspective involves providing information to patients and physicians and referring both to the appropriate specialties.

What we are really talking about is creating a new template for research that allows us to ask many pertinent questions. Why are the two genders different? What is the underlying mechanism of that difference? What do the differences tell us about the system as a whole and about how the system behaves? Are gender differences caused by genetic expression? If they are, when does the genetic expression affect the system—in utero or during growth? When is DNA imprinted differently in females and males, and how does this affect disease processes? Are there gender differences that play a role from conception to death? (See Table 15–1.) Was genetic expression altered because of the way the system reacts to different sex hormones? Are gender differences learned or hormonal; for example, what is the influence of steroidal sex hormones on the disparities between the genders in math ability? Can the differential genetic expression of diseases lead to understanding genetic mechanisms in gender, and can this understanding lead to different therapies? How do the early signs of disease, such as atherosclerosis, differ between women and men? What are the genetic factors that contribute to a long life?[1] With such basic questions, almost any system can be explored—which is why I believe it is time to test the power of this scientific approach in women's health research.

Let us look at some possible practical applications of this new template. For example, current thinking in research and patient care is often related to life phases so that new research subjects from the developmental stages of females and males are proliferating rapidly. In fact, a recent biomedical literature search of publications appearing between 1990 and 1994 found more than 5,000 citations referring to "gender differences" and revealed that gender differences are being examined across a broad spectrum of basic and clinical research.[2]

The primary differences between the genders occur, of course, during embryogenesis. Most basic is the expression of genetic sex, that is, the XX or XY chromosomal configuration. The genetic contribution from parent to child is important, but not just for the obvious reason that parental information passes on to each generation. It is crucial because

---

Table 15–1. Gender differences from conception to death

Genetic inheritance (parental inheritance/expression)
Growth pattern differences throughout life
Hormonal influences on systems throughout life

we have learned that a person expresses his or her genes differently, depending on whether they come from the mother or the father. This is called *imprinting* and is a fertile field for future research.

Following the early developmental stage is the effect of sex hormones—estrogen and progesterone in the female, testosterone in the male—on the genitals and other developing organs. Looking at differences between the sexes provides unlimited research possibilities. There is the primary effect of testosterone, estrogen, and progesterone on cells and then their impact on the organs that are produced. In fact, the potential for the future action of sex steroids occurs at this time.

Differences in sex hormone action can be seen at birth, with simple distinctions such as the average weight of babies, with boys being larger. Because the ovaries and testes are quiescent during childhood, the influence of sex hormones is secondary; in fact, the disparities we see between girls' intrauterine developments that play out in childhood. However, this changes dramatically at puberty and differences start to proliferate rapidly. The timing of puberty itself varies, with females becoming pubescent 2 years earlier than males, a striking example of a sexually dimorphic phenomenon. The major change of puberty occurs in the brain, which turns on various hormonal systems, not in the genitals. But why is there a difference in the timing? We know there is a disparity in brain development between females and males. Was this difference determined in utero, or was it already in the genes? How were maternal and paternal genes expressed differently?

The fact that the dissimilarity between male and female brains can be documented at an early age is not surprising. These variations will continue for the rest of a person's life. It is therefore vital that when studying any function or disease, researchers investigate and understand the effect of these gender discrepancies. That is why it is as crucial to look at organ systems that do not display sexual dimorphism as an obvious characteristic as it is to study those that do. Take, for example, the kidney and the liver, purportedly neutral organs. We know, however, that liver function in males and females is not the same. Women are exposed to fluctuating estrogen levels, and, as a result, the liver metabolizes many substances differently. Alcohol is a good example. Women end up with higher blood levels of alcohol even if they weigh as much as men and drink the same amount of liquor, beer, or wine—because the female body has more fat and less water, so there is less fluid in which alcohol can be distributed. Moreover, although both sexes have identical enzymes that break down alcohol in the stomach, women have fewer of them, get rid of less alcohol, and absorb more of it into the bloodstream. Some of these metabolic variations are probably related to developmental differences and to the presence of fluctuating estrogen levels; we know, for example, that women are more susceptible to alcohol's effects just before menses, when the oxidation of alcohol in the liver is at its slowest.

As far as the kidney is concerned, men and women have different risks of infection. Although women's kidneys appear similar to those of men, except that they are smaller, kidney function in some women is compromised simply because it is attached to a urinary system that is quite different from a man's. The much shorter female urethra allows bacteria easier access to the bladder, causing more urinary tract infections and a higher incidence of kidney disease (glomerulonephritis). Even though kidney failure may therefore occur earlier in women than in men, and could be explained simply on the basis of the female urinary tract, the impact of kidney disease is quite dissimilar in men and women. For example, for years nephrologists knew that a particularly virulent form of osteoporosis occurred in women in kidney failure. The culprit was estrogen loss as a result of ovarian dysfunction. Recently, nephrologists have decided that, because kidney failure makes osteoporosis a normal event for their female patients, this is a realistic research area to pursue.

Yet another area ripe for gender-based research centers on heart disease, specifically how lipids affect women differently than men. It has been known for some time that the incidence of heart disease rises sharply in women after menopause, presumably because of the severe drop in estrogen. Now research—the double-blind, randomized clinical trial known as the Postmenopausal Estrogen/Progestin Interventions (PEPI) Trial—shows that taking hormone replacement therapy increases the level of high-density lipoprotein cholesterol, the so-called good cholesterol, and decreases the level of low-density lipoprotein cholesterol, the "bad" guy in the cholesterol galaxy. What is interesting here—looking through the gender prism—is that high-density lipoprotein is a more potent risk factor in women than it is in men; low levels account for a sevenfold increase in heart disease risk. Conversely, whereas high levels of low-density lipoprotein markedly up the risk ante for heart disease in men, the same is not true in women.

Looking at drug reactions, we find evidence of gender-based differences in the action of psychoactive drugs such as antidepressants, which are clearly related to the menstrual cycle. Indeed, for many women, the only way to keep a constant blood level of these medications is to vary the dosage throughout the monthly cycle. Because depression is twice as frequent in women as men, this is a major consideration in the treatment of this condition.

If we examine overall systems rather than specific organs, drugs, or diseases, we also find gender disparities needing study. Why is the immune system in women stronger than in men? Is it to protect the species because women carry the greater responsibility for reproduction than do men? We already know that estrogen increases hormone activity in the immune system by increasing both prolactin and growth hormones, which increase the production volume of both T and B immune cells that fight disease. As future gender-based research teases out the entire mechanism explaining female immune stamina, it is possible that we will learn something to boost the male immune system.

If we cross the barrier from biology to sociology and examine the disabilities field, we find an example of research that has focused primarily on disabled youth, usually male accident victims. Here, as with acquired immunodeficiency syndrome (AIDS) patients, images of youthful suffering are heartbreakingly obvious. But if gender considerations were emphasized, a different focus would result. Elderly women make up the major disabled population in the United States. Why don't they get the attention? Because these women are hidden behind closed doors. A woman who is a respiratory or cardiac "cripple" is seldom seen in public. Her concerns are not addressed nor does she have a public voice. In addition, medicine has not studied the interrelationships among the various diseases that afflict elderly women. For these women to become the focus of additional research, they must be more active as voters and lobbyists. Perhaps as the field of disabilities research matures it will concentrate on disabled females.

Over the coming years, which may include severely restrictive budget reviews, it is important that women, policy makers, and scientists become aware of this rich field of investigational effort awaiting exploration. In gender-based biology, we have a research tool that is multidisciplinary in design, diagnostic in outlook, devised to bring new findings quickly into clinical practice, and geared to benefit both genders. Our job is to convince all interested parties of its value for society. I fear that, during the continuing rounds of funding evaluation, a knee-jerk response to any idea defined as "consumer driven" will appear tainted to the traditional establishment. The fact that the traditional science world was blind to women's health research in the past does not justify ignoring it now or in the future, particularly if we successfully create this new research template that is so much broader than our earlier approaches. We must not lose sight of the fact that, if scientists fail to keep up with current ideas in this vibrant area, they will fall behind other researchers. Should this occur, industry may wrest the initiative from traditional governmental funding sources, and government organizations will have a hard time proving that they should have the public trust to decide what research is worthwhile. This has already happened in the field of infertility research. Because research on contraception and infertility has always been held hostage to the conservative political atmosphere, infertility clinics mushroomed without any help from the federal research community. This meant that major advances in infertility occurred outside of the kind of peer review and oversight that the government-funded biomedical sciences enjoy. The result: the United States fell severely behind in research related to in vitro fertilization.

For all these reasons, it is vital for scientists and policy makers to understand that women's health research is not a passing fad and to acknowledge that it asks fundamental questions—questions that must be answered if women are to live out their extended lives in healthy and productive ways. The choice is between doing the research that will help create healthy women—particularly healthy older women—who can continue to contribute to society and the current situation of chronic disease that is bankrupting our national medical system.

Endnotes

[1]Haseltine F: Gender based biology—the next step. *Journal of Women's Health* 4(3):221–222, 1995. *Gender Differences: Known and Unknown.* Society for the Advancement of Women's Health Research Abstract, 1995

[2]LaRosa JH, Alexander L: *Gender Differences: Known and Unknown.* Prepared for the Fifth Annual Scientific Advisory Meeting of the Society for the Advancement of Women's Health Research on Gender Based Biology, 1995

Index

Page numbers in **boldface** *type refer to figures and tables.*

DATE DUE

DEC 10 1998		
MAR 05 1999		